Restorative Proctocolectomy

Restorative Proctocolectomy

Restorative Proctocolectomy

EDITED BY

JOHN NICHOLLS MChir, FRCS
Consultant Surgeon, St Mark's and St Thomas' Hospital, London,
and Dean of St Mark's Hospital

DAVID BARTOLO MS, FRCS
Consultant Colorectal Surgeon, Royal Infirmary of Edinburgh,
and Senior Lecturer, Department of Surgery,
University of Edinburgh

NEIL MORTENSEN MD, FRCS
Consultant Surgeon, Department of Colorectal Surgery,
and Clinical Lecturer, University of Oxford Medical School,
John Radcliffe Hospital

FOREWORD BY
ZANE COHEN
Surgeon in Chief, Mount Sinai Hospital,
University of Toronto, Faculty of Medicine,
Toronto, Canada

OXFORD

BLACKWELL SCIENTIFIC PUBLICATIONS

LONDON EDINBURGH BOSTON

MELBOURNE PARIS BERLIN VIENNA

© 1993 by
Blackwell Scientific Publications
Editorial Offices:
Osney Mead, Oxford OX2 0EL
25 John Street, London WC1N 2BL
23 Ainslie Place, Edinburgh EH3 6AJ
238 Main Street, Cambridge
  Massachusetts 02142, USA
54 University Street, Carlton
  Victoria 3053, Australia

Other Editorial Offices:
Librairie Arnette SA
2, rue Casimir-Delavigne
75006 Paris
France

Blackwell Wissenschafts-Verlag GmbH
Meinekestrasse 4
D-1000 Berlin 15
Germany

Blackwell MZV
Feldgasse 13
A-1238 Wien
Austria

First published 1993

Set by Excel Typesetters Company, Hong Kong
Printed and bound in Great Britain
at the University Press, Cambridge

DISTRIBUTORS

Marston Book Services Ltd
PO Box 87
Oxford OX2 0DT
(*Orders*: Tel: 0865 791155
          Fax: 0865 791927
          Telex: 837515)
USA
Blackwell Scientific Publications, Inc.
238 Main Street
Cambridge, MA 02142
(*Orders*: Tel: 800 759-6102
          617 876-7000)

Canada
Times Mirror Professional Publishing, Ltd
130 Flaska Drive
Markham, Ontario L6G 1B8
(*Orders*: Tel: 800 268-4178
          416 470-6739)

Australia
Blackwell Scientific Publications Pty Ltd
54 University Street
Carlton, Victoria 3053
(*Orders*: Tel: 03 347-5552)

A catalogue record for this title
is available from the British Library

ISBN 0-632-03333-9

Library of Congress
Cataloging-in-Publication Data

Restorative proctocolectomy/edited by
  R. John Nicholls, David C.C. Bartolo, Neil Mortensen.
        p.   cm.
    Includes bibliographical references
    and index.
    ISBN 0-632-03333-9
    1. Restorative proctocolectomy.   I. Nicholls, R.J.
    II. Bartolo, David C.C.   III. Mortensen, N.J. McC. (Neil J. McC.)
    [DNLM: 1. Proctocolectomy, Restorative—methods.
    WI 520 R436]
    RD544.R48   1993
    617.5'550592—dc20
    DNLM/DLC
    for Library of Congress

Contents

List of Contributors

D.C.C. BARTOLO MS, FRCS, *Consultant Colorectal Surgeon, Royal Infirmary of Edinburgh, Lauriston Place, Edinburgh EH3 9YW, UK, and Senior Lecturer, University Department of Surgery, University of Edinburgh*

G.S. DUTHIE MB, ChB, BMed Biol, FRCS (Ed), *Research Fellow, Department of Surgery, Royal Infirmary of Edinburgh, Lauriston Place, Edinburgh EH3 9YW, UK*

S. FASTH MD, *Department of Surgery II, University of Göteborg, Sahlgrenska Sjukuset, S-413 45 Göteborg, Sweden*

V.W. FAZIO MB, BS, FRACS, FACS, *Chairman, Department of Colorectal Surgery, The Cleveland Clinic Foundation, One Clinic Center, 9500 Euclid Avenue, Cleveland, Ohio 44195-5044, USA*

S.M. GOLDBERG MD, FACS, *Clinical Professor of Surgery, Division of Colon and Rectal Surgery, Department of Surgery, University of Minnesota Medical School, Minneapolis 55455, Minnesota, USA*

L. HULTÉN MD, PhD, *Professor of Surgery, Department of Surgery II, University of Göteborg, Sahlgrenska Sjukuset, S-413 45 Göteborg, Sweden*

I.C. LAVERY MB, BS, FRACS, FACS, *Staff Surgeon, Department of Colorectal Surgery, The Cleveland Clinic Foundation, One Clinic Center, 9500 Euclid Avenue, Cleveland, Ohio 44195-5044, USA*

M.V. MADDEN FRCS, *Senior Lecturer, Department of Surgery, University of Cape Town Medical School, 79 25 Cape Town, South Africa*

N.J. McC. MORTENSEN MD, FRCS, *Consultant Surgeon, Department of Colorectal Surgery, and Clinical Lecturer, University of Oxford Clinical Medical School, John Radcliffe Hospital, Oxford OX3 9DU, UK*

J.O. MYERS MD, *Fellow, Division of Colon and Rectal Surgery, Department of Surgery, University of Minnesota Medical School, Minneapolis 55455, Minnesota, USA*

D.G. NASMYTH MS, FRCS, *Consultant Surgeon, Department of Surgery, Furness General Hospital, Dalton Lane, Barrow in Furness, Cumbria LA14 4LF, UK*

R.J. NICHOLLS MChir, FRCS, *Consultant Surgeon, St Mark's Hospital, City Road, London EC1U 2PS, and St Thomas' Hospital, Lambeth Palace Road, London SE1 7EH*

T. ÖRESLAND MD, PhD, *Department of Surgery II, University of Göteborg, Sahlgrenska Sjukuset, S-413 45 Göteborg, Sweden*

J.H. PEMBERTON MD, *Associate Professor of Surgery, Mayo Medical School, and Consultant in Colon and Rectal and General Surgery, Mayo Clinic, 200 First Street SW, Rochester, Minnesota, USA*

D.A. ROTHENBERGER MD, FACS, *Clinical Professor of Surgery and Chief, Division of Colon and Rectal Surgery, Department of Surgery, University of Minnesota Medical School, Minneapolis 55455, Minnesota, USA*

N.A. SHEPHERD MB, BS, MRCPath, *Consultant Histopathologist, Department of Histopathology, Gloucestershire Royal Hospital, Great Western Road, Gloucester GL1 3NN, UK*

J.J. TJANDRA MB, BS, MD, FRACS, FRC, *Senior Lecturer, Department of Surgery, University of Wales, Cardiff, UK*

B.F. WARREN MB, ChB, *Lecturer in Pathology, Bristol Royal Infirmary, Malborough Street, Bristol BS2 8HW, UK*

N.S. WILLIAMS MS, FRCS, *Professor of Surgery, The Royal London Hospital, Whitechapel, London E1 1BB, UK*

Foreword

It is a great pleasure to be asked by colleagues to write a foreword for their literary work. In particular, this book entitled *Restorative Proctocolectomy*, edited by John Nicholls, David Bartolo and Neil Mortensen, is timely and covers in depth a subject matter which is highly significant. Surgery for selected patients – in particular with ulcerative colitis and familial polyposis – has evolved over the last three decades to the point where restorative proctocolectomy is a well accepted option in numerous centres around the world. There are still many questions to be asked regarding restorative proctocolectomy and there will most likely be further evolution of the procedure. However, at this particular time, the authors do an excellent job of explaining the evolution of the surgical procedure. The techniques of pouch construction are discussed as are the complications, management, failures and revisions of the procedures, and the controversies and practical aspects of problem solving. Some of their decision-making is based on physiological studies which are also well outlined. The significant complication of pouchitis in reservoir surgery is given a high priority as is the pouch ecology and pathology. The editors of this book are also authors of some of the chapters and together they have gathered other works from renowned authorities in the field of restorative proctocolectomy. Each author presents the subject matter of their own expertise and this is done in a way which allows easy flow from one chapter to another. All of the chapters are well written, illustrated and referenced. The subject matter is covered in detail and the choice of material allows almost complete coverage of all aspects of pouch surgery. All aspects necessary for surgical practice are available for consultation within this book not merely for in-hospital or Medical School libraries but also for the surgeon's own office and study.

This text represents a comprehensive coverage of the subject matter so that readers can feel familiar with the subject and feel confident that they can use it for consultation purposes, and receive good advice. That is why an up to date current review of the literature is so important and so well outlined in each of the chapters.

Often, a text that consists of a series of authors writing independent chapters on selected subtopics leaves gaps. However, this particular textbook provides a well integrated interpretation of the overall subject matter in a relatively unbiased way and thus can be presented as a personal reference volume.

In conclusion, I am honoured that the editors have asked me to write this foreword on a subject matter which also holds special interest for myself. On reading this text, I found it comprehensive and well presented, allowing for further questioning of the subject at hand which is in keeping with the exciting evolutionary nature of restorative proctocolectomy for future years. I have no hesitation in strongly recommending it as a reliable guide to the sound practice of contemporary colorectal surgery for patients with ulcerative colitis and familial polyposis.

ZANE COHEN

Preface

It is now just over 15 years since the introduction of restorative proctocolectomy. The operation has been one of the major developments in colorectal surgery and has transformed the management of ulcerative colitis and familial adenomatous polyposis. Its mortality is low, and while there is an appreciable morbidity, the ultimate outcome for patients is such that around 90% are well satisfied.

Numerous surgical variations have been reported and sometimes hotly discussed. Morbidity has fallen with experience and function has improved owing to developments in technique. There is, however, still room for further advance in clinical terms. In particular, salvage surgery and aspects of problem solving are growing areas. The application of tests of pelvic floor and visceral physiology has enhanced our knowledge of intestinal function and has enabled objective prediction and assessment of outcome. The indications now extend to selected patients with functional bowel disease and the application of restorative proctocolectomy has expanded also within the group of patients with ulcerative colitis and polyposis.

The operation has unwittingly produced a new disease. Pouchitis may resemble ulcerative colitis in many respects, but it is not known whether each has common aetiological factors. The study of pouchitis at the morphological, biochemical and microbiological level may lead to important discoveries of the evolution of inflammatory bowel disease. Changes occur in the pouch epithelium whether or not there are symptoms, and surgeons and gastroenterologists must have a lifelong commitment to this unique group of patients.

We have attempted to deal with all these aspects through the contributions of experts in the field. They rightly do not always agree in detail but this reflects a relatively new and developing area. The fundamental principles are generally accepted, however, and it is at the sharp edge of progress that there is polemic. We hope that the reader will find that such discussion will increase his or her knowledge and understanding and be useful for the clinical management of patients undergoing restorative proctocolectomy.

JOHN NICHOLLS
DAVID BARTOLO
NEIL MORTENSEN

Chapter 1
The Evolution of Surgical Procedures for Anal Preservation

JAMES O. MYERS, DAVID A. ROTHENBERGER
AND STANLEY M. GOLDBERG

History and background

Restorative proctocolectomy is an evolutionary step in the surgeon's attempt to remove either precancerous or severely diseased colonic and rectal mucosa while maintaining anal continence. The history of the ileoanal pouch is inseparably bound to the surgeon's attempt to deal with ulcerative colitis and its complications. At the turn of the century, appendicostomy, and later, caecostomy were performed to irrigate the colon with various fluids to control the inflammation of severe ulcerative colitis (Brown, 1913; Brooke, 1954). As operations became safer and more invasive, bypass and excisional procedures followed and with them better long-term management of the disease (Cahel, 1935). It was realized that by removing the colon and rectum in patients with ulcerative colitis and familial adenomatous polyposis syndrome, the risk of large bowel cancer was eliminated.

Proctocolectomy with permanent ileostomy

Although relatively safe intra-abdominal surgical techniques had been developed in the late 19th and early 20th centuries with the advent of asepsis and anaesthesia, it was not until 1944 that Strauss and Strauss introduced proctocolectomy in the management of ulcerative colitis (Strauss & Strauss, 1944). There was major morbidity related to the ileostomy until the 1950s when Brooke (Fig. 1.1) and later Turnbull (Fig. 1.2) described the everted ileostomy to minimize nutrient and fluid loss and avoid serositis (Brooke, 1952; Turnbull, 1953).

The development of rubber adhesives and stoma bags in the 1940s replaced bandage truss and corset contraptions which were unreliable at holding the small bowel effluent. In 1944 a flat light-weight rubber appliance was first described by Strauss and Strauss which bonded and sealed to the skin with rubber adhesives and was supported by a lightweight belt. For the first time the stoma patient had a reasonably reliable device that allowed an active lifestyle and minimized excoriation of peristomal skin.

In 1958 Dr Rupert B. Turnbull Jr, of the Cleveland Clinic enlisted an interested ostomy patient, Norma Gill, to aid in counselling and advising future stoma patients and to help in the rehabilitation of former stoma patients. Out of their interest and the reputation that they gained in the effective management of ostomies and ostomy appliances, they developed a fund of knowledge that was eventually transmitted to other interested individuals, and was formalized as a school of enterostomal therapy at the Cleveland Clinic. The cooperation of physicians, enterostomal therapists and patients resulted in the rapid development, not only of lighter, more effective stoma devices, but also of techniques of complicated ostomy care which have made life for the ostomy patients approach normality. Intersphincteric proctectomy and primary perineal wound closure were also key events in the decreased morbidity and mortality of total proctocolectomy. The technical advances in ostomy appliance management have brought proctocolectomy with permanent ileostomy to the end of its evolution.

Continent permanent ileostomy

In an effort to construct a continent ileostomy, that is, an ileostomy that requires no stoma appliance and may be irrigated at a convenient place and time, Kock developed the 'intra-abdominal reservoir' in the late 1960s at Sahlgren's Hospital in Göteborg, Sweden (Kock, 1969). In 1972, Kock introduced a nipple valve in his ileal reservoir which created a leak-proof one-way valve system (Faren et al., 1973). However, nipple valve failure required further valve modifications with revision being necessary in over 50% of patients. By 1985 valve construction had improved such that valve revision was necessary in only 10% of patients (Dozois et al., 1980; Gerber et al., 1983).

This reservoir and permanent ileostomy procedure survives to this day. High complication rates make it

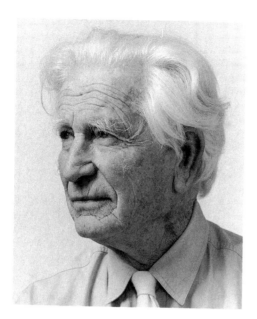

Fig. 1.1 Professor Bryan Brooke.

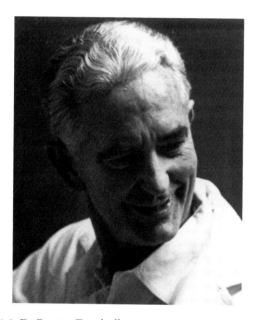

Fig. 1.2 Dr Rupert Turnbull.

a compromise operation which preserves continence and function at the risk of leaving diseased rectal mucosa. It was first described by Devine and Devine (Devine & Devine, 1957). Parc *et al.* (1985) reviewed 17 studies comprising 1206 patients undergoing ileorectal anastomosis for ulcerative colitis and found that patients averaged four to five bowel motions per day and that 99% of the patients had normal continence. In this review, 15% of patients eventually required bypass or completion proctectomy. The risk of cancer developing in the remaining rectum is real and appears to be

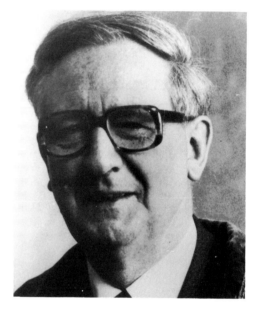

Fig. 1.3 Sir Alan Parks.

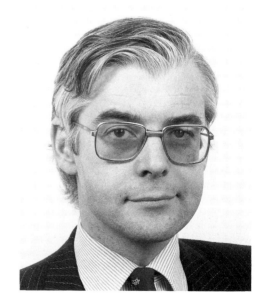

Fig. 1.4 Mr John Nicholls.

suitable to be done only by specialized institutions in which the operation is commonly performed. The ileoanal pouch procedure has, however, largely replaced the technically demanding continent ileostomy procedure.

Total colectomy with ileorectal anastomosis

Total colectomy and ileorectal anastomosis for mucosal ulcerative colitis and familial adenomatous polyposis is

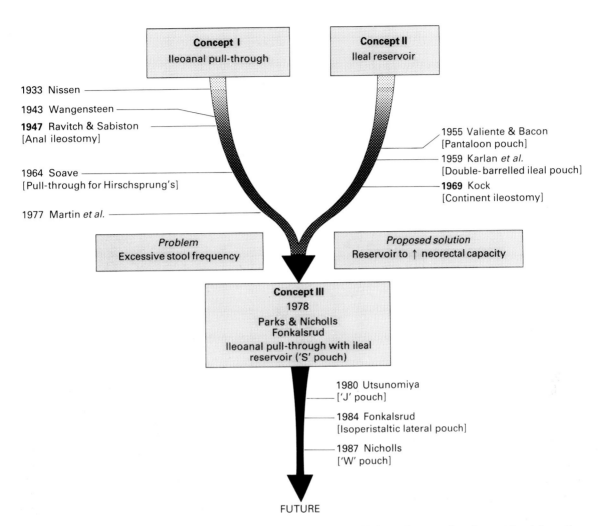

Fig. 1.5 Evolution of restorative proctocolectomy. The ileal pouch–anal pull-through procedure has evolved from the amalgamation of two concepts: (I) the ileoanal pull-through, which incorporated a total colectomy, rectal mucosectomy and pull-through of the distal ileum with anastomosis to the anus, and (II) an ileal reservoir. From Wong *et al.* (1985) with permission.

in the range of 2–20% depending on the institution reporting and the length of follow-up. Close surveillance of the remaining cancer-prone rectal mucosa in both ulcerative colitis and familial adenomatous polyposis is required.

Colectomy with ileorectal anastomosis remains an attractive option in patients with minimal rectal disease providing they are available for regular follow-up to minimize the chance of developing undiagnosed cancer of the rectum. Careful patient follow-up is also required to change medical and surgical management as necessary if disease in the remaining rectal segment progresses or is unremitting.

Restorative proctocolectomy

Total colectomy, with full-thickness proximal proctectomy, distal mucosal proctectomy and ileoanal anastomosis with ileal reservoir is the operation that has evolved as the procedure that most ideally maintains bowel function and removes diseased large bowel and rectal mucosa. The operation as described by Parks (Fig. 1.3) and Nicholls (Fig. 1.4) in 1978, is the amalgamation of the ileal reservoir procedure with the earlier described straight ileoanal anastomosis in rectal mucosal stripping procedures (Parks & Nicholls, 1978).

As early as 1900 and 1912, Hochenegg and Vignolo attempted ileoanal anastomosis (Hocheregg, 1900).

The normal defaecation pathway was maintained with removal of the diseased colon and rectum. Poor functional results and high morbidity prevented widespread adoption of these techniques. These lessons were relearned in 1933 by Nissen and in 1947 and 1948 by Ravitch and Sabiston, who studied the concept of mucosectomy prior to anal ileostomy in dogs and later in a limited number of humans (Nissen, 1933, Ravitch & Sabiston, 1947; Ravitch, 1948). A colonic pull-through procedure with coloanal anastomosis after mucosal stripping of the distal rectum was described in a case of megacolon by Yancey *et al.* (1952), but was popularized by Soave (1964) who described a colonic pull-through procedure after distal rectal mucosectomy for Hirschsprung's disease and had good results in children. Though morbidity and mortality decreased, an increase in stool frequency and unpredictable continence problems prevented widespread acceptance of this operation in adults. The application of distal rectal mucosal stripping was combined with a total colectomy and a straight ileoanal anastomosis by Safaie-Shirafi and Soper (1973) in four young patients with familial adenomatous polyposis coli. In 1977, Martin *et al.* reported satisfactory results in young patients with ulcerative colitis. Early postoperative stool frequency, urgency and incontinence, particularly at night, plagued early attempts at straight ileoanal anastomosis in adults.

The idea of decreasing stool frequency by construction of an ileal reservoir attached to the low rectum or anal canal actually antedated the operations by Safaie-Shirafi and Soper (1973) and Martin *et al.* (1977). Valiente and Bacon (1955) described the construction of a triple limb (pantaloon) ileal pouch in dogs combined with an ileoanal anastomosis. Karlan *et al.* (1959) attempted a double-barrel isoperistaltic pouch and demonstrated its effectiveness in dogs. It was Parks & Nicholls (1978) who combined ileal reservoir with distal rectal mucosal stripping and pouch-anal anastomosis and demonstrated acceptable results in adults. The main steps in the Parks' procedure included total abdominal colectomy, proximal proctectomy, mucosal stripping of the distal rectum, construction of an ileal S pouch, and an ileoanal anastomosis. Technical modifications of this operation have been performed at various institutions, but the individual components remain essentially the same (Fig. 1.5).

Modification of the original Parks pouch

Technical modifications – pouch configuration

The various reservoir designs, have their proponents throughout the world. Utsunomiya (Fig. 1.6) of Japan described the J pouch (Utsunomiya *et al.*, 1980). Fonkalsrud (Fonkalsrud & Ament, 1978) (Fig. 1.7) from the United States described the lateral side-to-side ileal pouch, and Nicholls (Nicholls & Lubowski, 1987) from England, the W pouch. The J pouch is easily con-

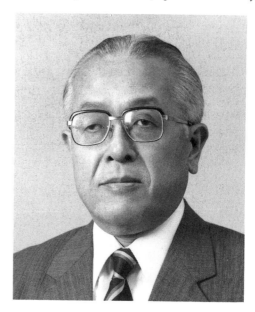

Fig. 1.6 Professor Utsunomiya.

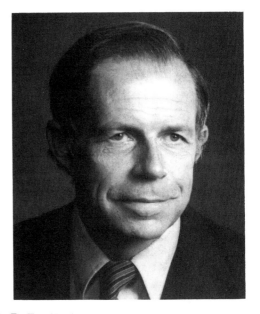

Fig. 1.7 Dr Eric Fonkalsrud.

structed with conventional stapling devices. It fits into the true pelvis and empties easily since it lacks the efferent limb of some other pouch types. Proponents of the more difficult to construct S pouch claim that it more easily reaches the perineum and has a lower stricture rate with a higher volume than the J pouch (Smith *et al.*, 1984). Champions of the W pouch note the highest volumes, but it may not fit into a small pelvis. Provided adequate volume is achieved, a tension-free anal anastomosis is constructed, and the reservoir is placed in the true pelvis with a short outflow tract; each of these pouch designs appears to have similar functional results.

Mucosal stripping

Over the years most surgeons performing restorative proctocolectomy have decreased the length of remaining rectal muscular cuff. An area of intense debate is whether to begin mucosal stripping at the dentate line or above the so-called transitional zone between the dentate line and rectal mucosa. Proponents of the former, claim that by removing all diseased rectal mucosa they prevent any likelihood of recurrent ulcerative colitis, adenomatous disease or cancer. Advocates for leaving the anal transitional tissue claim better functional results although the patients may have to accept a more frequent follow-up to maintain adequate surveillance of the remaining potentially diseased rectal mucosa. An area of debate is whether to strip the mucosa at all. Some authors claim improved continence without mucosectomy and are making the pouch-anal anastomosis 1–2 cm above the dentate line. When prospective, comparative studies are reported, these areas of debate should be resolved.

Summary

Surgeons have modified the original restorative proctocolectomy as described by Parks in an attempt to decrease surgical morbidity and to make the procedure technically less demanding. A greater appreciation of anal and rectal functional anatomy and physiology has aided optimal patient selection, as well as improving the postoperative management of these patients. It has been a decade since this procedure has gained widespread acceptance and the long-term natural history of the 'pouch' is just beginning to be appreciated.

Today restorative proctocolectomy with ileal reservoir stands as an acceptable alternative to conventional proctocolectomy and ileostomy in selected patients with ulcerative colitis and familial adenomatous polyposis. As understanding of anal and rectal continence improves, the operation will continue to evolve and better functional results can be expected.

References

Brooke BN (1952) The management of ileostomy. *Lancet* ii:102–104.

Brooke BN (1954) *Ulcerative Colitis and its Surgical Treatment* (original source by Keetly). Edinburgh, E & S Livingstone.

Brown JY (1913) Value of complete physiological rest of large bowel in treatment of certain ulcerations and obstetrical lesions of this organ. *Surg Gynecol Obstet* 16:610–616.

Cahel RB (1935) The surgical treatment of colitis. *JAMA* 104:104–109.

Devine H, Devine J (1957) Subtotal colectomy and colectomy in ulcerative colitis. *Br Med J* 1:489–492.

Dozois RR, Kelly KA, Beart RW, Beahrs OH (1980) Improved results with continent ileostomy. *Ann Surg* 192:319–324.

Faren A, Kock NG, Sundin T (1973) The long-term functional results after ileocystoplasty. *Scand J Urol Nephrol* 7:127–130.

Fonkalsrud EW, Ament ME (1978) Endorectal mucosal resection without proctocolectomy as an adjunct for abdomino-perineal resection for non-malignant condition: clinical experience with five patients. *Ann Surg* 67:533–538.

Gerber A, Apt MK, Craig PH (1983) The Kock continent ileostomy. *Surg Gynecol Obstet* 156:345–350.

Hochenegg J (1900) Meine operationerfolge bei rectum carcinoma. *Wein Klin Wocheschr* 13:394–404.

Karlan M, McPherson RC, Watman RN (1959) An experimental evaluation of fecal continence – sphincter and reservoir in the dog. *Surg Gynecol Obstet* 108:469–475.

Kock NG (1969) Intra-abdominal 'reservoir' in patients with permanent ileostomy; preliminary observations on a procedure resulting in fecal 'continence' in five ileostomy patients. *Arch Surg* 99:223–231.

Martin LW, LeCoultre C, Shubert WK (1977) Total colectomy and mucosal proctectomy with preservation of continence in ulcerative colitis. *Ann Surg* 186(4):477–480.

Nicholls RJ, Lubowski DZ (1987) Restorative Proctocolectomy: the four loop (W) reservoir. *Br J Surg* 4:564–566.

Nissen R (1933) Meeting of the Berlin Surgical Society. *Zentralb. Chirurgie* 15:888.

Parc R, Levy E, Frileux P, Loygue J (1985) Current results: ileorectal anastomosis after total abdominal colectomy for ulcerative colitis. In *Alternatives to Conventional Ileostomy*, RR Dozois (ed). Chicago, Year Book Medical Publishers, pp. 81–99.

Parks AG, Nicholls RJ (1978) Proctocolectomy without ileostomy for ulcerative colitis. *Br Med J* 2:85–88.

Ravitch MM (1948) Anal ileostomy with sphincter preservation in patients requiring total colectomy for benign conditions. *Surgery* 24:170–187.

Ravitch MM, Sabiston DC (1947) Anal ileostomy with preservation of the sphincter: a proposed operation in patients requiring total colectomy for benign lesions. *Surg Gynecol Obstet* **84**:1095–1099.

Safaie-Shirafi, Soper RT (1973) Endorectal pull through procedure in the surgical treatment of familial polyposis coli. *J Pediatr Surg* **8**(5):711–716.

Smith LE, Friend WG, Medwell SJ (1984) The superior mesenteric artery: the critical technical factor in the ileal pouch pull through operation. *Dis Colon Rectum* **27**:741–744.

Soave F (1964) A new surgical technique for treatment of Hirschsprung's disease. *Surgery* **56**:1007–1014.

Strauss AA, Strauss SF (1944) Surgical treatment of ulcerative colitis. *Surg Clin North Am* **24**:211–224.

Turnbull RB (1953) Management of an ileostomy. *Am J Surg* **86**:617–624.

Utsunomiya AJ, Iwama T, Imajo M, Matsuo S, Sawai S, Yalgashi K, Hirayama R (1980) Total colectomy, mucosal proctectomy and ileoanal anastomosis. *Dis Colon Rectum* **23**:459–466.

Valiente MA, Bacon HE (1955) Construction of pouch using 'pantaloon' technique for pull-through following total colectomy. *Am J Surg* **90**:6621–6643.

Wong WD, Rothenberger DA, Goldberg SM (1985) Ileoanal pouch procedures. *Curr Problems in Surg* **22**(3):1–18.

Yancey AG, Cromartie JE, Ford JR, Nichols RR, Saville AF (1952) A modification of the Swenson technique for congenital megacolon. *J Natl Med Assoc* **44**(5):356–363.

Chapter 2
Patient Selection for Restorative Proctocolectomy

NEIL J. McC. MORTENSEN

Introduction

In some ways the pouch operation has made the task of the gastroenterological surgeon or physician easier. When faced with a patient with ulcerative colitis or familial adenomatous polyposis there is an alternative to a permanent ileostomy. At first sight this may seem an unmissible opportunity, but the pouch is not a return to normal, and great care must be taken to explain carefully the alternatives and disadvantages to any potential candidate. There is a whole range of considerations including subsequent employment prospects, fertility and pregnancy, ageing and compliance with future follow-up schemes, in addition to any purely technical ones like physical build, continence or frequency. This chapter discusses the indications for restorative proctocolectomy as they best apply to each individual patient. To put this in context the advantages and disadvantages of the three currently used operations for ulcerative colitis are compared in Table 2.1. Conventional proctocolectomy and ileostomy has the advantage that all the disease is excised during one operation, it removes the risk of cancer and it is a well tried and usually uncomplicated technique. The patient is left, however, with a permanent ileostomy with its social and psychological consequences. With the advent of restorative proctocolectomy the indications for this procedure would now be elderly patients especially those with a weak sphincter and those unwilling to have a more complex operation which holds the possibility of more morbidity and a longer hospital stay. In Oxford, less than one-quarter of our patients now elect to have a conventional proctectomy.

General

Restorative proctocolectomy is a complex procedure with a complication rate in the region of 25–40% (Dozois *et al.*, 1986). There is a re-operation rate of 15–25% and in those patients suffering major post-operative complications there can be a protracted postoperative stay.

For this reason patients must be fit for such a major procedure psychologically and physically. We would not carry out a restorative proctocolectomy in a patient having urgent surgery for severe colitis or toxic megacolon. Here the operation of choice is a total abdominal colectomy with preservation of the rectal stump and an ileostomy. This allows for subsequent checking of the histological diagnosis, and for the patient to recover physically and nutritionally. Steroids *per se* are not a contraindication but as far as possible we try to wean patients off any immunosuppressants prior to surgery. Nutritional status should be assessed by weight loss, serum albumin and general clinical wellbeing, and if necessary nutritional supplements are given prior to surgery. In borderline cases we would put in a central line at the time of surgery to anticipate any problems.

Extra-intestinal manifestations of ulcerative colitis include arthritis, iritis and pyoderma gangrenosum. They are not a contraindication to the procedure, but there does seem to be an increased risk of pouchitis in these patients (Lohmuller *et al.*, 1990; de Silva *et al.*, 1991), and the operation may not cure their extra-intestinal manifestations.

Anatomy

As with any operation there are anatomical considerations. The short obese subject can prove a formidable technical challenge. The mesentery of the small intestine in these patients is also short and fat and this may give less length and reach into the pelvis (Smith *et al.*, 1984). A very tall subject may also have a limited length of small bowel mesentery. In patients who have had a previous ileal resection there is not only the potential physiological effect on function but the added problem of reach. After previous surgery for colitis there can also be dense adhesions and all these factors should be taken into account.

Table 2.1 Comparison of the three operations most commonly used in treatment of ulcerative colitis.

	Conventional proctocolectomy and Brooke ileostomy	Colectomy with ileorectal anastomosis	Restorative proctocolectomy
Advantages	Curative, one operation	One operation; sphincter unchanged; evacuation 2–4 times/day; no stoma; no bladder or sexual dysfunction	Curative; anal function preserved
Disadvantages	Ileostomy appliance; need to empty 4–8 times/day	Not curative; cancer risk persists; late proctectomy for cancer or inflammatory disease in 5–50%	Failure 10%; need to evacuate 3–8 times/day; two operations usually
Complications	Stoma revision 10–25%; perineal wound problems 10–25%; small bowel obstruction 10–20%; bladder dysfunction minimal; sexual dysfunction minimal	Small bowel obstruction 10–20%; potential anastomotic leak	Pouch fistulae; ileoanal anastomotic sepsis; stenosis; small bowel obstruction 10–20%; pouchitis; bladder dysfunction minimal; sexual dysfunction minimal; anal excoriation
Contraindications	Strong desire to avoid ileostomy	Sphincter incompetence; severe rectal disease; rectal dysplasia; rectal cancer	Crohn's disease; rectal cancer in distal half; no objection to ileostomy

It is for this reason that patients should always be told that there is a remote possibility that the operation may not be possible and that they could find themselves with a permanent ileostomy. At the very least, surgeons undertaking the operation in a difficult patient should have a number of pouch techniques at their command. For example, in the thick-set male pelvis an eversion technique (Goligher, 1984) may be more feasible than a conventional one; in the short obese subject, restorative proctocolectomy with an ileo upper anal anastomosis may be easier for reach, or mesenteric vessels may have to be divided, or an S configuration used.

Age

The elderly

There is no absolute contraindication to pouch surgery on the grounds of age at either extreme. Patients as young as 3 years of age have had the operation, and there are reports of patients in their late 70s or early 80s having a successful pouch. Early in the experience of the operation, many centres placed the upper age limit at an arbitrary 55 years. Continence disturbances are known to be more common after restorative proctocolectomy in those over 50 years old (Dozois, 1985). There is a correlation between electromyographic abnormalities which are more common in patients over 40 years of age and continence after restorative proctocolectomy (Stryker *et al.*, 1985).

Several studies have shown a decrease in resting and squeeze anal pressures with increasing age particularly in women over 60 years of age (Matheson & Keighley, 1981; McHugh & Diamant, 1987), so special care must be taken in the selection of this group. Restorative procedures for rectal cancer are regularly carried out in patients in their seventh or eighth decade and similar considerations can be used when selecting the elderly for a pouch operation. In suitably motivated elderly patients who understand the risks and problems it is certainly feasible, but many surgeons would feel that an ileostomy would be a more reliable and predictable option. In the elderly there must obviously be no cardiovascular or respiratory risk factors as morbidity will be less well tolerated. Since the possibility of future dysplasia or cancer is unlikely to be so important in the much older patient, this is the ideal situation for an ileoanal operation making the anastomosis at the upper anal canal level where there may be better sphincter function.

Paediatric

There are to date only a few studies on the use of restorative proctocolectomy in children. The paediatric surgical service at the Mayo Clinic have reported 121 patients with a restorative proctocolectomy (Telander *et al.*, 1990). The mean age was 15, the youngest 3 and, surprisingly, the oldest was 29 years of age which must weaken the paediatric emphasis of the paper. Of the 114 available for follow-up, 49 had a straight ileoanal anastomosis, whilst 72 had a J pouch and anastomosis. One hundred and one of these were for chronic ulcerative colitis, 19 had familial adenomatosis and one had whole bowel aganglionosis.

There was no mortality. Three (2%) out of 121 had a septic episode postoperatively, but only one out of 121 (0.5%) had pelvic sepsis. Stool frequency in those with a straight ileoanal was six in daytime and one at night in the J pouch patients. Daytime incontinence was rare, but 14 patients noted some smearing once a week. Six (3%) out of the 121 failed the operation, four had Crohn's disease, one had a fistula which could not be dealt with surgically and one had intense perianal irritation. Pouchitis occurred in 40% of patients with a straight ileoanal anastomosis and 22% in those with a J pouch, but diagnostic criteria were not stated. Comparing the results with a larger group of adults, adults tended to have more sepsis, strictures and more pouchitis than the paediatric group. Nearly all paediatric patients now have a J pouch constructed.

In a small group of eight children and teenagers having straight ileoanal anastomosis and 10 having ileoanal reservoir were compared (Odigwe *et al.*, 1987). Two of the children in the first group developed intractable diarrhoea that persisted despite revision to an ileoanal pouch, and ileostomies were necessary in both cases. One patient in the second group had a diversion for anastomotic sepsis. Despite a longer period of follow-up (49 vs. 12 months) the remaining patients in the first group had greater frequency (7.8 vs. 4.8 stools/day). Faecal incontinence persisted in two and six patients in each group, and perianal dermatitis in two and four respectively. Attendance at school and participation in social activities was greater postoperatively when compared with the 6-month period prior to surgery in both groups. To date there is too little information on function after restorative proctocolectomy with ileal reservoir in children, but in the Oxford experience of four cases, morbidity has been minimal and function excellent with a frequency of defaecation of no more than 5/24 h. Clearly further studies of the long-term functional results are required before its true place can be assessed. Until such data become available the operation of choice in children should perhaps be an ileorectal anastomosis wherever possible. Where the severity of rectal disease excludes this option, then a colectomy with ileostomy and rectal preservation should be seriously considered. In either case, a decision can then be made later in teenage or early adult life as to the best long-term choice.

Anal sphincter

Since the ileal pouch contents remain liquid or at best semi-formed even in the best functioning pouch, a good anal sphincter is essential for satisfactory function. Any past history of anal sphincter injury, fistula or previous anal surgery should be noted. While this would not necessarily exclude a pouch operation, it must be taken into account when weighing up the pros and cons in the individual case. In young patients it is unusual to find any suggestion of weakness on routine digital examination, but the anus should be carefully examined for scars or tears. Anorectal physiology studies including manometry and sensory studies are advisable though these are not mandatory. It has been very useful to have preoperative test results with which to compare postoperative values in elucidating the problem of poor or imperfect continence after pouch surgery.

With age the sphincter may deteriorate. In women this is more apparent than in men and tends to become significant in the sixth or seventh decade (Matheson & Keighley, 1981; Neill *et al.*, 1981; McHugh & Diamant, 1987). Both maximal resting and maximal squeeze pressures decline, and although this may not be apparent in elderly patients with constipated stools, the pouch contents of a 70-year-old may prove to be more of a challenge to the ageing sphincter. For this reason there has been a sensible degree of caution in recommending the procedure to elderly females. The changes are less marked in males.

Pregnancy

In women considering pregnancy, careful thought should be given to the danger of damage to the anal sphincter during vaginal delivery. It is usual in British centres to advise pouch patients to have a Caesarian section rather than risk a traumatic or prolonged delivery, but in the Mayo series successful vaginal deliveries have been reported. In their first report Metcalf *et al.* (1986) described six successful pregnancies all carried to term. Three had transient deterioration of anorectal function during the third trimester which resolved after delivery. Four patients were delivered vaginally without any alteration in subsequent continence. In a further report from the Mayo Clinic, Nelson *et al.* (1989) described 20 of their 354 pouch patients who had had one or more pregnancy. Eleven were delivered per vaginam, and nine by Caesarian section. The method of delivery had no effect on sphincter function, but there was an increase in nocturnal frequency during pregnancy which persisted for 3 months after delivery. They felt that the route of delivery could be safely individualized for each patient.

Snooks *et al.* (1984) have shown, however, that pudendal nerve motor latency can be prolonged after vaginal delivery, especially if there is a long second stage, or in those who require a forceps delivery. It would seem reasonable therefore to recommend that at least those patients with a pre-existing continence deficit, those with a short perineal body and those with cephalopelvic disproportion should have an elective Caesarian section.

Fertility

There have been few papers reporting the fertility of patients after proctocolectomy. Metcalf *et al.* (1986) looked at sexual function in 50 female patients after a Kock pouch, and 50 after an ileoanal pouch. In both groups there was an increase in the frequency of intercourse and a decrease in dyspareunia. In one patient in each group there was a decrease in the quality of orgasm. There was no change in the menstrual cycle and a minimally impaired fertility with six out of eight ileoanal pouch patients and 10 out of 12 Kock pouch patients trying for a pregnancy being successful. Thus there is no strong evidence to suggest that the operation leads to reduced fertility.

Sexual function in males

Damage to the pelvic autonomic nerves in the course of a rectal excision can impair bladder and sexual function. The reported incidence of impotence ranges from 5 to 17% after proctocolectomy, and depends to some extent on the age of the patient (Williams & Johnson, 1985). Close rectal dissection (Lee & Dowling, 1972) and intersphincteric excision of the anus (Lyttle & Parks, 1977) may well have reduced the incidence, but there continues to be a small risk whether the patient has a restorative procedure or a permanent ileostomy. In pouch patients, the incidence of impotence postoperatively is very low following close rectal dis-

section (Nicholls, 1987), whereas with dissection in the mesorectal plane, three men (1.5%) had erectile dysfunction and seven (4%) retrograde ejaculation (Pemberton *et al.*, 1987). Where a particular problem is anticipated or the patient has a preference, facilities for preoperative storage of a semen specimen should be made available.

Previous surgery

As experience has grown with restorative proctocolectomy, surgeons have become more bold in using the procedure in situations previously thought to be a contraindication. Remarkably Pearl *et al.* (1985) have reported a successful restorative proctocolectomy 24 years after total proctocolectomy for ulcerative colitis. Two similar cases have been reported by Ryan and Fink (1988). In these cases and one by Parker and Nicholls (1992) the functional outcome must rely upon the intact external anal sphincter, the internal sphincter having been removed. In a case reported by Hulten *et al.* (1988) a mucosal proctectomy had been carried out at the original operation 5 years previously. They were able to take down a Kock pouch and successfully anastomose it to the anal sphincter. All these authors have claimed a good functional outcome, but imperfections of continence might be expected to be more common after these procedures.

Previous abdominal surgery involving the upper small bowel could compromise mesenteric length. Parker and Nicholls (1992) have reported successful pouch surgery in two patients who had undergone total gastrectomy and a Whipple's procedure, but there is otherwise little in the literature on this point. In such a situation it would be prudent to make a very careful check for mesenteric length before constructing a pouch.

In the rare situation of a pouch having to be resected early in the postoperative period, for ischaemia for example, a further attempt at pouch surgery is reasonable despite the decreased distal small bowel length, but the patient should be warned of the possibility of technical failure and poorer function in terms of increased frequency. Similar considerations apply to those patients who have had laparotomies for adhesion obstruction. Previous pelvic surgery will also present technical problems but is not necessarily a contraindication.

Indications

Inflammatory bowel disease – Crohn's disease

Ulcerative colitis is the principal indication for restorative proctocolectomy. Although Crohn's disease is generally regarded as a contraindication some have suggested that patients with Crohn's disease may be suitable. Kock reported a series of continent ileostomies in patients with Crohn's disease (Kock & Myrvold, 1980). Out of 52 patients, 26 (53%) developed recurrent Crohn's disease in the reservoir. There were three deaths (two late) and eight patients had the reservoir removed. Out of the remaining 41 patients, 37 were continent and of these 35 led a healthy life. With an incidence of major postoperative complications of 26% and a failure rate of 16%, they concluded that the operation was not recommended for Crohn's disease patients although many had a satisfactory long-term outcome.

The experience has been similar if not worse in patients with Crohn's disease who have a restorative proctocolectomy. Deutsch *et al.* (1991) found Crohn's disease in nine (3.5%) out of 272 pouch patients. In five the diagnosis was made after excision of the rectum, and in four it developed a mean of 2.5 years after the pouch procedure. Overall four had the pouch removed, two had persisting perianal disease and three were well. In the first 210 patients operated on at St Mark's Hospital, there were 12 (6%) failures. Out of these, five were patients with Crohn's disease, and in each case progressive disease in the reservoir or the anal region was the prime cause of failure. Thus, nearly half the failures were due to Crohn's disease. Furthermore, in the whole group of 210 patients, there was no patient known to have Crohn's disease who had not failed (Nicholls, 1987). More recently Grobbler *et al.* (1991) have reported 80 patients having restorative proctocolectomy for inflammatory bowel disease; out of these, 20 were said to have Crohn's disease or indeterminant colitis. Of these, 40% failed within 18 months; it is very likely that some of the remainder will do so as time progresses. Hyman *et al.* (1991) found 25 patients out of 362 pouch procedures who eventually had a diagnosis of Crohn's disease. Sixteen had a functioning pouch, seven required pouch excision, one was diverted and one had died. Only one out of nine patients in whom there was a preoperative clinical feature suggesting Crohn's disease had a functioning pouch. At the very least, the prognosis after restorative proctocolectomy in Crohn's disease is bad. It must be remembered that failure, that is the removal of the reservoir with establishment of a permanent ileostomy, involves considerable suffering by the patient over a sustained period of time. Jobs are lost, careers impaired and family life is disrupted. Wexner *et al.* (1990) while showing that most failures occur within 2 years of operation, pointed out that only one-third did so within the first year. Thus suffering may be drawn out before failure is acknowledged. In their series, in one-third of all failures, Crohn's disease was the reason.

If Crohn's disease is contraindicated, how often is the diagnosis of ulcerative colitis mistaken? In the series of Myrvold and Kock (1981), 36 out of the 52 Crohn's patients had a preoperative diagnosis of ulcerative colitis. Reported incidences of Crohn's disease masquerading as ulcerative colitis range from less than 5 to 25%. Why should this be so? Crohn's disease is diagnosed on the basis of clinical, radiological and histological criteria. In excluding it, the most important clinical factors include absence of small bowel and anal disease, and the presence of rectal disease. The presence of any clinical factor should raise suspicion of Crohn's disease whatever the histology shows. (Anal disease does not necessarily mean Crohn's disease. Around 10% of patients with ulcerative colitis coming to proctocolectomy have an anal lesion.) In a retrospective review of 112 such patients with ulcerative colitis at St Mark's Hospital, 12 had an anal lesion. In these the lesions were minor and included low fistulae and fissure (Springall R., personal communication). However, rectovaginal fistulae occasionally occur, but are more likely to be due to Crohn's disease (Radcliffe *et al.*, 1988). A high fistula or ulceration should also be regarded clinically as more likely to be associated with Crohn's disease (Morson & Dawson, 1990).

Indeterminate colitis

Patients with so-called indeterminate colitis present a difficulty in case selection. A report of indeterminate colitis on a histological section only expresses the pathologist's unwillingness to commit him or herself to a specific diagnosis. About 10–15% of cases fall into this category (Price, 1978; Lee *et al.*, 1979). Essentially it means that the pathologist is unable to identify features strongly in favour of either ulcerative colitis or Crohn's disease. On receiving such a report, the clinician must place it within the general context of the case. This includes clinical and radiological factors. Sometimes despite considering all features, it is still not possible to be sure of the diagnosis. Patients in this category probably form a distinct entity. From the pathologist's point of view, a histological diagnosis of indeterminate colitis is more likely in patients with severe acute disease where the magnitude of inflammatory changes may obscure discriminating histological features (Price, 1978). Thus it is essential to take further rectal biopsies in patients who have had a previous colectomy with ileostomy and preservation of the rectal stump for acute disease, in order to establish the true diagnosis as far as possible, but bearing in mind that the changes of defunctioned colitis can further add to the confusion. Despite such precautions, some patients will still be unclassifiable and will therefore have a diagnosis of indeterminate colitis.

The long-term natural history of indeterminate colitis is of considerable importance when considering restorative proctocolectomy. Pezim et al. (1989) reported the outcome in 25 patients with indeterminate colitis having a restorative proctocolectomy. They were followed for a mean of 38 months. All had been thought preoperatively to have ulcerative colitis and the diagnosis of indeterminate colitis was made on the postoperative histological examination of the resected specimen. The results were excellent in terms of function and a low failure rate.

In a recent retrospective study of 46 patients diagnosed between 1960 and 1983, clinical, radiological and histological features were reviewed. They were placed in three groups: probable Crohn's disease (19 patients), probable ulcerative colitis (11 patients) and 'true' indeterminate colitis (16 patients). The patients were then followed by further clinical and histological assessment over a median period of 10 years (range 2.5–28 years). Out of the 16 patients with true indeterminate colitis, three were subsequently classified as ulcerative colitis and only one as Crohn's disease (Wells et al., 1991). If these observations are true, then it is reasonable to conclude that indeterminate colitis behaves more like ulcerative colitis than Crohn's disease.

A diagnosis of indeterminate colitis may, however, sway the decision towards colectomy with ileorectal anastomosis in patients in whom the rectum is not excessively inflamed or contracted. Some surgeons even advocate an initial colectomy with ileostomy and preservation of the rectal stump as routine in order to

be as sure as possible of the diagnosis. There is as yet no information on whether this approach reduces the incidence of a false positive diagnosis of ulcerative colitis. Certainly there is no evidence that morbidity of the pouch operation itself or function after closure of the ileostomy are any different whether or not a previous colectomy has been performed.

In summary, unequivocal Crohn's disease is a contraindication to restorative proctocolectomy. Those with indeterminate colitis can be safely offered the operation, but where there is serious doubt, a colectomy should be carried out first and the rectum subsequently biopsied repeatedly in an attempt to exclude Crohn's disease.

Familial adenomatous polyposis

Restorative proctocolectomy might seem the ideal operation for familial adenomatous polyposis. By removing all large bowel mucosa, the risk of cancer in that organ should be completely avoided. However, there are disadvantages in its routine use. The most important include the morbidity and duration of convalescence when compared with colectomy and ileorectal anastomosis. There is a small but significant chance of failure which would then leave the patient with a permanent ileostomy after months of suffering from the very surgical complications that were responsible for failure. It would be wrong to subject all affected adolescents to such a procedure given that the cancer risk at that age is low. On the other hand ileorectal anastomosis has been reported to be followed by a high incidence of carcinoma developing in the rectal stump (Bess et al., 1980). The cumulative incidence of cancer in this study was 32%, out of 143 patients followed up 20 years after the colectomy. There was a lower incidence of cancer in the rectal stump in the St Mark's Hospital series of 214 cases (14 (6.5%) cancers) (Thomson, 1990) with a cumulative risk of about 10% at 25 years from colectomy (Bussey et al., 1985). Explanations might include a less well controlled follow-up, a longer length of distal large bowel preserved in the Mayo Clinic series and possibly a greater propensity for cancer in the United States compared with the United Kingdom. Whatever the reasons, it has to be acknowledged that colectomy with ileorectal anastomosis is a compromise procedure aimed to achieve a satisfactory clinical outcome with the minimal risk of morbidity to the patient.

Pouch or ileorectal anastomosis?

There is now a well-established observation that polyposis patients have fewer postoperative complications than those having the procedure for colitis (Dozois, 1988). In a recent comparison of the morbidity following restorative proctocolectomy and colectomy with ileorectal anastomosis for polyposis treated at one institution between 1976 and 1990, there were also marked differences. When the complications of 37 patients having restorative proctocolectomy and closure of the temporary ileostomy were combined, the re-operation rate was 18% compared with only 2% among 62 patients having ileorectal anastomosis during the same period. Total hospital stay was 25 days and 11 days, respectively, and the interval between the operation and return to normal activity was 31 weeks and 14 weeks, respectively (Madden et al., 1991). These differences were statistically significant. To some extent they could be ascribed to the temporary ileostomy which was responsible for significant complications in six patients, including intestinal obstruction in five. The stoma was also responsible for a longer treatment time. It may be that an ileostomy is not necessary in these cases as advocated by Everett and Pollard (1990), in which case restorative proctocolectomy would perform better in terms of treatment time and stoma related complications. There would however be patients developing pelvic sepsis who would suffer a significant morbidity without an ileostomy. The question of ileostomy is discussed more fully in Chapter 5.

As regards ultimate function, there appears to be little to choose between restorative proctocolectomy and colectomy with ileorectal anastomosis. After an ileorectal anastomosis, median frequency was 3/24 hours and urgency (unable to wait 15 minutes) occurred in 50% compared with 4.5/24 hours and 17% after restorative proctocolectomy. Night evacuation occurred

in 10 and 43% respectively (Madden et al., 1991). The choice between restorative proctocolectomy and colectomy with ileorectal anastomosis will depend on the perceived risk of carcinoma in the rectal stump (Table 2.2). This is largely related to the age of the patient. In persons below 20 years, carcinoma is exceedingly rare, whereas it is common in patients presenting with symptoms. This generally occurs in the third to fourth decades of life and about one-third of patients presenting at this age will already have an invasive neoplasm. In the adolescent, therefore, it is reasonable to recommend colectomy with ileorectal anastomosis provided that follow-up is likely to be good. Conversely, a restorative proctocolectomy would seem to be the safer procedure in older patients, certainly those over 30 years. For those in between, it is not possible to be dogmatic. The clinician will have to base a decision on factors which include the behaviour of other members of the same pedigree in terms of cancer formation, the patient's wishes, availability for follow-up and the extent of rectal involvement, for example, those with large or confluent polyps. Since rectal adenomas regress after colectomy with ileorectal anastomosis this last criteria is by no means absolute. However, in patients who still have uncontrollable rectal adenomas after colectomy with ileorectal anastomosis, there is evidence that the risk of cancer is increased (Moertel et al., 1970). In these, proctectomy with ileoanal anastomosis should be advised. In those who have already formed a carcinoma of the colon, the chance of carcinoma subsequently developing in the rectum is increased (Shepherd & Bussey, 1990). Thus established malignancy in a polyposis patient should be an indication for restorative proctocolectomy (Taylor et al., 1988).

Desmoid disease

The presence of intra-abdominal desmoid disease is probably a contraindication to restorative proctocolectomy. This is certainly so if the lesion is large where diffuse desmoidosis has reduced the mobility of the mesentery. Desmoids occur in 8–15% of patients with polyposis (Phillips et al., 1991, unpublished observations) and may be related to kindreds. There is a high incidence of previous abdominal operations in these patients, in line with the anecdotal impression that their growth may be encouraged by surgery. Where desmoid disease is present, colectomy with

Table 2.2 Surgical options in familial adenomatous polyposis.

Ileorectal anastomosis	Restorative proctocolectomy
Under 20 years of age	Over 30 years of age
Good follow-up	Poor follow-up
Controllable polyps	Large or confluent rectal polyps
No established cancer	Established cancer
Desmoid disease	No desmoid disease

Table 2.3 Preferences in 55 patients who have undergone restorative proctocolectomy with ileal reservoir (including four failures).

	Stoma preferred	No difference	Reservoir preferred
Feel more natural	4	0	51 (92.7%)
Feel more confident	6	1	48 (87.32%)
Easier to keep clean	6	0	49 (89.1%)
Feel 'cleaner'	6	0	49 (89.1%)
Feel more sexually attractive	6	1	48 (87.3%)
Less time to manage	9	1	45 (81.8%)
Less interference with work	7	2	46 (83.6%)
Less interference with social activities	7	1	47 (85.4%)
Less interference with sports activities	6	7	42 (87.5%)
Less interference with clothing	5	1	49 (89.1%)
Less odour between emptying	6	3	46 (83.6%)
Less odour during emptying	5	5	45 (81.8%)
Less diet restriction	19	8	28 (50.9%)
Overall preference	6	1	48 (87.3%)

From Pezim & Nicholls (1985) with permission.

ileorectal anastomosis is probably to be preferred unless there is severe rectal disease. In this circumstance, particularly if it is invasive, a rectal excision will be necessary either with restoration of the intestinal continuity or not as is feasible.

Functional bowel disease

This is a controversial indication for the operation but its use in functional bowel disorders is likely to increase. In patients with Hirschsprung's disease or an idiopathic megacolon a segmental resection of colon is usually sufficient, but in the rare case of universal colonic involvement perhaps after previous less radical surgery has failed a restorative proctocolectomy may be indicated.

In the group of patients with slow transit constipation, restorative proctocolectomy can be used as a second line procedure after a failed ileorectal anastomosis, but great care must be taken with case selection. There is some evidence that the motility disorder which may be responsible for delayed colonic transit could also affect the small bowel. Psychological assessment is crucial in these patients. Hosie et al. (1990) have reported 13 cases, eight with slow transit and five with mega bowel. Complications were common and two patients required a permanent ileostomy. In the short term, 85% were improved. In a small series of four patients Nicholls and Kamm (1988), found acceptable results in two patients who had had a

failed ileorectal for slow transit constipation, and the author has had similar results in two patients. Since there is no concern about mucosal disease, an ileo-upper anal anastomosis can be used in these patients but care must be taken in using staplers on the abnormal megarectum group owing to the large diameter of the rectum.

If restorative proctocolectomy is being considered for this difficult group of patients it should be reserved for those cases where the more conventional procedures have failed and the patient is still very opposed to the idea of an ileostomy.

Quality of life and occupation

There is little published information on the effects of pouch function as related to occupation. However there are studies which have looked at quality of life after pouch surgery. Pezim and Nicholls (1985) sent 55 patients a questionnaire. The reservoir was preferred to their previous ileostomy with regard to confidence (87%), cleanliness (89%), sexual self-image (87%), social reasons (85%) and sport activities (87%) and ease of carrying out work (84%). The overall preference was 87% (Tables 2.3 and 2.4). Thirty-four (66.7%) felt there was no significant disadvantage associated with the reservoir, while 10 (19.6%) saw the long convalescent period and nine (17.6%) the requirement for catheterization as drawbacks. Pemberton et al. (1989) compared the performance status of 406 Brooke

Table 2.4 Disadvantages of the reservoir operation reported by 51 patients.

No significant disadvantage	34 (66.7%)
Long convalescence period	10 (19.6%)
Requirement for catheter	9 (17.6%)
Faecal leakage	4 (7.8%)
Perianal irritation	4 (7.8%)
Reservoir inflammation	2 (3.9%)
Mucous leakage	2 (3.9%)
Perianal pain during healing	2 (3.9%)
Dietary restriction	1 (2.0%)
Urgency	1 (2.0%)
Abdomen appears distended with reservoir full	1 (2.0%)

From Pezim & Nicholls (1985) with permission.

ileostomy patients with 298 pouch patients. A great majority of patients in each group were satisfied (93% Brooke ileostomy; 95% pouch). Thirty-nine percent of Brooke ileostomy patients, however, desired a change in the type of ileostomy they had. In each performance category, the performance score discriminated between operations in favour of the pouch procedure, indicating a better quality of life in this group.

There is a world of difference between the patient with a sedentary job at a desk within easy reach of toilet facilities, and the builder on a site going up and down scaffolding. Provided that the appropriate steps have been taken to ensure good sphincter function, there is no reason to be concerned that heavy manual labour or vigorous sporting activity would be a contraindication, and indeed there are successful pouch patients in both these occupational groups. For those with a long history of colitis the effects of frequent bowel actions on their work and life-style will be only too well known. What can be explained to the pouch candidate is that although frequency may be even as high as that with their colitis, the major difference is that there is no longer the urgency of colitis and that evacuation can be deferred for up to 3 or 4 hours in many cases. Although there are the obvious advantages of not having an appliance there are still some patients who decide on the grounds of their occupation that the pouch is not for them. Here again is another reason for trying to match patients by occupation when arranging preoperative counselling.

The other important consideration is the effect of a potentially long and complicated postoperative course on sickness, absentee rates and job security. It is always worth asking patients about their employer's attitude to their condition and any delay in return to work. For the self-employed this is a key issue which needs to be discussed in detail.

Psychological considerations

In most major series there are one or two eventual failures on the grounds of psychological unsuitability. This is a difficult area in which to give clear cut advice, but patients with major psychiatric disorders should probably not be offered the procedure. Those with a very limited intelligence quotient or understanding of the anatomy need plenty of time with careful counselling. It may be the scale of the procedure or the frequency of evacuation which they find unacceptable. Whatever the reason, extreme caution is advised in these patients.

Counselling

Candidates for restorative proctocolectomy should have as much information as possible to help them make a decision about the operation. There should be at least two interviews with the surgeon prior to surgery to cover all the pros and cons of the procedure. Multiple sources of information should be provided including published literature, patient information booklets, videotapes and diagrams. At the Mayo Clinic, the stoma therapist acts as an independent counsellor and previous pouch patients matched for age, sex and occupation can be helpful volunteers in preoperative counselling. We have also set up a 'pouch group' of patients to provide continuing support for pouch patients and their families. This is potentially a very useful vehicle for offering advice to prospective patients, continuing education and fund-raising.

References

Bess MA, Adson MA, Moertel CG (1980) Rectal cancer following colectomy for polyposis. *Arch Surg* **115**:460–467.

Bussey HJR, Eyers AA, Ritchie JK, Thomson JPS (1985) The rectum in adenomatous polyposis – the St Mark's policy. *Br J Surg* **72**(suppl):S29–31.

de Silva HJ, De Angelis CP, Soper N, Kettlewell M, Mortensen NJ, Jewell DP (1991) Clinical and functional outcome following restorative proctocolectomy. *Br J Surg* **78**:1039–1044.

Deutsch A, McLeod RS, Cullen J, Cohen Z (1991) Results of the pelvic pouch procedure in patients with Crohn's disease. *Dis Col Rect* **34**:475–477.

Dozois RR (1985) Ileal 'J' pouch-anal anastomosis. *Br J Surg*

72(suppl):580–582.

Dozois RR (1988) Surgical aspects of familial adenomatous polyposis. *Int J Colorectal Dis* 3:1–16.

Dozois RR, Goldberg SM, Rothenburger DA *et al.* (1986) Restorative proctocolectomy with ileal reservoir (Symposium). *Int J Colorectal Dis* 1:2–19.

Everett WG, Pollard SG (1990) Restorative proctocolectomy without temporary ileostomy. *Br J Surg* 77:621–622.

Goligher JC (1984) Eversion technique for distal mucosal proctectomy in ulcerative colitis: a preliminary report. *Br J Surg* 71:26–28.

Grobbler S, Affice E, Keighley MRB, Thompson H (1991) Outcome in patients with restorative proctocolectomy and a suspected diagnosis of Crohn's disease. *Br J Surg* 78:729.

Hosie KB, Kmiot WA, Keighley MRB (1990) Constipation; another indication for restorative proctocolectomy. *Br J Surg* 77:801–802.

Hulten L, Fasth S, Nordgren S, Oresland T (1988) Kock's pouch converted to a pelvic pouch. *Dis Colon Rectum* 31:467–469.

Hyman NH, Fazio VW, Tuckson WB, Lavery IC (1991) The consequences of ileal pouch-anal anastomosis for Crohn's colitis. *Dis Colon Rectum* 34:653–657.

Kock NG, Myrvold HE (1980) Progress report on the continent ileostomy. *World J Surg* 4:143–148.

Lee ECG, Dowling BL (1972) Perimuscular excision of the rectum for Crohn's disease and ulcerative colitis. *Br J Surg* 59:29–32.

Lee KS, Medline A, Hockey S (1979) Indeterminate colitis in the spectrum of inflammatory bowel disease. *Arch Pathol Lab Med* 193:173–176.

Lohmuller JL, Pemberton JH, Dozois RR, Ilstrup D, Van Heerden J (1990) Pouchitis and extraintestinal manifestations of inflammatory bowel disease after ileal pouch anal anastomosis. *Ann Surg* 211:622–629.

Lyttle JA, Parks AG (1977) Intersphincteric excision of the rectum. *Br J Surg* 64:413–416.

McHugh SM, Diamant NE (1987) Effect of age, gender and parity on anal canal pressures. Contribution of impaired anal sphincter function to faecal incontinence. *Dig Dis Sci* 32:726–736.

Madden MV, Neale KF, Nicholls RJ *et al.* (1991) Comparison of morbidity and function after colectomy with ileorectal anastomosis or restorative proctocolectomy for familial polyposis. *Br J Surg* 78:789–792.

Matheson DM, Keighley MRB (1981) Manometric evaluation of rectal prolapse and faecal incontinence. *Gut* 22:126–129.

Metcalf AM, Dozois RR, Kelly KA (1986) Sexual function in women with proctocolectomy. *Ann Surg* 204:624–627.

Moertel CG, Hill JR, Adson MA (1970) Surgical management of multiple polyposis. *Arch Surg* 100:521–526.

Morson BC, Dawson IP (1990) *Gastrointestinal Pathology*, 3rd edn. Oxford, Blackwell Scientific Publications.

Myrvold HE, Kock NG (1981) Continent ileostomy in patients with Crohn's disease. *Gastroenterol* 80:1237–1239.

Neill ME, Parks AG, Swash M (1981) Physiological studies of the anal sphincter musculature in faecal incontinence. *Br J Surg* 68:531–534.

Nelson H, Dozois RR, Kelly KA, Malkasian GD, Wolff BG, Ilstrup DM (1989) The effect of pregnancy and delivery on the ileal pouch anal anastomosis functions. *Dis Colon Rectum* 32:384–388.

Nicholls RJ (1987) Restorative proctocolectomy with various types of reservoir. *World J Surg* 11:751–762.

Nicholls RJ, Kamm MA (1988) Proctocolectomy with restorative ileo-anal reservoir for severe idiopathic constipation. *Dis Colon Rectum* 31:12; 968–969.

Odigwe L, Sherman PM, Fillerr R, Shandling B, Wesson D (1987) Straight, ileoanal anastomosis and ileal pouch anal anastomosis in the management of idiopathic ulcerative colitis and familial polyposis coli in children: follow up and comparative analysis. *J Paediatr Gastroenterol Nutr* 6:426–429.

Parker MC, Nicholls RJ (1992) Restorative proctocolectomy in patients after previous intestinal or anal surgery. *Dis Colon Rectum* 37(7):681–684.

Pearl RK, Nelson RL, Prasad ML, Abcarian H, Schuller N (1985) Ileoanal anastomosis 24 years after total proctocolectomy for ulcerative colitis. *Dis Colon Rectum* 28:180–182.

Pemberton JH, Kelly KA, Beart RW, Dozois RR, Wolff BG, Ilstrup DM (1987) Ileal pouch, anal anastomosis for chronic ulcerative colitis. Long term results. *Ann Surg* 206:504–511.

Pemberton JH, Phillips SF, Ready RR, Zinsmeister AR, Beahrs OH (1989) Quality of life after Brooke ileostomy and ileal pouch-anal anastomosis – *Ann Surg* 209:620–628.

Pezim ME, Nicholls RJ (1985) Quality of life after restorative proctocolectomy with pelvic ileal reservoir. *Br J Surg* 72:31–33.

Pezim ME, Pemberton JH, Beart RW *et al.* (1989) Outcome of 'indeterminate' colitis following ileal pouch-anal anastomosis. *Dis Colon Rectum* 32:653–658.

Price AB (1978) Overlap in the spectrum of non-specific inflammatory bowel disease – 'colitis indeterminate.' *J Clin Pathol* 31:567–577.

Radcliffe AG, Ritchie JK, Hawley PR, Lennard-Jones JE, Northover JMA (1988) Anovaginal and rectovaginal fistulas in Crohn's disease. *Dis Colon Rectum* 31:94–99.

Ryan P, Fink R (1988) New rectum and new anal canal: two cases of ileal reservoir – cutaneous anastomosis. *Aust N Z J Surg* 58:161–165.

Shepherd NA, Bussey HJ (1990) Polyposis syndromes – an update. *Curr Top Pathol* 81:323–351.

Smith LE, Friend W, Medwell S (1984) The superior mesenteric artery: the critical factor in pouch pull-through procedures. *Dis Colon Rectum* 27:741–744.

Snooks SJ, Setchell M, Swash M, Henry MM (1984) Injury to the innervation of the pelvic floor sphincter musculature in childbirth. *Lancet* (ii):546–550.

Stryker SJ, Daube JR, Kelly KA *et al.* (1985) Anal sphincter electromyography after colectomy, mucosal rectectomy, and ileo anal anastomosis. *Arch Surg* 120:713–716.

Taylor BA, Wolff BG, Dozois RR, Kelly KA, Pemberton JH, Beart RW Jr (1988) Ileal pouch-anal anastomosis for chronic ulcerative colitis and familial polyposis coli complicated by adenocarcinoma. *Dis Colon Rectum* 31:358–362.

Telander RL, Spencer M, Perrault J, Telander D, Zinsmeister AR (1990) Long term follow up of the ileoanal anastomosis in children and young adults. *Surgery* **108**:717–725.

Thomson JPS (1990) Familial adenomatous polyposis: the large bowel. *Ann R Coll Surg Engl* **72**:177–180.

Wells AD, McMillan I, Price AB, Ritchie JK, Nicholls RJ (1991) Natural history of indeterminate colitis. *Br J Surg* **78**: 179–181.

Wexner SD, Wong WD, Rothenburger DA, Goldberg SM (1990) The ileoanal reservoir. *Am J Surg* **159**:178–185.

Williams NS, Johnson D (1985) The current status of mucosal proctectomy and ileo-anal anastomosis in the surgical treatment of ulcerative colitis and adenomatous polyposis. *Br J Surg* **72**:159–168.

Chapter 3
Techniques of Pouch Construction

VICTOR W. FAZIO, JOE J. TJANDRA AND IAN C. LAVERY

Introduction

In this chapter the technical aspects of the restorative proctocolectomy procedure are discussed. There are few, if any, surgeons who in current times use exactly the same procedure as the one they started with or the one observed or performed in their training. This is perhaps true of any surgical procedure, but is especially so with restorative proctocolectomy, as the modern operation has really emerged only since the mid 1970s. Many lessons have been learned since the modern pioneers, the late Sir Alan Parks (Parks & Nicholls, 1978) Lester Martin (Martin & Fischer, 1982) and Eric Fonkalsrud (Fonkalsrud & Ament, 1978), reported their early experience; these lessons will be discussed in this chapter. A few examples of such lessons quickly spring to mind. It is now clear that in addition to ileoanal anastomosis, a pelvic ileal pouch is needed for optimal function. Secondly, much of the pelvic sepsis and intra-operative bleeding associated with restorative proctocolectomy occurred as the result of preservation of a long rectal cuff ranging in length from 7 to 10 cm, yet this cuff preservation adds nothing to functional improvement and the procedure is facilitated by its exclusion. Thirdly, the poor to indifferent function following S pouch construction in early studies was found to be related to excessive length of the exit conduit of ileum, leading to outlet obstruction and evacuation difficulties. This has been obviated by using a shorter exit conduit of ileum from 0 to 2 cm.

The search for the ideal pouch technique goes on (Table 3.1), especially advanced by the increasing body of knowledge relating to factors influencing faecal continence, and one must admit, the occasional serendipitous benefit of empiric procedure.

Since 1984, 605 cases of restorative proctocolectomy have been performed in the Department of Colorectal Surgery at the Cleveland Clinic Foundation, utilizing the J or S pouch configuration. Our preferred methods are indicated, although, given the present controversies, these procedures may well change with time.

Goals of surgery with restorative proctocolectomy

Removal of all large bowel epithelium

Exceptions to this are discussed below with the procedures in which the anal transitional zone (ATZ) is preserved (Lavery et al., 1990). Yet the disadvantages of the latter (possibility of continued inflammatory activity, risk of significant dysplasia or cancer, recurrence or persistence of certain extra-intestinal manifestations) have to be weighed against the claims of the protagonists of ATZ removal (Beart et al., 1985; Lavery et al., 1990; O'Connell & Williams, 1991). ATZ preservation is associated with improved anal sphincter function, greater ease and speed of the operation, and lessened rates of anastomotic complications.

Radical colectomy if there is synchronous colonic dysplasia or cancer

Since occult carcinoma can be present in patients in whom dysplasia is found preoperatively, high ligation of the colonic blood supply along with wide mesenteric resection is strongly recommended (Fazio, 1991). Radical rectal resections, on the other hand, with wide lateral and radial margins, are rarely necessary even with synchronous dysplasia, unless an upper rectal or high midrectal cancer is diagnosed.

Fashioning an ileal reservoir

The goal here is to construct a compliant sac of two or more loops of terminal ileum. This has been shown to be superior to straight ileoanal anastomosis in terms of function (Parks & Nicholls, 1978). The techniques of pouch construction are discussed below. Clearly there is a minimum and a maximum capacity of such a reservoir, yet there are few data on what is and is not a satisfactory volume capacity. In practice, this is a moot point as different dimensions of the intestinal loops

Table 3.1 Variables in pelvic pouch procedures.

Pouch design	J, S, W, H
Dimensions	12–20 cm limbs
Limb anastomosis	Handsewn vs. stapled
Mucosectomy	Quadrant, tube *In situ* vs. eversion Endoanal vs. abdominal
Preservaton of anal transitional zone	
Ileal pouch anal anastomosis	Handsewn vs. stapled

Stapled ileal pouch anal anastomosis	Side-to-end vs. end-to-end
	Purse-string suture:
	  transabdominal vs.
	  transanal
	Double-stapled technique
	Stapler calibre: 28, 29, 31,
	  33 mm

Diversion of pouch	Loop vs. end ileostomy vs. no diversion
Drains	Presacral Intrapouch

used in the published literature, with all the variations reported, appear to give comparable outcome.

Preservation of a continence mechanism

Since the anal sphincter function is critical, all possible measures are taken to avoid injury to such structures. Most clinicians assess preoperative status of the sphincter muscles on clinical grounds, this assessment being critical in the selection process for restorative proctocolectomy. Anal manometry is useful in patients where function is or may be questionable or when studies are being done for analysis of results. Older age (over 50 years old), a history of multiparity or possible sphincter injury, e.g. birth trauma or previous perianal surgery, may highlight potential inadequacy of the sphincters. There can be a surprising lack of correlation between a history of incontinence preoperatively and manometric findings (either pre- or postoperatively). Such incontinence may be due to severe urgency secondary to an inflamed rectum, the removal of which almost always produces excellent functional results when sphincter pressure measurement is in the normal range.

Provision of a tension-free and well-vascularized bowel anastomosis

This holds as an imperative for all anastomoses and is discussed below.

Others

The need for avoidance of injury to important structures in the course of pelvic dissection and bowel anastomosis is self-evident. Nonetheless, particular attention is given to avoiding injury to the nervi erigentes, presacral nerves, ureters, bladder base, posterior vaginal wall and presacral vessels. Too much emphasis cannot be placed on acquisition of perfect haemostasis as pelvic haematomas are vulnerable to infection with abscess formation and delayed anastomotic dehiscence. Integrity of the completed anastomosis is critical and should be tested by pouch insufflation. Such anastomoses are vulnerable to leakage and, as such, at least at the present time, temporary faecal diversion is recommended routinely unless there is a total absence of adverse factors relevant to healing (see pp. 29, 65).

Before the operation

Selection of patients for restorative proctocolectomy

This procedure is covered in Chapter 2. Patients usually excluded from consideration are those with: toxic colitis (fever, leukocytosis, tachycardia, hypotension) with or without megacolon; history of ileal resection; desmoid tumour; Crohn's disease diagnosed pre- or intra-operatively; poor sphincter function; medical ill health; and patients with low rectal cancer. In the past, exclusion of patients on grounds of age was common, but several centres have reported successful outcome in patients in their 60s, provided sphincter function is normal. Significant malnutrition is also a contraindication to restorative proctocolectomy, but a modest degree of hypoalbuminaemia (e.g. 30 mg/l) is not a contraindication. Colonic haemorrhage requiring pre-operative blood transfusion, in the absence of toxicity, is likewise not a contraindication *per se*.

Preoperative work-up

This includes an assessment of the patient's fitness for surgery and anaesthesia and assessment of the extent and nature of the inflammatory bowel disease and the sphincter function. Thus the patient will undergo a blood count and biochemistry analysis, coagulation profile, chest X-ray, colonoscopy with biopsies (to detect Crohn's disease or dysplasia), small bowel roentgenographic studies and nutritional assessment. Other tests are performed as needed for assessment of concurrent illness. At the Cleveland Clinic, we routinely perform manometric studies; this is not essential if clinical assessment indicates satisfactory anal sphincters.

Timing of surgery

Restorative proctocolectomy is an elective operation. A proportion of patients will have undergone a previous abdominal colectomy. In these patients, we favour a delay of 6 months from the time of colectomy before the pouch procedure. This is to minimize the difficulties of the second procedure, in as much as adhesions can be particularly formidable (especially within the first 2–4 months).

Another circumstance is that of a patient who has been successfully managed conservatively during a bout of toxic colitis/megacolon. At what time following this successful management is surgery appropriate? We know of no good data on this but provided the features of toxicity are absent, and the nutritional state is reasonable, there seems to be no special reason to delay restorative proctocolectomy if the patient so desires. This is true even when daily prednisone doses are in the 40–60 mg range.

Regarding timing of closure of temporary diverting ileostomy, there seems to be decided value in waiting 2–3 months following ileostomy construction. Ostomy closure is easier at 3 months than at 6 weeks. At the Cleveland Clinic, current rate of bowel obstruction after ileostomy closure was reduced compared to our earlier practice of closure at 6 weeks (van de Pavoordt, 1987). An exception to this 'rule' is when the patient with a temporary ileostomy develops bowel obstruction requiring surgery. Here we recommend assessment of the pouch anal anastomotic integrity by endoscopy and gastrografin enema. If satisfactory, then after the adhesive band/adhesions have been dealt with, the ileostomy is closed at the same procedure.

Preparation for surgery

There are few operations where discussion with the patient and their family is so extensive. A complete and factual discussion of the indications for surgery, alternative treatments, sequelae and complications and anticipated or possible outcomes is held. Commonly, this requires two meetings with the surgeon and is facilitated by such aids as diagrams, booklets, tapes, and discussions with enterostomal therapists and former patients of similar age, gender and life-style.

Mechanical bowel preparation is provided using polyethylene glycol. Rectal washout with saline is given in the operating room until the effluent is clear. Intravenous antibiotics, usually metronidazole and a third generation cephalosporin, are given at induction and continued postoperatively for 2–5 days depending upon degree of intraoperative contamination and risk of postoperative sepsis. A urethral Foley catheter and a nasogastric tube are inserted after induction of anaesthesia. Compression stockings to the calf are used intra- and postoperatively and one of us (VWF) uses mini-heparinization. Preoperative stoma marking is done.

Positioning of the patient

Techniques differ in the order of operative steps and the need for mucosal proctectomy. Rothenberger et al. (1983) and Utsunomiya et al. (1980) begin with the mucosal proctectomy in the prone jack-knife position and abdominal dissection in the supine position. Our practice, and that of many others, is to place the patient in the Lloyd-Davies position and carry out the abdominal procedure first (Nicholls, 1987; Beart, 1988; Lavery et al., 1989). The right hip is not flexed (to allow easy distraction of the self-retaining retractor) and the left hip is flexed to about 30°. Special care is taken to ensure there is no compression to the calf and peroneal nerve by using 'egg crate' foam padding.

Operation techniques

Abdominal dissection

The abdomen is opened through a midline incision and a thorough exploration of the abdomen is performed, noting in particular any evidence of small bowel disease, which may then suggest Crohn's disease. The colon is then mobilized from the ileocaecal junction to the rectum. The terminal ileum is divided flush with the caecum to preserve length. Conservative ligation and division of the mesenteric vessels are performed. However, in the presence of high grade dysplasia in mucosal ulcerative colitis, radical colectomy is recommended as occult carcinoma can be present.

Technique of proctectomy

This was partly addressed on p. 19. With respect to the rectal resection, the aim is to provide a bloodless dissection and at the same time avoid injury to other pelvic structures. We do not use ureteric stents and have not encountered a ureteric injury in over 600 pelvic pouch operations. The presacral space is entered between the investing layer of fascia propria of the rectum and Waldeyer's fascia after preliminary identification of the ureters. This entry corresponds to the bifurcation of the superior rectal artery. The presacral nerves can be identified easily at the pelvic brim and preserved. This dissection is continued in the midline posteriorly to the level of the levators. Care is taken not to breach Waldeyer's fascia posteriorly where the nervi erigentes and presacral veins are vulnerable. Most of this dissection is done with the cutting cautery and is practically bloodless. We believe this technique does not risk development of impotence, and lessens blood loss and operating time considerably, compared to the traditional method of dissecting close to the rectal wall inside the superior rectal vessels posteriorly throughout its course (see p. 55). This is an experience equally shared by others (Rothenberger *et al.*, 1983; Beart, 1988).

Laterally, the pelvic peritoneal incisions are made with the cautery, uniting these on the anterior rectal wall about 1 cm above the peritoneal reflection. It is at this point that close rectal dissection is carried out. The assistant and the surgeon alternately 'trade' retraction of the rectum, long tissue forceps and a Kelly clamp depending on the side of the rectum being dissected. In essence, all tissues are placed under significant traction by placing the Kelly clamp beside the rectal wall itself and then retracting the pararectal tissues with opening of the clamp. The lateral ligaments are divided close to the rectum. Coagulating dissection is used. On occasion, coagulation is not enough and these pararectal pedicles (in particular, the middle rectal vessels) require suture or clip ligation. Lighted retractors are particularly advantageous. Anteriorly the dissection is carried to the lower border of the prostate (or lower one-third of vagina) while operating directly against the rectal wall. At no time should the seminal vesicles be seen. This will ensure dissection posterior to Denonvilliers' fascia. As the autonomic plexus lies immediately anterior to that fascia, this will minimize sexual dysfunction. In our experience of 293 male patients having restorative proctocolectomy, only one patient and three patients suffered impotence and retrograde ejaculation, respectively.

The next step will depend on the plans for the anastomosis, namely, anorectal mucosectomy and handsewn anastomosis vs. stapled technique. At this point, the rectum will have been completely mobilized, the rectum tied off in its midportion with a stout ligature and the rectal stump irrigated from below. With the handsewn anastomosis, the rectum is transected using a combination of cutting/coagulation at the anorectal ring (upper border of the levators).

With the stapled technique, the surgeon checks the level of the planned distal anastomosis by placing his or her arm between the patient's legs (previously prepared and draped) and inserts an index finger into the anus. With the proximal interphalangeal joint resting at the anal verge, the tip of the digit corresponds to the level of the anorectal ring. From the abdominal side, the surgeon uses the other hand to palpate the tip of the finger in the patient's anus. The finger is removed, the glove is changed and a new sleeve provided. At this point the level is marked on the anterior surface of the rectum and this corresponds to the level of the planned purse-string suture (or linear stapler). Subsequent anastomosis with a circular stapler will remove, in addition, a distal ring doughnut of 1.0 cm in diameter.

Technique of distal stump preparation

Our practice has changed from doing routine mucosectomy and handsewn anastomosis to stapled pouch-anal anastomosis using the circular stapler with a detachable anvil. This is based on our belief that improved anal function occurs from the avoidance of excessive manipulation of the anal canal and dilatation of the anal sphincters (Lavery *et al.*, 1989; Tuckson *et al.*, 1991). With mucosectomy and a sometimes lengthy handsewn anastomosis, a significant stretch injury of the sphincters can occur. Resting anal canal pressure is lower after mucosectomy than after stapled anastomosis without mucosectomy. This may not recover in the

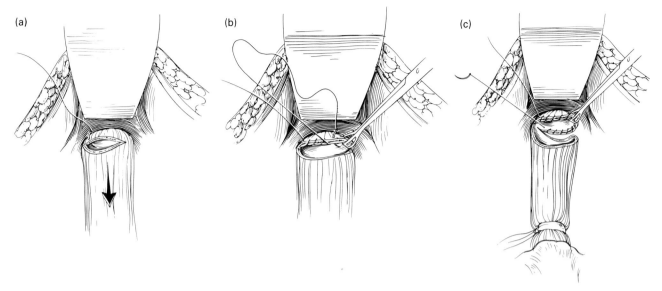

Fig. 3.1 Complete rectal excision and techniques of insertion of distal purse-string suture. The rectal purse-string suture is inserted just above the anorectal ring. (a) An incision is made in the anterior wall of the rectum whilst applying traction upwards. The purse-string suture is placed in one corner.

(b) The incision is enlarged and the over and over purse string suture continued to the opposite corner. (c) The posterior rectal wall is then divided piecemeal and the purse string completed in short stages.

short term or for several years. Further, we have shown that functional outcome may suffer as compared to non-manipulative techniques like stapling (Lavery *et al.*, 1989; Tuckson *et al.*, 1991). We reserve handsewn techniques for patients with ulcerative colitis and synchronous colon cancer, rectal mucosal dysplasia or patients with familial adenomatous polyposis where polyps approach the anal canal. Others hold the view that anorectal mucosectomy should be performed in all patients with familial adenomatous polyposis because of the higher incidence of dysplasia in the anorectum (O'Connell & Williams, 1991).

The importance of sensory receptors in the anorectal transitional zone in the differentiation between faeces and flatus has been recently emphasized, but this is controversial (Lavery *et al.*, 1990; O'Connell & Williams, 1991). As a result, there is an increasing tendency to preserve the anorectal transitional zone (Fonkalsrud, 1980). This had led to improved continence, greater ease and speed of the operation and a safer anastomosis, compared to sphincter stretching techniques as are necessary with mucosectomy (Lavery *et al.*, 1990; Tuckson *et al.*, 1991). There is a risk of continued inflammation, persistence of extra-intestinal manifestations and cancerous change of the remaining mucosa (Beart *et al.*, 1985). Longer follow-up will be necessry to clarify these issues. So far, problems with subsequent inflammation of the anal transitional zone are few and

minor and the risk of cancer in this remnant is probably very low. In one study (Tsunoda *et al.*, 1990), dysplasia of anorectal mucosa was found in only 3 (2.5%) of 118 mucosectomy specimens in patients with ulcerative colitis who underwent restorative proctocolectomy. Dysplasia was only found when it was also widespread within the colon and rectum.

For stapled anastomoses, we use one of two basic techniques for preparing the distal stump (Lavery *et al.*, 1989) and the one with which we have most experience, is that of application of a hand-placed whip stitch of 0 proline across the anorectal ring. With good retraction and lighting, an incision is made across the anterior half of the anorectum (Fig. 3.1). The surgeon, standing on the patient's left side, then starts the purse-string suture at the left anterolateral aspect of the distal segment (backhand sutures). As the stitch approaches the midline or right side, the sutures are placed forehand, taking small bites of the muscularis and minimal bites of the mucosa at 7-mm intervals. Strategic placing of Babcock clamps and/or guy sutures facilitate the process. Thereafter, sutures are placed and cautery/division of the bowel is done sequentially, so that at all times cephalad traction of the rectum can be done to facilitate accurate suture placement. At completion of transection, the specimen is opened and examined to rule out Crohn's disease. The pelvis is irrigated with saline and a dry gauze pack placed in position.

(a)

(b)

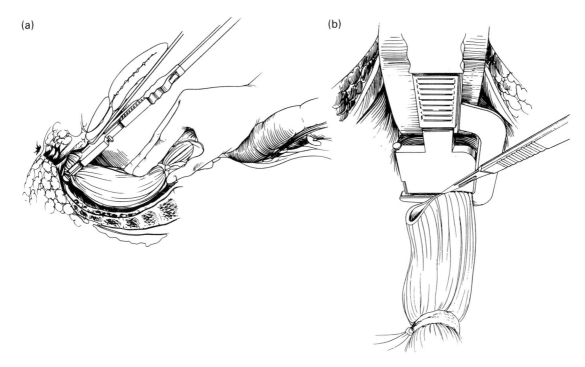

Fig. 3.2 (a) The PI-30 instrument (3M)® is applied at the lower limit of resection and a double row of staples placed. (b) An occluding tape is placed proximal to the staple line and the rectum divided along the edge of the staples.

The alternative to proline purse-string sutures is the linear stapler if the double-stapling technique is used (Knight & Griffen, 1990). We have used the PI-30 instrument (3M)®. Unlike the Roticulator TA-linear stapler, this has a substantive 'feel', allowing for easier closure of the jaws and can be applied in almost all circumstances (Fig. 3.2). For the obese male patient, where the symphysis pubis can limit the 'angle of attack' in placing a linear stapler, the PI-30 has the added advantage of having a detachable anvil. The detached anvil can be put in place in the deep narrow pelvis and then attached to the shaft/firing mechanism. After firing, a long-handled knife severs the bowel above the staple line. On withdrawing of the stapler, the transverse staple line commonly withdraws into the levators, resting at a level below the superior border of the levators. Indeed, a potential hazard in patients with an 'easy' pelvis, e.g. in young women, is that of applying the linear stapler too low, i.e. at or even below the dentate line. (The same caution has to be exercised with choosing the level for Proline purse-string suture placement.) This could lead to excision of a significant amount of internal sphincter when subsequent anastomosis using circular stapler is performed.

Technique of mucosectomy

In anorectal mucosectomy, the mucosa is stripped from the muscle wall from the dentate line to the level of rectal division. This is performed in many centres and the technique varies with excision as a complete cylinder transabdominally (Keighley, 1987); endoanal excision (Vasilevsky et al., 1987), or a combination of both approaches (Johnston et al., 1981). Goligher (1984) everted the rectal stump to facilitate mucosectomy, whereas others removed the mucosa entirely from below in strips (Parks & Nicholls, 1978). None of these different approaches appears to confer any particular advantage, but reduced sphincter damage has been demonstrated with abdominal mucosectomy compared with the endoanal approaches (Keighley, 1987). A simultaneous decrease in rectal cuff length may have accounted for some of the decreased morbidity.

Our preferred technique is hereby described. As can be gathered from our technique of rectal transection at the anorectal ring, there is no muscular 'sleeve' of rectum left save for the 2 or 3 cm of internal anal sphincter remaining. The perineal team prepares the area for surgery. In the past, we have used the lighted bi-valve Pratt retractor because of the excellent exposure provided. However, because of the significant sphincter stretch, we now use a medium sized lighted Fergusson anal retractor. The anal canal mucosa is elevated with submucosal injection of 1:200 000 adrenaline using a total of 10–15 ml. The injection is started at the dentate line. A tube excision is preferred rather than quadrant excision starting at the level of the dentate line. There is probably a greater risk of leaving islands of mucosa with quadrant excision compared to tube excision, with consequent increased risk of sinus or sepsis, as well as risk of leaving large bowel mucosa no longer amenable to surveillance. Indeed, islands of mucosa may remain on the anorectal muscular cuff despite seemingly complete mucosectomy (O'Connell et al., 1987). An adenocarcinoma has been reported in the rectal cuff of a patient 4 years after restorative proctocolectomy with anorectal mucosectomy, severe dysplasia being present in the mucosectomy specimen at the time of original surgery (Stern et al., 1990).

Cautery provides haemostasis. Sutures (2/0 Vicryl) are then placed radially at the dentate line incorporating a small amount of internal sphincter. Too deep a stitch, especially into the rectovaginal septum, may cause anastomotic–vaginal fistula. The needles are left attached to the sutures and are attached to the drapes. These sutures will then be used later to be passed through full thickness of the emerging ileal spout of the S pouch or apex of the J pouch at the appropriate compass points when the ileum is delivered through the anus.

The alternative technique of mucosectomy from the abdominal aspect was in vogue especially in paediatric patients and subsequently performed in adults (Keighley, 1987). This approach usually leaves a variable amount of rectal sleeve or cuff. Specifically, when done from the abdominal approach, there seemed to be no deleterious functional outcome compared to reported results where anal transitional zone was preserved. In this regard, avoidance of sphincter stretch in abdominal mucosectomy is probably a more important factor than preservation of anal transitional zone. In our experience, abdominal mucosectomy is tedious, lengthy, difficult and often bloody and has no place in our current practice.

In Goligher's technique (1984), the rectal stump is everted on to the perineum with mucosectomy done somewhat more easily than endoanal techniques because of improved exposure. However there is significant sphincter stretch that occurs with this procedure and functional results are likely to be no better, and possibly worse, than with endoanal mucosectomy. Using the biological analogue, the Turnbull–Cutait pull-through as a similar model (Cutait & Figliolini, 1961; Turnbull & Cuthbertson, 1961), it would not be surprising to see greater degree of pelvic bleeding from manipulation of the rectal cuff in everting the stump through the anus.

In earlier series that practised anorectal mucosectomy, a long rectal muscular cuff (up to 10 cm) used to be made in the belief that it will enhance continence (Utsunomiya et al., 1980; Johnston et al., 1981). This has been found to be associated with increased intra-operative bleeding, to be a major source of septic complications such as cuff abscess and subsequent fibrosis and decreased pouch compliance. Current practice is to leave a shorter rectal muscular cuff of no more than 1–2 cm above the levators. Comparative study of long and short cuffs has confirmed similar functional results and a decreased complication rate with the short cuff (Fonkalsrud, 1980; Grant et al., 1986; Nicholls, 1987). There has been a trend towards removing the entire rectum leaving no muscular cuff with equally good functional results. This suggests that receptors for sensation in the neorectum do not lie predominantly in the rectal mucosa or muscle.

Techniques of pouch construction

Small bowel mobilization

With completion of colonic mobilization, the terminal ileum is transected flush at the ileocaecal valve and a non-crush clamp applied. The small bowel mesentery is totally mobilized up to the third part of the duodenum and inferior border of the pancreas. One of us (VWF) routinely excises the ileocolic vessels at their origin to provide greater mobilization of the small bowel. For others, this is a more selective process, preserving the ileocolic vessels and superior mesenteric vessels when a J pouch can be anastomosed without tension to the upper anal canal. One of the mechanisms cited as a factor in late pouchitis is that of relative mucosal ischaemia of the pouch, possibly minimized by avoiding division of the ileocolic vessels.

In obese patients, patients with extensive adhesions from previous surgery or patients with previous small bowel resection, attaining of sufficient viable small bowel to reach the anus can be a problem. The segment of ileum requiring greatest mobility differs

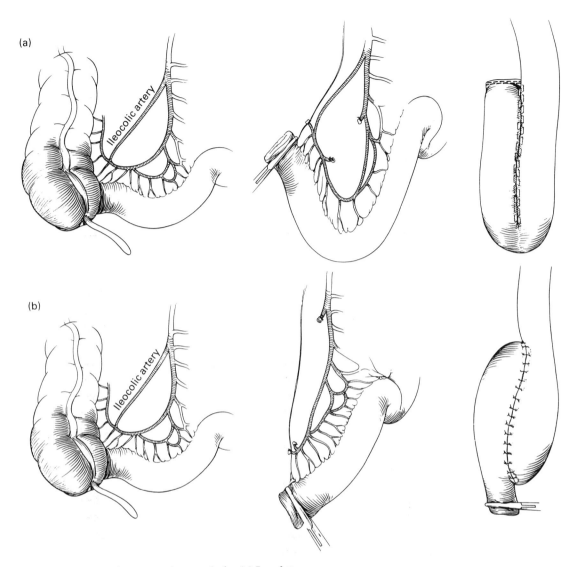

Fig. 3.3 Site of division of mesenteric vessels for (a) J and (b) S pouches, when further mobilization is necessary.

according to the pouch design and to the type of anastomosis (Fig. 3.3). A number of manoeuvres may prove valuable. First, one can estimate the potential 'reach' problem by placing a Babcock clamp on the apex of the intended pouch, about 15 cm from the end of bowel in the J pouch and at the bowel end in the S pouch. If this can be made to reach 2–3 cm beyond the symphysis pubis, it is unlikely that anastomotic tension will be a problem. Our preference is to place the clamped bowel end into the deep pelvis, getting the instrument to abut against the top of the levator muscles.

When these manoeuvres fail to give a clear indication that mobilization is adequate, excision of all peritoneal tissue to the right of the superior mesenteric vessels, leaving a 0.5 cm edge of peritoneum lateral to these vessels, may provide added mobility. This is facilitated by using transillumination of the small bowel mesentery. Preservation of the terminal arcades of the mesenteric vessels is important. With similar back lighting it is usually feasible to divide small arcadal branches (not vasa recti), 5–10 cm from the terminal ileum. This usually adds at least 2–3 cm or so to mobility. Whenever in doubt about the effect of division of any vessels that supply the ileum, one can always apply a temporary clamp such as a bulldog clamp, and observe for any ischaemic effects. A further manoeuvre that is helpful is the making of a series of transverse 1–2 cm peritoneal incisions over the superior mesenteric vessels. These are done anteriorly and posteriorly at

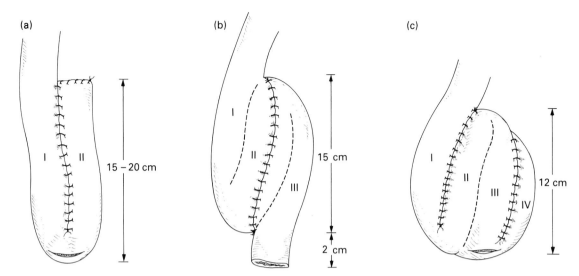

Fig. 3.4 Various pouch designs: (a) Double (J) (b) Triple (S) (c) Quadruple (W).

about 1–2 cm intervals. Indeed, for that extra difficult case, and again using transillumination, radial peritoneal incisions can be made between the vasa recti supplying that part of the ileum which will be most dependent.

Even when all these manoeuvres have been done, and even when one knows that enough bowel has been mobilized, there are still occasions when a bulky pouch (e.g. S pouch) in a narrow pelvis, where the levator muscles are particularly prominent, where the anal canal is longer than usual, will lead to difficulty in fashioning a tension-free anastomosis. In this case, there is one further manoeuvre, of great value and importance, that will help the surgeon. A long Babcock clamp is passed transanally, and used to grasp the end of the exit conduit of an S pouch, and a bi-manual manoeuvre applied. Here the operator's abdominal hand is passed behind the pouch, in the curve of the sacrum while exerting modest traction on the Babcock clamp from the perineal aspect. The abdominal hand helps 'seat' the pouch into position, in effect coaxing the junction of the pouch fundus and exit conduit to lie more freely between the levators. The exit conduit is then anastomosed to the dentate line. With our technique, which uses modern circular stapling devices and preserves the anal transitional zone, these manoeuvres are now less frequently required.

Pouch construction, principles and rationale

The goal is to construct a compliant sac of two or more loops of terminal ileum. This has been shown to be superior to straight ileoanal anastomosis in terms of function. The four most common pouch designs (Fig. 3.4) are the triple loop or S pouch, the two loop or J pouch, the four loop or W pouch and the lateral isoperistaltic or H pouch, using either sutures or stapled techniques (Parks & Nicholls, 1978; Fonkalsrud, 1980; Utsunomiya et al., 1980; Nicholls & Pezim, 1985). The functional results of these various pouch designs appear to be comparable (Keighley et al., 1988; Everett, 1989), despite claims that the W pouch has a lower frequency of defaecation than the J pouch (Nicholls & Lubowski, 1987). Factors other than pouch designs, such as bacterial overgrowth, gut motility and transit probably play a more important role in deciding the functional outcome.

Firstly, the terminal ileum is quarantined by liberal and strategic placement of packs. The terminal ileum is irrigated through its open end with saline until clear effluent is obtained and evacuated. At this point a decision is made regarding shape of pouch and dimensions of limbs to be used. While the H pouch (isoperistaltic) has been advocated by Fonkalsrud (1980), one is concerned by the fact that the ensuing exit conduit is rather long and can produce obstructive defaecation and outlet angulation. The W pouch is discussed in Chapter 5. This is associated with excellent functional results, but we have seen no clear advantage to this model which is more complex to construct than other models. The preferred technique used at the Cleveland Clinic is either the S pouch or J pouch. The S pouch usually reaches 2–4 cm farther than the J pouch and this additional length is invaluable in avoiding anastomotic tension (Smith *et al.*, 1984). The J pouch has the advantage of ease of construction using stapling techniques requiring much less operating time. At the Cleveland Clinic, we have performed approximately equal numbers of S and J pouches. While we have shown a marginal advantage favouring S pouches over J pouches (better compliance and fewer bowel movements (Tuckson & Fazio, 1991)), much of this advantage was realized when mucosectomy was routine, a practice that led to increased tension in J pouch anastomoses compared to S pouches. This advantage has largely been nullified by use of the circular stapled anastomoses. Since the J pouch can be fashioned quickly with linear stapler GIA-90 (United States Surgical®) or ILA (3-M Health Care® 100-mm) applied twice, this has some advantage over the S pouch which requires hand-suturing and takes an additional 40-minutes to construct. Bleeding from the linear staple line can occasionally be a problem and may require reinforcement with haemostatic suture.

Thus, at this time, with stapled restorative proctocolectomy, the J pouch is perhaps the preferred procedure using two limbs of 15 cm. However, if there is any question of adequate reach of the bowel to the anus, e.g. in obese patients or patients for whom mucosectomy is performed, then the S pouch is favoured.

Technique of pouch construction

J pouch

The J shaped ileal reservoir is made from the terminal 30–40 cm of small bowel folded into two 15–20-cm segments (Fig. 3.5). The end of the divided ileum is closed by a linear stapler and oversewn with 3/0 Vicryl sutures for reinforcement. The J pouch is created by side-to-side anastomosis of two limbs of the ileum, using the linear stapler through the apical enterotomy.

Note that when one applies two passes of the 100-mm ILA stapler, this will produce 20-cm limbs of the J pouch, even though one has made the apical enterotomy in the flaccid ileum some 15 cm from the end of the bowel. Cutting cautery is used to make a linear 2.5-cm enterotomy at the apex. The J limbs are approximated on their antimesenteric surface; the ILA instrument is passed to its full length, the assistant checks that no mesentery is interposed between anvil and cartridge and the instrument is fired. A second staple line is made similarly. Care is taken that no gap

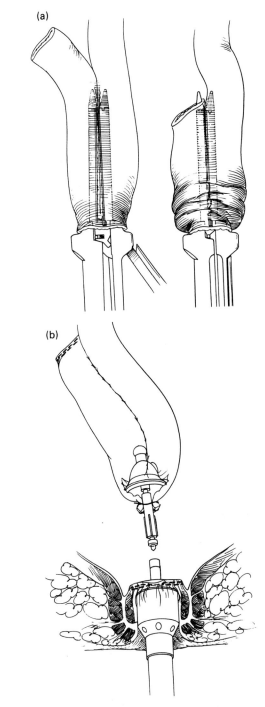

Fig. 3.5 (a) Stapled J pouch with (b) the detachable anvil/shaft complex in the apical enterotomy.

is left between consecutive stapler lines. The pouch is inflated with saline to check for leaks and the staple line checked for haemostasis. The detachable anvil is then placed in the apical enterotomy and a 0 proline purse-string suture is applied and tied.

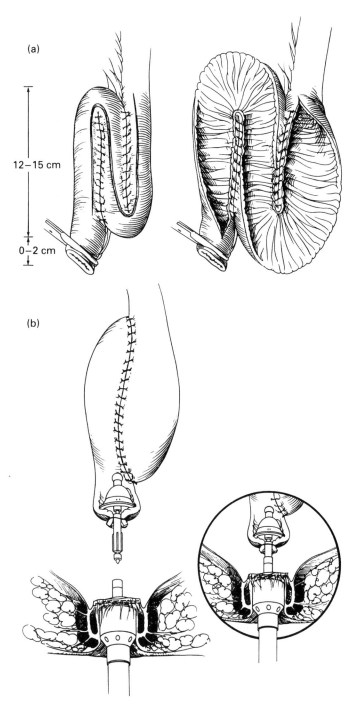

Fig. 3.6 The S pouch. (a) The distal ileum is aligned in an S shape and the limbs approximated by continuous seromuscular sutures. The antimesenteric surfaces are opened by an S-shaped enterotomy and the posterior anastomotic lines closed from inside the pouch. (b) The S pouch is completed after closure of the anterior layer. The detachable anvil/shaft complex of premium CEEA is placed in the exit conduit and then 'mated' with the shaft protruding from the anorectal stump.

S pouch

Three limbs of 12–15 cm of ileum are aligned using a 2-cm exit conduit (Fig. 3.6). In Parks' early series, the distal ileal spout was longer, measuring 5 cm. This was associated with evacuation problems that required the use of a catheter (Parks *et al.*, 1980) and led to subsequent modification with shortening of the distal ileal segment to 2-cm or less (Rothenberger *et al.*, 1983). Continuous seromuscular sutures of 3/0 Vicryl approximate the loops. An S-shaped enterotomy is made. The two posterior anastomotic lines are closed from inside the pouch using 3/0 Vicryl. The anterior layer is closed in the same way. If a stapled anastomosis is planned, the detachable anvil is placed into the exit conduit, and a purse-string suture applied, provided the conduit will accept at least a size 29 stapler. Otherwise, the anvil is placed in the most dependent part of the pouch and interrupted Vicryl sutures are used in lieu of a purse-string suture on the anterior layer. In this case, the exit conduit is sealed with a linear stapler, and a side of pouch to end of anal canal anastomosis is made. Prior to completion, intactness of the pouch is tested by insufflation with normal saline.

Technique of anastomosis

Before construction of the anastomosis, total haemostasis is achieved in the pelvis. Anastomotic complications appear to be fewer with stapled compared with handsewn anastomosis and this is our preferred method. The premium CEEA stapler® is used for ileoanal anastomosis because of its detachable anvil/shaft complex.

With stapled anastomoses two basic techniques are used. With the double-stapling technique (Knight & Griffen, 1990), the cartridge end of the circular stapler is introduced into the anus, and the trocar point is advanced through the centre of the linear staple line (Fig. 3.7). The trocar is then removed and the anvil/shaft (emerging from the pouch) 'mated' with the shaft protruding from the anorectal stump. The mesentery must be carefully inspected to ensure no twisting has occurred. The ends are approximated, care being taking to avoid extraneous tissue being included in the staple line, especially posterior vaginal wall, and the anastomosis is completed. The double-stapling technique obviates the technical frustrations involved in placing the lower purse-string suture and permits an adequately low anastomosis. As the anorectal stump

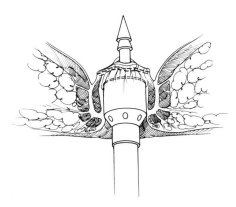

Fig. 3.7 In double-stapling techniques, the trocar point on the shaft should traverse the staple line itself or in its immediate proximity.

is not opened, it also minimizes intraoperative contamination. Disparity of size of the bowel segments is also avoided. There has been some concern that the intersecting staple lines might increase the risk of anastomotic leak (Fazio, 1988). However, experimental work and clinical experience have attested to the safety of the procedure (Feinberg *et al.*, 1986; Trollope *et al.*, 1986; Julian & Ravitch, 1988). One might predict that the double-stapling technique will become the procedure most used in the 1990s for restorative proctocolectomy because of its relative simplicity.

For stapled anastomoses where a proline purse-string suture has been applied, there is no need for a trocar. Basically, the instrument is advanced as described above, the shaft is advanced beyond the distal purse-string suture which is then tied. The anastomosis is then completed. In cases where the anal canal is narrowed, trauma to mucosa is possible during insertion of the stapling instrument. Here, one needs gently to distract the four corners of the anal verge with Babcock clamps to allow easy passage of the stapling instrument.

The handsewn anastomosis is used when mucosectomy has been performed. A Pratt bi-valve or lighted Fergusson retractor (our preference) is placed in the anal canal. The apex of the J loop or end of exit conduit of the S pouch is delivered via a Babcock clamp on to the anal verge. The previously placed sutures in the dentate line are now serially placed through full-thickness of ileum and tied after removal of the retractor. Vicryl 2/0 suture mounted on a heavy-duty 25-mm needle which will not bend when placed in tissue is suitable. Some anchor the small bowel with seromuscular sutures at this level before opening the

reservoir (Beart *et al.*, 1985). The anastomosis is then tested for integrity by inflation of dilute betadine, while checking the pelvis for evidence of leak.

Technique of ileostomy construction

In view of the large number of suture or staple lines and the fact that many patients are on steroids and malnourished, a temporary defunctioning ileostomy has been used. This could be in the form of a loop ileostomy or divided end ileostomy. Our favoured approach is to exteriorize the most proximal loop of ileum (usually 20–25 cm proximal to the pouch) that can be brought through the right lower quadrant of the abdominal wall without tension. This can be in a previously marked stoma site or at the site of the previous ileostomy. The loop ileostomy procedure has been previously described (Fazio, 1986). No rotation is necessary as the ileostomy seems to lie best with the dominant functional end being located in the cephalad position. Others (Rothenberger *et al.*, 1985) prefer to divide the ileum and construct an end stoma. This may allow for lessened tension in the functioning ileostomy, but usually mandates a midline laparotomy and formal end-to-end anastomosis at the time of ileostomy closure. We have found this to be a more involved procedure than loop ileostomy closure, which can be closed with a peristomal incision in more than 95% of cases (van de Pavoordt, 1987).

There is increasing interest and experience with avoidance of use of a covering temporary ileostomy. Early experience with this approach was disappointing and septic complications were considerable (Wong *et al.*, 1985). In that early study, an S pouch had been constructed by one-layer hand-sutured stitches. With the use of stapled anastomoses, there is a common view, shared by our group, that such anastomoses are more secure than with handsewn techniques, so there is less trepidation about leaving stapled anastomoses unprotected. Some (Everett, 1989; Matikainen *et al.*, 1990) feel that this one-stage procedure is now the rule rather than the exception. At this time, we feel it is perhaps premature to regard omission of faecal diversion as the standard approach. Certainly, a strong case can be made for one-stage procedures: (1) when the operation has gone particularly smoothly, there is a lack of features adverse to anastomotic healing (toxicity, malnutrition, high-dose steroids, imperfect haemostasis, pelvic contamination, anastomotic tension, incomplete tissue rings); (2) when ileostomy construction would be especially difficult; and (3) when the patient has been appraised of the risks involved. In these cases, the pouch is drained by a catheter introduced through the anus for 4 days and the small bowel is decompressed by a gastrostomy tube until the return of bowel function. Anastomotic leak occurred in two out of 25 patients managed in this way, and only one patient required surgery to provide drainage and proximal defunctioning.

Certain cases can pose problems in ileostomy construction, especially obese patients or those in whom the superior mesenteric vessels produce excessive tethering of the ileum. In these cases, it may be best treated by dividing the ileum and performing end ileostomy. The somewhat flush stoma thus produced may be more difficult to manage, but with good counselling by the enterostomal therapy nurse, patients can usually make do for the relatively short interval prior to closure. In extreme cases one might resort to higher placement of the stoma, both in terms of a higher level in the small bowel where there is less tension, as well as a supra-umbilical right upper quadrant location. When the ileostomy pouch distance exceeds 70–80 cm, patients will have excessive ileostomy effluent requiring considerable anti-diarrhoeal medications and increased fluid intake, and are vulnerable to dehydration.

The covering loop ileostomy does carry a morbidity of its own. Complications related to the stoma occurred in as many as 41% of patients and serious morbidity after ileostomy closure occurred in 30% of cases (Keighley & Kmiot, 1990). In addition, a second operation is needed to close the stoma. However, use of a covering stoma is the safest option especially in the early learning phase of the surgeon.

Drains

We practise routine drainage of the presacral space using sump suction drains. Opinion is divided about the value of saline irrigation as well as suction. In one study, we found no advantage adding irrigation to suction (Galandiuk & Fazio, 1991). The drains are left for 3–5 days or until drainage is less than 50 ml/day. No tubes or drains are left in the pouch itself, except when an ileostomy is not used.

Some have used the intraluminal colo-shield (Ravo tube), as a means of avoiding temporary ileostomy with reported success (Ravo et al., 1987).

Pelvic reservoir procedure in Crohn's disease

Pouch procedures are not recommended in Crohn's colitis because of the likelihood of recurrence and loss of a large amount of valuable small bowel. However, if the diagnosis is made only after pouch construction, one would still proceed to ileostomy closure after advising the patient of possible sequelae. Pouch complications in Crohn's colitis appear to be related to precolectomy features that are suggestive of Crohn's disease, in particular, the presence of perianal disease. Outcome of patients who lack preoperative features of Crohn's disease in the short term (up to 4–5 years) is similar to patients with ulcerative colitis or indeterminate colitis (Hyman et al., 1991).

Follow-up and management

Patients are advised to take a low residue diet. Bulk agents of the psyllium group are used together with anti-diarrhoeal agents such as Lomotil (diphenoxylate hydrochloride with atropine sulphate) or Imodium (loperamide hydrochloride). Re-measurement of the stoma site is done at the first postoperative visit usually in 6 weeks' time. Pouch endoscopy is done at this time. Any web effect producing anastomotic narrowing is easier to deal with at this time than at 12 weeks following discharge (when the ileostomy is closed). Prior to closure of the ileostomy, pouch endoscopy is repeated to check the anastomosis. Gastrografin enema is done routinely to check anastomotic and pouch integrity.

Functional adequacy of the sphincters is confirmed by the patient's ability to control mucus drainage from the pouch. Manometric or functional testing of the sphincters (ability to hold 100-ml saline enema) is useful if there is any question about continence. In questionable cases, continued sphincter exercise with deferment of ileostomy closure may be appropriate. Efficacy of such exercises is by no means a certainty. In selected cases, even sphincter plication may be considered, if incontinence appears to be a likely sequel.

Ileostomy closure

This is done on the day of admission and the mean hospitalization time is 5 days. Preparation consists of oral liquids only the day preceding surgery, and prophylactic perioperative antibiotics are given for 24 hours. In most cases, a parastomal incision is made at the mucocutaneous junction, followed by intraperitoneal mobilization, excision of scar at the edges of the afferent and efferent ends of the loop, and a one layer interrupted 3/0 Vicryl suture closure. A check is made for inadvertent enterotomy by irrigation of afferent and efferent limbs. Care is taken to divide any adhesive peritoneal band that tends to keep the closed loop in a hairpin configuration. Closure of the abdominal wall defect is done using a mass closure of peritoneum, fascia and rectus muscle with interrupted 1 Vicryl sutures. The skin defect is left open.

Post-ileostomy closure follow-up

Patients are discharged on the same programme as that following the earlier admission. In both cases, if steroid preparation has been used, a graduated tapering of steroid amounts is used, the duration depending upon dosage amounts and duration of steroid use preoperatively.

Patients are seen 4–6 weeks postoperatively and adjustments made as necessary to anti-diarrhoeal medications. By this time, function is usually satisfactory. A more liberal diet is usually initiated by the patient, but many will observe some dietary restriction depending upon perceived or real intolerance of particular foods.

In patients in whom the anal transitional zone has been preserved, we recommend lifetime annual pouch endoscopy and biopsy of the ATZ and pouch. In our experience, occurrence of dysplasia in ATZ has rarely been encountered in the short term (3-year follow-up). We have not observed persistent dysplasia, i.e. dysplasia present on consecutive biopsies. In the event that this was seen, and verified as significant on histological review, one would then recommend transanal mucosectomy and pouch advancement to the dentate line with neo-ileal pouch anal anastomosis.

Experience at the Cleveland Clinic

A total of 605 pouches have been performed at the Cleveland Clinic since 1984. Despite the complex nature of the procedure, the mortality was 2 out of 605 (0.3%). Morbidity is more common, averaging 28%. Common morbidity includes pelvic sepsis (5%) and small bowel obstruction from adhesions requiring laparotomy (12%). Pouch failure as defined by the need to excise the pouch occurred in 3% of cases with a median follow-up of 3 years. Major contributing factors to pouch failure were Crohn's disease, poor sphincter function and pelvic sepsis.

Anastomotic stricture also occurred frequently but most of these responded to dilatation, which can be performed in the office. Several dilatations are usually necessary and surgical 'plasty' procedures were needed in only one out of 605 cases. Pouchitis occurred in 18% of patients and was much more common in patients with ulcerative colitis than those with familial adenomatous polyposis. Bladder dysfunction occurred in 4% of cases and was mostly transient. Sexual dysfunction was uncommon (<1.4%). Normal faecal continence was achieved in 80% of patients after pouch surgery, although the quality of continence was variable. Major faecal incontinence was uncommon and occurred in <5% of patients. Functional results including anal sensation and discriminatory function are significantly better after stapled anastomosis without mucosectomy than after mucosectomy with endoanal handsewn anastomosis. These findings are reflected in improved continence, particularly at night.

Summary

Restorative proctocolectomy has become an important part of the treatment of diffuse mucosal colonic disease. The principle of the procedure is established and refinements of surgical technique will continue. Until a few years ago, patients with ulcerative colitis and familial adenomatous polyposis, who were unsuitable for colectomy with ileorectal anastomosis, would have been offered a conventional proctocolectomy with a permanent ileostomy as the main surgical option. It is now possible to treat many of these patients with a continence saving procedure. Considerable technical advance has taken place as a result of the lessons learned over the last decade. As a result, restorative proctocolectomy with ileal reservoir has become a relatively safe procedure.

References

Beart RW Jr (1988) Proctocolectomy and ileoanal anastomosis. *World J Surg* **12**:160–163.

Beart RW Jr, Metcalf AM, Dozois RR, Kelly KA (1985) The J-ileal-pouch-anastomosis. The Mayo Clinic experience. In *Alternatives to Conventional Ileostomy*, RR Dozois (ed). Chicago, Year Book Medical Publishers, pp. 384–387.

Cutait DE, Figliolini FJ (1961) A new method of colorectal anastomosis and abdomino-perineal resection. *Dis Colon Rectum* **4**:335–342.

Everett WG (1989) Experience of restorative proctocolectomy with ileal reservoir. *Br J Surg* **76**:77–87.

Fazio VW (1986) Loop ileostomy and loop-end ileostomy. In *Smith's Atlas of General Surgery*, 4th edn, H Dudley, DC Carter, RCG Russell (eds). London, Butterworths, pp. 448–456.

Fazio VW (1988) Cancer of the rectum – sphincter-saving operation. *Surg Clin North Am* **68**:1367–1381.

Fazio VW, Tjandra JJ (1991) Primary therapy in large bowel carcinoma. *World J Surgery* **15**:568–575.

Feinberg SM, Parker F, Cohen Z, *et al.* (1986) The double stapling technique for low anterior resection of rectal carcinoma. *Dis Colon Rectum* **29**:885–890.

Fonkalsrud EW (1980) Total colectomy and endorectal ileal pull-through with internal ileal reservoir for ulcerative colitis. *Surg Gynecol Obstet* **150**:1–8.

Fonkalsrud EW, Ament ME (1978) Endorectal mucosal resection without proctocolectomy as an adjunct for abdomino-perineal resection for non-malignant condition: clinical experience with five patients. *Ann Surg* **67**:533–538.

Galandiuk S, Fazio VW (1991) Postoperative irrigation–suction drainage after pelvic colon surgery. *Dis Colon Rectum* **34**:223–228.

Goligher JC (1984) Eversion technique for distal mucosal proctocolectomy in ulcerative colitis: a preliminary report. *Br J Surg* **71**:26–28.

Grant D, Cohen Z, McHugh S, McLeod R, Stern H (1986) Restorative proctocolectomy clinical results and manometric findings with long and short rectal cuffs. *Dis Colon Rectum* **29**:27–32.

Hyman NH, Fazio VW, Tuckson WB, Lavery IC (1991) The consequences of ileal-pouch-anal-anastomosis for Crohn's colitis. *Dis Colon Rectum* **34**:653–657.

Johnston D, Williams NS, Neal DE, Axon ATR (1981) The value of preserving the anal sphincter in operations for ulcerative colitis and polyposis: a review of twenty-two mucosal proctectomies. *Br J Surg* **68**:874–878.

Julian TB, Ravitch MM (1988) Evaluation of the safety of end-to-end (EEA) stapling anastomoses across linear stapled closures. *Surg Clin North Am* **68**:1367–1381.

Keighley MRB (1987) Abdominal mucosectomy reduces the incidence of soiling and sphincter damage after restorative proctocolectomy and J-pouch. *Dis Colon Rectum* **30**:386–390.

Keighley MRB, Kmiot W (1990) Surgical options in ulcerative colitis: Role of ileo-anal anastomosis. *Aust NZ J Surg* **60**:835–848.

Keighley MRB, Yoshioka K, Kmiot WA (1988) Prospective randomised trial to compare the stapled double lumen pouch and the sutured quadrupled pouch for restorative proctocolectomy. *Br J Surg* **75**:1008–1011.

Knight CD, Griffen FD (1990) An improved technique for low anterior resection of the rectum using the EEA stapler. *Surgery* **88**:710–714.

Lavery IC, Fazio VW, Oakley JR, Milsom JW (1990) Pouch surgery – the importance of the transitional zone. *Can J Gastroenterol* **7**:428–431.

Lavery IC, Tuckson WB, Easley KA (1989) Internal anal sphincter function after total abdominal colectomy and stapled ileal pouch-anal anastomosis without mucosal

proctectomy. *Dis Colon Rectum* **32**:950–953.

Martin LW, Fischer JE (1982) Preservation of anorectal continence following total colectomy. *Ann Surg* **196**:700–704.

Matikainen M, Santavirta J, Hiltunen KM (1990) Ileoanal anastomosis without covering ileostomy. *Dis Colon Rectum* **33**:384–388.

Nicholls RJ (1987) Restorative proctocolectomy with various types of reservoir. *World J Surg* **11**:751–762.

Nicholls RJ, Lubowski DZ (1987) Restorative proctocolectomy the four loop (W) reservoir. *Br J Surg* **74**:564–566.

Nicholls RJ, Pezim ME (1985) Restorative proctocolectomy with ileal reservoir for ulcerative colitis and familial adenomatous polyposis: A comparison of three reservoir designs. *Br J Surg* **72**:470–474.

O'Connell PR, Williams NS (1991) Mucosectomy in restorative proctocolectomy. *Br J Surg* **78**:129–130.

O'Connell PR, Pemberton JW, Weilano LH, *et al.* (1987) Does rectal mucosa regenerate after ileoanal anastomosis? *Dis Colon Rectum* **30**:1–5.

Parks AG, Nicholls RJ (1978) Proctocolectomy without ileostomy for ulcerative colitis. *Br Med J* **2**:85–88.

Parks AG, Nicholls RJ, Belliveau P (1980) Proctocolectomy with ileal reservoir and anal anastomosis. *Br J Surg* **67**:533–538.

Ravo B, Michrick A, Addei K, *et al.* (1987) The treatment of perforated diverticulitis by one-stage intracolonic bypass procedure. *Surgery* **102**:771–776.

Rothenberger DA, Buls JG, Nivatvongs S, Goldberg SM (1985) The Parks' S-ileal pouch-and anal anastomosis after colectomy and mucosal proctectomy. *Am J Surg* **149**:390–394.

Rothenberger DH, Vermeulen FD, Christenson CE, *et al.* (1983) Restorative proctocolectomy with ileal reservoir and ileoanal anastomosis. *Am J Surg* **145**:82–88.

Smith LE, Friend W, Medwell S (1984) The superior mesentric artery: the critical factor in pouch pull-through procedure. *Dis Colon Rectum* **27**:741–744.

Stern H, Walfisch S, Mullen B, McLeod, Cohen Z (1990) Cancer in an ileoanal reservoir. A new late complication? *Gut* **31**:473–475.

Trollope ML, Cohen RG, Lee RH, *et al.* (1986) A 7-year experience with low anterior sigmoid resections using the EEA stapler. *Am J Surg* **152**:11–15.

Tsunoda A, Talbot IC, Nicholls RJ (1990) Incidence of dysplasia in the anorectal mucosa in patients having restorative proctocolectomy. *Br J Surg* **77**:506–508.

Tuckson WB, Fazio VW (1991) Functional comparison between double and triple ileal loop pouches. *Dis Colon Rectum* **34**:17–21.

Tuckson WB, Lavery IC, Fazio VW, Oakley JR, Church JM, Milsom JW (1991) Manometric and functional comparison of ileal-pouch-anal-anastomosis with and without anal manipulation. *Am J Surg* **161**:90–96.

Turnbull RB Jr, Cuthbertson AM (1961) Abdomino-perineal pull-through resection for cancer and for Hirschsprung's disease. *Cleve Clin Q* **28**:209–115.

Utsunomiya J, Iwama T, Imajo M, *et al.* (1980) Total colectomy, mucosal proctectomy and ileoanal anastomosis. *Dis Colon Rectum* **23**:459–466.

van de Pavoordt HDWM, Fazio VW, Jagelman DG, *et al.* (1987) The outcome of loop ileostomy closure in 293 cases. *Int J Colorectal Dis* **2**:214–217.

Vasilevsky CA, Rothenberger BA, Goldberg SM (1987) The S-ileal-pouch-anal anastomosis. *World J Surg* **11**:742–750.

Wong WD, Rothenberger DA, Goldberg SM (1985) Ileoanal pouch procedures. *Curr Probl Surg* **22**:9–18.

Chapter 4
Complications, Management, Failure and Revisions

JOHN H. PEMBERTON

Introduction

Although experimental just a short time ago, restorative proctocolectomy has become the standard surgical approach recommended to most patients, particularly younger ones, who face proctocolectomy for either chronic ulcerative colitis or familial adenomatous polyposis. Indeed, the indications, patient selection procedures, operative techniques and routines of postoperative care are today relatively straightforward, thus reducing the potential serious problems patients might encounter postoperatively.

Moreover, in most major institutions, the 'learning curve' has been negotiated successfully and experience has matured. For example, among the first 200 patients at the Mayo Clinic the difficult problem of pelvic sepsis occurred in 15%. Today that rate is less than 5%.

Restorative proctocolectomy is a complex, sophisticated operation, and complications occur with some frequency. The overall rate of morbidity for all patients still hovers between 25 and 30%. Failure however is rare, even with those who suffer a postoperative complication. In our experience, 94% of patients have a successful outcome. It is just as important to understand the complications of restorative proctocolectomy, how to avoid them and what to do if they occur as it is to know how to select appropriate patients and how to perform the procedure rapidly and accurately. Although it will not be discussed any further here, the key to a successful outcome after restorative proctocolectomy is a surgeon who performs the operation effortlessly; the operation struggled through is the one fraught with complication and sometimes failure.

The aim of this chapter is to report upon the experiences at the Mayo Clinic with problems associated with restorative proctocolectomy based upon a series of slightly more than 1200 patients operated upon over a 10-year period of time between 1981 and 1991, and at appropriate junctures, to compare these results with the literature.

The Mayo series

Between January 1981 and June 1991, 1218 patients underwent restorative proctocolectomy at the Mayo Clinic. The operation was done for chronic ulcerative colitis in 89% of the patients and for familial adenomatous polyposis in 11%. Four patients underwent the operation for motor disorders of the gut. Out of all the patients; 52% were men, 48% women. The mean age of the patients was 32 years, while the age range was 12–64 years.

Among these patients, an initial group of 390 patients was identified who had a J restorative proctocolectomy performed for chronic ulcerative colitis. These patients were followed from 6 months to 5 years postoperatively. This study (Pemberton *et al.*, 1987) serves as foundation for the following presentation of the clinical and functional outcomes after restorative proctocolectomy.

Patient selection

General

A centrally important element in determining outcome is the fitness of the patient; the candidate must be able to endure a complex, multiple stage operation. Most patients facing *emergency* colectomy, therefore, are poor candidates for restorative proctocolectomy. Patients with a carcinoma, however, are good candidates, provided the cancer is above the mid-rectum. Severe extra-intestinal manifestations do not, *per se*, render patients ineligible for restorative proctocolectomy. These patients should be warned, however, that inflammatory changes in the pouch may occur with greater frequency after restorative proctocolectomy than if they did not have extra-intestinal manifestations, and that restorative proctocolectomy may not cure the extra-intestinal manifestations at all.

Sclerosing cholangitis is likewise not a contraindication to restorative proctocolectomy. Patients with indeterminate colitis appear to behave in the same way as patients with chronic ulcerative colitis and therefore are candidates for the operation. Patients with familial adenomatous polyposis who have mesenteric fibromatosis or desmoid tumours concomitantly, however, are usually rendered anatomically unfit for restorative proctocolectomy.

Age *is* an issue. Stool frequency and incontinence, after restorative proctocolectomy, increase as age increases and thus we have arbitrarily set 60–65 years as an upper limit, especially for women. McHugh and Diamant's (1987) careful studies showed that decline of resting and squeeze pressure was associated with ageing and female gender. In order to improve results in the elderly, perhaps a modified restorative proctocolectomy could be performed, sparing the distal rectal mucosa and upper anal canal as suggested by Johnston and others (1987).

Short, obese patients are poor candidates for the operation because the mesentery of the small bowel is short and fat and because the retroperitoneal fat bulges anteriorly, effectively increasing the distance between the root of the mesentery and the anal canal. Very tall patients have a similar problem in that their mesentery may not reach far enough to permit the ileal anal anastomosis to be performed. If such patients are operated upon, modification of the operation, such as construction of an S pouch or stapling the pouch to the top of the anal canal should be considered.

Nearly all of our chronic ulcerative colitis patients had been receiving steroids preoperatively, and steroid use therefore, is definitely not a contraindication to the operation. Poor nutritional status and general inanition, however, are relative contraindications.

Although rarely discussed, a further relative contraindication is that some people are psychologically unfit to undergo this operation. Patients should be bright, have an appreciation of their underlying disease, be able to follow instructions, be compliant and compulsive about follow-up. Every centre has at least several people who fail the operation for psychological reasons.

Absolute contraindications, those that, if present, would likely guarantee complications and ultimate failure, are: Crohn's disease, cancer of the distal rectum or anal canal, damaged anal sphincters, history of faecal incontinence, poorly repaired episiotomies and patients who are elderly, debilitated and non-active.

Special situations

Concomitant colorectal carcinoma

Restorative proctocolectomy should probably not be carried out if the cancer is located in the distal half of the rectum. However, a more favourable cancer located higher in the rectum *does not* preclude restorative proctocolectomy. Seventeen patients (13 with chronic ulcerative colitis, four with familial adenomatous polyposis) had a concomitant adenocarcinoma of the colon or rectum at the time of restorative proctocolectomy (Taylor *et al.*, 1988.) The stage of the tumours were: A = 5%, B1 = 32%, B2 = 18%, C1 and C2 = 45%. There were no operative deaths. The rate of pelvic sepsis was 18%, compared to 5% for all other restorative proctocolectomy patients. Both the cancer and non-cancer patients had the same daytime and night-time stool frequencies: six stools during the day/one stool during the night. The rate of daytime and night-time seepage was also the same: cancer – 17% daytime / 50% night-time incontinence; no cancer – 23%/47%. We concluded that restorative proctocolectomy is not contraindicated in patients with resectable colorectal cancer.

In colitis patients with cancer, the ileocolic vessel should be ligated higher, there should be greater lymphatic clearance for caecal cancer and rectal mobilization should be wider than commonly accomplished during restorative proctocolectomy.

Severe extra-intestinal manifestations of chronic ulcerative colitis

Extra-intestinal manifestations of ulcerative colitis, such as pyoderma gangrenosum, erythema nodosum, polyarterritis nodosum, arthritis and uveitis sometimes prompt colectomy, even if the chronic ulcerative colitis is quiescent. These conditions usually improve after colectomy. In contrast, ankylosing spondylitis and primary sclerosing cholangitis may not be affected at all by proctocolectomy; they may instead progress after operation. Interestingly, sometimes these manifestations may appear for the first time *after* proctocolectomy has been performed.

Sclerosing cholangitis is a chronic cholestatic disease frequently associated with chronic ulcerative colitis (LaRusso *et al.*, 1984). Progression may result in liver failure. Proper management of the ulcerative colitis in these patients is most important because patients with primary sclerosing cholangitis are often candidates for liver transplantation. While proctocolectomy cures the colitis, it should be reserved for the usual indications for colectomy and *not* for the liver disease itself, because proctocolectomy does not affect the progression of the liver disease (Cangemi *et al.*, 1989).

When proctocolectomy is indicated, restorative proctocolectomy should be performed, and not a Brooke ileostomy; if a stoma is established, approximately one-half of the patients will bleed from peristomal varices (Wiesner *et al.*, 1986.) While the risk of colon surgery in patients with cirrhosis is substantial, mortality was zero among the 40 patients with primary sclerosing cholangitis. Moreover, no patient has bled from the anal anastomosis.

Indeterminate colitis

Patients with Crohn's disease fare poorly after restorative proctocolectomy (Deutsch *et al.*, 1991.) However, distinguishing Crohn's disease from chronic ulcerative colitis is difficult, even in the pathology laboratory. Patients who harbour macroscopic and microscopic features of both chronic ulcerative colitis and Crohn's have 'indeterminate colitis'. This diagnosis is established in about 10% of patients with inflammatory bowel disease who come for proctocolectomy, not an insignificant number.

Out of 514 consecutive restorative proctocolectomy patients operated upon between January 1981 and June 1986, 25 had features of indeterminate colitis: unusual distribution of inflammation, deep linear ulcers, neural proliferation, transmural inflammation, fissures and creeping fat (Pezim *et al.*, 1989). We compared the functional outcome of these 25 indeterminate colitis patients to the outcome of the remaining 489 chronic ulcerative colitis patients and found no significant difference in rates of complications, pouch function, incidence of pouchitis, or requirement for pouch excision. These findings have been confirmed and extended in a recent report of 46 patients followed for a median 10 years after proctocolectomy (Wells *et al.*, 1991).

It is centrally important to keep in mind that only patients who are diagnosed preoperatively as having typical chronic ulcerative colitis, but at the time of operation are found to possess histologic features overlapping with those of Crohn's disease, are properly labelled as having 'indeterminate colitis.' On the other hand, when the pathologist hesitates to classify the colitis as 'typical' on preoperative biopsies and some clinical features are worrisome, such as a history of complex perianal suppuration, restorative proctocolectomy should not be performed. In this way, fewer patients with Crohn's disease will undergo restorative proctocolectomy mistakenly.

The operation

The mucosal resection

At the Mayo Clinic all diseased mucosa in patients with ulcerative colitis and familial adenomatous polyposis is removed. This includes the zone of transitional epithelium. Leaving the transitional mucosa of the anal canal in place, as some have advocated, leaves disease behind (Emblem *et al.*, 1988; King *et al.*, 1989; Tsunoda *et al.*, 1990; Ambrose *et al.*, 1991b; Sugerman *et al.*, 1991; Tuckson *et al.*, 1991) and predisposes the patient to the need for continued surveillance, the risk of symptoms, and the possible necessity of further therapy. Also, the risk of cancerous degeneration of the residual mucosa remains (Emblem *et al.*, 1988; King *et al.*, 1989; Tsunoda *et al.*, 1990), although the chance admittedly is very small.

The muscular 'cuff'

A rectal muscular 'cuff' of 3–5 cm in length results in satisfactory anal function. Longer cuffs were made initially, but the dissections were tedious, and the long cuff sometimes obstructed outflow during defaecation. Short muscular cuffs decrease operating time, decrease bleeding and minimize contamination. In addition, the likelihood of leaving rests of mucosa behind (O'Connell *et al.*, 1987) is less if the cuff is short. Short muscular cuffs, however, may be associated with loss of the rectal inhibitory reflex (Becker, 1984), but this does not appear to affect function adversely (Beart *et al.*, 1985). In contrast, Chaussade and others (1989) have proposed that a cuff is not necessary to ensure good clinical results and thus resect all rectal muscle. We, however, continue to preserve a 3–5 cm rectal cuff which appears to provide adequate protection of the anal sphincter.

The reservoir

At the Mayo Clinic, we have used the J shaped ileal pouch (Utsunomiya, 1980) almost exclusively (Fig. 4.1).

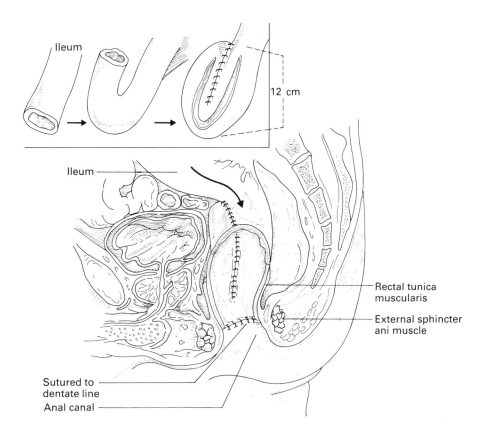

Ileum

12 cm

Ileum

Rectal tunica
muscularis

External sphincter
ani muscle

Sutured to
dentate line
Anal canal

Fig. 4.1 J shaped ileal pouch used for restorative proctocolectomy. From Taylor *et al.* (1983) with permission.

The pouch is made from the terminal 30 cm of ileum. It is easy to construct, provides an adequate reservoir, and empties readily.

Other pouch designs, such as the S, W and K, have also been satisfactory. Initially, functional results appeared to be better with the J pouch than with the S pouch. This was probably because a long efferent limb obstructed outflow from the S pouch; as the S pouch procedure has evolved, the efferent limb has been shortened, and results of the S pouch have become similar to those of the J pouch.

The S, W and K pouches, however, do provide a larger reservoir which should lower the stool frequency. Indeed, there is some evidence that this occurs (Nasmyth *et al.*, 1986; Harms *et al.*, 1987). However, reservoir function has not been improved dramatically. Importantly, these pouches are not as easy to construct with staples as is the J pouch and so require increased operative time. In the Mayo series, the J pouch has been the predominant pouch configuration, because it is easy to construct and functional results are excellent.

The Anastomosis

At the Mayo Clinic, a handsewn anastomosis of the pouch to the anal canal using absorbable sutures is preferred. Others have described satisfactory results with a stapled technique (Peck, 1988; Williams *et al.*, 1989; Wexner *et al.*, 1991). There is some concern, that the stapler may damage the anal sphincter, particularly when the anastomosis is performed at the level of the mid anal canal; in this situation, the proximal two-thirds of the internal anal sphincter will be included in the distal doughnut of tissue.

The temporary ileostomy

Although most surgeons use a temporary diverting ileostomy constructed proximal to the pouch, some authors have reported good results in patients in whom no diverting stoma was used (Kmiot & Keighley, 1989; Sugerman *et al.*, 1991). We have found that the ileostomy protects the pouch and anastomosis from the faecal stream, thus promoting healing. Although the ileostomy does cause morbidity (Metcalf *et al.*, 1986; Everett & Pollard, 1990), it is easier and far more successful to treat complications associated with the diverting stoma than those which occur as a result of pelvic sepsis. Interestingly, patients diverted with a conventional Brooke ileostomy appeared to experience a higher rate of obstruction than those with a loop ileostomy (12.5% Brooke vs. 4.6% loop, $p = 0.07$) (Francios *et al.*, 1989).

Two- vs. three-staged restorative proctocolectomy

At the Mayo Clinic, restorative proctocolectomy is performed as a two-staged operation: colectomy and ileoanal anastomosis as one stage and closure of the temporary ileostomy as the second stage. Some surgeons have advocated that an additional stage, colectomy and ileostomy and Hartmann pouch be performed first, followed by construction of the pouch as stage two and closure of the ileostomy as stage three. The rationale is that patients on high doses of steroids, who are nutritionally depleted and who are generally ill, may be poor candidates for ileoanal anastomosis.

To determine whether an additional stage might be beneficial, we reviewed 871 patients who underwent restorative proctocolectomy between January 1981 and September 1989 and identified 95 patients who had had a three stage procedure. The mean delay between stage one (colectomy) and stage two (construction of pouch) was 24 months. Patients in the three-stage group had a lower incidence of small bowel obstruction, 7%, compared to patients after the two stage operation, 15% ($p < 0.05$). However, patients in the three-stage group had a significantly higher rate of pelvic sepsis than did those in the two-stage group (11% vs. 5%, respectively, $p < 0.05$). The frequency of all complications, as well as the long-term clinical and functional results, were similar in both groups. We concluded that three-stage procedures probably added little benefit compared to two-staged procedures in patients not requiring emergency colectomy.

Clinical results

Clearly, the results of restorative proctocolectomy have been analysed carefully by authors everywhere; the operation has been examined from almost every possible point of view. This section examines published reports, using data from the Mayo Clinic as a baseline.

Early results

Mortality

At the Mayo Clinic only two out of 1218 patients died postoperatively; one from massive pulmonary embolus and one from complications of a perforated, steroid-induced gastric ulcer. Certainly, the literature and our experience support the conclusion that the operation is safe. The greatest mortality reported after restorative proctocolectomy was by Morgan *et al.* (1987) and that was only 1.5%; normally, mortalities range from 0–1% (Cohen *et al.*, 1985; Nicholls & Pezim, 1985; Becker & Raymond, 1986; Nasmyth *et al.*, 1986; Schoetz *et al.*, 1986; Pemberton *et al.*, 1987). Although complex, ileoanal anastomosis is nearly always performed electively, under controlled operative and anaesthetic conditions with few patients in critical distress. In addition, there is no doubt that as results have steadily improved over the years patients are being referred earlier in the course of their disease, before they become debilitated rendering them poor candidates for this type of aggressive surgical management.

Morbidity

In distinct contrast to mortality, morbidity after restorative proctocolectomy remains considerable. The reported overall complication rates vary between 13 and

Table 4.1 Postoperative morbidity after restorative proctocolectomy and after closure of the ileostomy in 390 patients.

Complication	Patients with complication (%)
After ileal pouch anal anastomosis	
Small bowel obstruction	13
Transient	8
Required reoperation	5
Pelvic sepsis	5
Antibiotics alone	3
Required reoperation	2
Wound infection	3
Urinary retention	7
Transient	5
Required catheterization	2
After closure of ileostomy	
Small bowel obstruction	9
Transient	4
Required reoperation	5
Anastomotic leakage	2
Longer term	
Anastomotic stricture	5
Pouchitis	31

From Pemberton JH (1992) with permission.

54% (Williams & Johnston, 1985; Nasmyth *et al.*, 1986; Harms *et al.*, 1987; Morgan *et al.*, 1987; Pemberton *et al.*, 1987). Restorative proctocolectomy is therefore certainly not trouble-free. Patients should be so informed. To be perfectly accurate, most complications occur early after operation and do *not* result in long-term disability or loss of the pouch.

Complications

Complications immediately after restorative proctocolectomy

Table 4.1 lists the incidence of the early postoperative complications which have occurred after restorative proctocolectomy at the Mayo Clinic. The most frequent problem was small bowel obstruction, which occurred in 13% of our patients. About one-half of patients with obstruction required reoperation to relieve the obstruction. Importantly, this rate of small bowel obstruction is in keeping with the literature describing the complications occurring after *conventional* Brooke ileostomy (Watts *et al.*, 1966; Roy *et al.*, 1970; Pemberton *et al.*, 1985).

Pelvic sepsis, clearly an early problem with restorative proctocolectomy (Williams & Johnston, 1985) occurred in only 5% of patients with chronic ulcerative colitis at the Mayo Clinic. Fever, leukocytosis, suprapubic or left lower quadrant fullness and tenderness hailed the onset of pelvic sepsis. A CT scan was often used to confirm the presence of an abscess or of oedematous tissues. One-third of patients, specifically those with phlegmons, were treated by antibiotics alone successfully. Those with organized abscesses underwent CT-guided transperineal or transabdominal drainage. The incidence of pelvic sepsis has decreased dramatically, probably because the muscular cuff is now quite short (Becker & Parodi, 1989) and because the operation is more expertly performed.

Overall, the incidence of abdominal sepsis was 6% (Scott *et al.*, 1988). Interestingly, of patients who required laparotomy to control sepsis, 41% lost the pouch ultimately and only 29% ever recovered ileoanal function. However, if no reoperation was required, 92% of patients with sepsis eventually had a functioning pouch.

Deep and/or superficial wound infections occurred in 3%. Seven percent of the patients had transient urinary retention, while 2% required intermittent catheterization upon dismissal. Importantly, no patient had to have a catheter in place permanently.

Stricturing of the ileoanal anastomosis *before* ileostomy closure occurred commonly and was treated simply by digital dilatation. This soft stricturing was actually a web of tissue which formed at the anastomosis. This type of stricture did not recur.

Complications after ileostomy closure (Table 4.1)

Again, small bowel obstruction was the most common complication after closure of the ileostomy. Nine percent of patients had small bowel obstruction, one-half of whom required reoperation. The incidence then of early *and* late obstruction was fully 22%. This overall rate of obstruction is greater than that reported after proctocolectomy and Brooke ileostomy, although not much greater, and does indeed remain a problem.

Anastomotic leakage at the site of closure of the ileostomy occurred in about 0.5–1.0% of patients. This incidence of leakage appears to have decreased after we abandoned the 'fold-over' ileostomy closure technique in favour of resecting all extraperitoneal bowel and performing an end-to-end anastomosis.

Comparing complications: proctocolectomy with Brooke ileostomy and restorative proctocolectomy

As hinted above, proctocolectomy combined with Brooke ileostomy is not complication free. The incidences and types of complications after this more conservative operation are, like those after restorative proctocolectomy, moderate in frequency. In an interesting study, Phillips and co-authors (1989) surveyed results in 70 patients who underwent proctocolectomy and Brooke ileostomy in the recent past (1976–1986.) The mean age was higher than that of most ileoanal series (49 years); 39% suffered immediate postoperative complications. Major complications occurred in 17%. Eleven percent were related to a persistent perineal wound. During follow-up, 36% of patients were readmitted to hospital and 21% were reoperated upon. The cumulative probability of readmission at 6 years was 45%. Twenty-five patients had either ileostomy dysfunction or small bowel obstruction. This risk of complication, 39%, is not different from that reported after restorative proctocolectomy. It seems fair to conclude that proctocolectomy with Brooke ileostomy and restorative proctocolectomy have similar rates of complication.

Table 4.2 Functional results of restorative proctocolectomy from 6 months to 6 years postoperatively in 389 patients.

Parameter	Follow-up					
	6 months	1 year	2 years	3 years	4 years	5 years
No. of stools (mean ± SD)						
Daytime	5 ± 2	5 ± 3	6 ± 3	6 ± 2	6 ± 3	6 ± 2
Night-time	1 ± 1	1 ± 1	2 ± 2	2 ± 1	1 ± 1	2 ± 1
Able to discriminate gas from stool (% of patients)	69	77	73	84	77	86
Lomotil (% of patients)	26	19	17	25	6	4
Metamucil (% of patients)	43	36	40	38	30	27

From Pemberton JH (1992) with permission.

Late results

Function

Table 4.2 and Fig. 4.2 detail the stool frequency, patterns of continence, ability to discriminate gas from stool and the use of medications for 6 months to 5 years after ileoanal anastomosis. The daytime and night-time stool frequency remained stable and did not change over time. The incidence of night-time incontinence and dependence on medication, however, declined (Fig. 4.2). For comparison, Table 4.3 lists the stool frequency of several large series. Using the stool frequency as a determinant of outcome is somewhat suspect, principally because patients do not themselves use stool frequency to describe their functional status.

Faecal incontinence does occur after restorative proctocolectomy. Daytime incontinence is uncommon in any reported series. In contrast, occasional (once per week) night-time spotting occurs in about 20–30% of patients at greater than 12 months after operation.

Trying to determine the rate of nocturnal incontinence by reporting the frequency of pad use is also highly suspect; about 60% of all female patients will use a pad sometimes at night but mostly for peace of mind. Fortunately, the incidence of nocturnal incontinence and dependence on medication declines as time passes after operation (Fig. 4.2).

We found among 390 patients after restorative proctocolectomy that older patients had more daytime stools than younger patients (≤50 years, 6 ± 3 stools/day; >50 years, 8 ± 4 stools/day; $p = 0.05$). Women and men had the same number of stools each day, but women had more episodes of occasional faecal spotting than men, both during the day and night (day: women 33% vs. men 14%, $p < 0.001$; night: women 56% vs. men 44%, $p < 0.02$). Interestingly, the frequency of faecal spotting after ileoanal anastomosis was affected significantly by the *preoperative* stool frequency; the greater the number of stools before ileoanal anastomosis, the more likely patients were to be incontinent after the operation ($p < 0.03$).

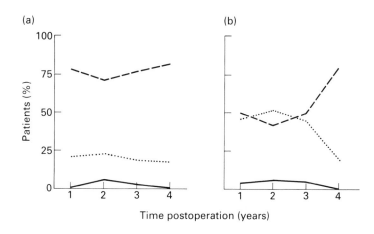

(a)   (b)

Time postoperation (years)

Fig. 4.2 (a) Daytime and (b) night-time continence after restorative proctocolectomy against the year after operation. Data points are connected for illustrative purposes only. ———, perfect, no faecal leakage; ·····, spotting, faecal spotting of underclothes, 3 cm or less in diameter, two times or less/week; —, gross, gross faecal incontinence more than two times/week. From Pemberton *et al.* (1987) with permission.

Table 4.3 Stool frequency of patients with ileal pouch anal anastomosis.

Series	No. of stools/24 hours	
	Early	Late
Cohen *et al.* (1985)	7	5
Nicholls & Pezim (1985)	3–4	–
Becker & Raymond (1986)	6	6
Nasmyth *et al.* (1986)	6	6
Schoetz *et al.* (1986)	7	5
Pemberton *et al.* (1987)	5	6

Quality of life

These data support the observation that restorative proctocolectomy is safe, effective and achieves its goals of restoring faecal continence. This would be relatively meaningless if patients were dissatisfied with the operation or in some way had a less than optimal quality of life. We therefore surveyed 298 ileal pouch patients and 406 Brooke ileostomy patients who had the operations performed for chronic ulcerative colitis or familial adenomatous polyposis (Pemberton *et al.*, 1989). After adjusting for age, diagnosis and reoperation rate, logistic regression analysis of performance scores of seven different daily activity categories: sexual activity, sports, social activities, recreation, family relationships, work around the house, and travel was used to discriminate between operations. Median follow-up was longer in Brooke ileostomy patients than in ileal pouch patients (104 months vs. 47 months, respec-

tively), and Brooke ileostomy patients were slightly older (38 years vs. 32 years).

The great majority of patients in each group were satisfied (93% Brooke ileostomy; 95% restorative proctocolectomy). In each performance category, the performance score *did* discriminate between operations; the probability of having had a restorative proctocolectomy increased with improvement in performance scores ($p < 0.05$) (Fig. 4.3). We concluded that restorative proctocolectomy patients experienced significant advantages in performing daily activities compared to patients with Brooke ileostomy, and thus experienced a better quality of life. These results largely agree with those of other authors who have studied the functional outcome of the operation (McHugh *et al.*, 1987; Becker & Parodi, 1989). This study also establishes that patients not only regain health predictably and quickly, but are satisfied with the operation and perform daily activities with little compromise.

Sexual function

The median age of our patients was 32 years. Potency and sterility were the main issues raised by the male patients while the future ability to conceive and to carry a pregnancy to term was the predominate concern of women.

We observed that sexual activity *increased* dramatically after restorative proctocolectomy compared with preoperative levels. This was most likely due to improvement in general health (Metcalf *et al.*, 1986). *Preoperatively*, 49% of patients reported problems

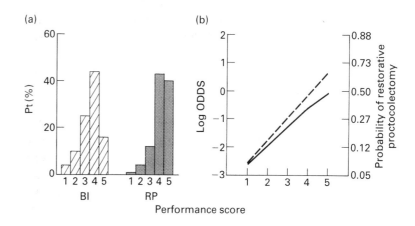

Fig. 4.3 Comparison of performance status; category: sports. (a) Overall distribution of patient performance scores for Brooke ileostomy (BI) and restorative proctocolectomy (RP). The data indicate higher scores among RP patients. (b) Plots of estimated log probability of having had the RP operation (log ODDS). ---, 35-; —, 45-year-old patients with chronic ulcerative colitis, and no reoperation. The rising lines (positive slopes) indicate that an improving performance score is associated with an increased probability of having had the RP operation in both age groups. From Pemberton *et al.* (1989) with permission.

with sexual activity. In contrast, *postoperative* sexual dysfunction occurred in 11% of the men and 12% of the women overall (Pemberton *et al.*, 1987). Three men (1.5%) were impotent and seven or 4% had retrograde ejaculation. The remainder reported that 'lack of motivation' or 'fatigue' were the principle causes of sexual dysfunction. In women, dyspareunia was the primary complaint in 7%, while 3% feared leakage of stool during intercourse. Other authors report very similar rates of sexual problems in men and women after this operation (Williams & Johnston, 1985; Wong *et al.*, 1985).

Pregnancy and delivery, even per vaginam, were quite safe after restorative proctocolectomy. Among Mayo Clinic patients, 40 women have had at least one successful pregnancy and delivery. We studied the effect of pregnancy and delivery on function in 20 of these patients (Nelson *et al.*, 1989). Eleven deliveries were vaginal with an episiotomy, and nine were by Caesarean section. No maternal deaths occurred. One child died of hyaline membrane disease. The reason given for the type of delivery used was patient preference in the vaginal delivery group and obstetrical reasons or 'protection of the pouch' in the Caesarean section group.

Function was altered minimally during and immediately after pregnancy. The frequency of daytime stooling and the incidence and degree of daytime and night-time incontinence were not significantly changed by pregnancy or delivery. The frequency of nocturnal stooling, however, did increase during pregnancy, and the increase persisted for approximately 3 months postpartum. Importantly, long-term pouch function was not influenced by the type of delivery.

Late complications (general)

Stricturing of the anastomosis is usually caused by tension (with and without ischaemia) and/or sepsis. If the pouch is on tension and if anchoring sutures either were not placed or broke and the anastomosis pulled apart, then the pouch retracts to the top of the anal canal, leaving the underlying denuded internal anal sphincter exposed: heavy scarring and a localized long, dense stricture inevitably result. If perianastomotic sepsis occurs and the anastomosis breaks down, the anal canal as well as the pelvic floor becomes fibrotic. The result is dense pelvic floor scarring. The tissues lose their compliance, resulting in a stricture. Patients with strictures may complain that they are having

increased difficulty with straining at stool, or alternatively, that they have a high stool frequency (>10–12 stools/day), and feel as if they never empty the pouch completely.

These kinds of strictures are difficult to treat successfully. Repeated dilatation keeps the stricture from progressing, and patients sometimes do well (Galandiuk *et al.*, 1990). Often, however, such strictures must be treated aggressively. One approach is to incise and loosen the stricture and advance pouch mucosa distally. Concomitantly, the perianal skin is elevated as an advancement flap and moved cephalad into the anal canal to abut the pouch mucosa at mid-sphincter level. The most aggressive operation is to remove the pouch from the pelvis, repair it or construct another, excise the pelvic floor scarring carefully (hopefully leaving the internal anal sphincter intact) and re-anastomose the pouch to the dentate line. The chances that good control can be achieved after such a procedure are slim but if the patient understands the risk, then it may be worth the effort to try.

Fistula/sinus

There are several different types of fistula and sinus tracts which occur after restorative proctocolectomy (Dozois, 1988).

Asymptomatic

Small radiographic leaks are not worrisome and are treated usually by deferring closure of the ileostomy for 2–4 *additional* months. Nearly always, the fistula disappears.

Symptomatic

Pouch or anastomotic – perianal

Perineal fistulae occur in less than 1% of patients at some time after closure of the stoma. If superficial, they are treated by fistulotomy. If this involves the sphincter mass, then a seton is used slowly to perform the fistulotomy over several weeks. If anterior in a female patient, the secondary site should be excised down to the sphincter and a flap of pouch mucosa advanced over the primary site. Diversion in these patients is prudent.

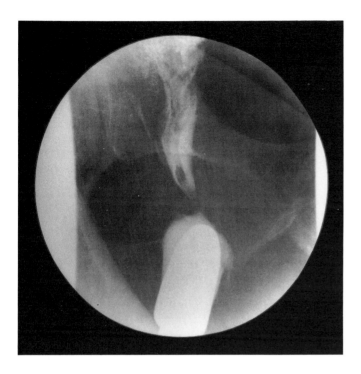

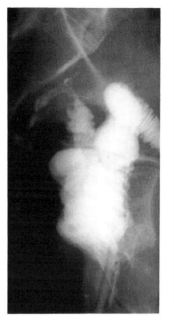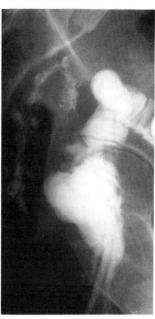

Fig. 4.5 Pouchogram showing leakage and a sinus tract from the posterior ileal pouch staple line to the presacrum.

Fig. 4.4 Pouchogram showing anastomotic–pelvic sinus tract and an associated short stricture of the ileoanal anastomosis.

Anastomotic – pelvic

Pelvic sinus tracts occur in about 2% of patients. Pouchograms usually show a small tract extending from the anastomosis towards the sacrum. Figure 4.4 shows such a tract and an associated short stricture of the anastomosis. Under anaesthesia, the tract should be curetted and packed and the patient placed on an antibiotic such as metronidazole. Using this approach, symptoms in most patients will almost always resolve. Closure of the temporary ileostomy should be delayed.

Anastomotic – vaginal

Vaginal fistulae are fortunately a rare event. Often the only noticeable symptom is increased mucous discharge from the vagina. Once again, delaying the ileostomy closure usually results in resolution of this fistula. If not, then transvaginal or transperineal approaches may be used to repair the fistula. Interestingly, only about one-half of such patients will have a good result, even without evidence of Crohn's disease. Overall, about 55% of all fistulae after restorative proctocolectomy are anastomotic in origin whereas 45% are from the pouch (Ambrose *et al.*, 1991a).

Leaks from the pouch (Fig. 4.5)

This difficult problem occurred early after the first descriptions of J pouches had been published. The nature of the staple lines is such that if they overlap imprecisely, a posterior hole in the pouch is created which, if not recognized and sutured, leads invariably to a persistent sinus or abscess, often causing failure of the operation. The conservative approach to treatment of this problem is prolonged diversion, while aggressive management is accomplished by elevating the pouch, repairing the hole and re-anastomosing the pouch to the anal canal.

Long efferent limb (S pouch)

Impaired defaecation was the primary symptom of this complication. Schoetz *et al.* (1988) described that the septum between the elongated efferent limb and the pouch could be stapled and divided readily, thus resolving the obstruction in nearly all patients. Nicholls and Gilbert (1990), however, used a transabdominal route to resect the redundant efferent limb and perform an endoanal re-anastomosis (Fig. 4.6); about one-half of the patients who underwent this procedure were converted to spontaneous stooling while the rest continued to intubate the pouch.

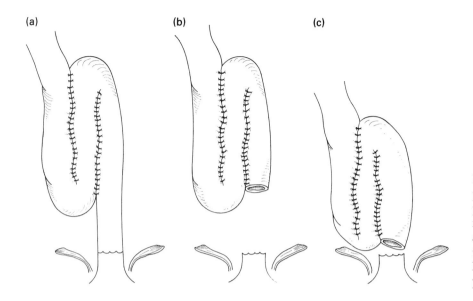

Fig. 4.6 Diagram of reconstructive surgery performed for a long efferent limb in a patient with an S pouch. (a) The pouch is mobilized completely; (b) the limb is amputated; and (c) the shortened outflow tract re-anastomosed to the anal canal. From Nicholls RJ *et al.* (1990) with permission.

J pouch septum

Patients with a retained apical septum experience obstructed defaecation and sometimes bleeding. The septum is stapled easily through the anus using a GIA® stapler; almost all symptoms resolve immediately.

Cancer

A disturbing report was recently published by Stern *et al.* (1990). They reported a patient who developed an adenocarcinoma in the rectal muscular cuff *4 years* after restorative proctocolectomy. This observation lends credence to our recommendation that the rectal cuff should be as short as possible, thus reducing the amount of rectal muscular cuff at risk of incomplete rectal mucosal excision (O'Connell *et al.*, 1987). After a mean follow-up of 17 months (range 2–48 months), we found residual rests of rectal mucosa between the muscular cuff and the serosa of the pouch in 14% of patients who had failed the operation. These rests were microscopic in size and showed no evidence of inflammation or proliferation; proliferation or sheeting likely being limited by the severe surrounding fibrosis. None of these patients had any evidence of neoplastic growth and no patient in our series had a 'cuff' cancer. This is a potentially serious problem for two reasons. One is that there may be implications for follow-up; should all patients after restorative proctocolectomy undergo anal canal palpation and random biopsy yearly? The other is that if there was a cancer in the rectal cuff *following mucosectomy*, what is the fate of the retained mucosa in the operation advocated by Johnston *et al.* (1987)?

The possibility that a cancer might occur in the pouch itself is quite remote; cancer has not been observed in patients with Kock pouches during extended periods of follow-up.

The role of pouchography

About half of our patients undergo pouchography using gastrografin prior to closure of the ileostomy. In a recent study, our aim was to determine if pouchography was useful in predicting clinical outcome (Tsao *et al.*, 1991). Pouchograms were abnormal in 16% of patients. The incidence of subsequent complications such as persistent stricture was much higher in the abnormal pouchography group (33%) than in the normal group (4%) ($p < 0.05$). More importantly, the overall rate of failure in the abnormal pouchogram group was 23% while it was only 6% in the normal group ($p < 0.05$). We concluded that pouchography predicted those patients at increased risk of long-term complications and failure after restorative proctocolectomy.

Reoperation for late complications

Out of 114 patients reoperated upon for pouch specific complications and not to the colectomy, ileostomy closure was delayed in 33 (25%) and the complications occurred after ileostomy closure in 68 (60%) (Galandiuk, 1990). Several different approaches were used to salvage these patients (Table 4.4).

Table 4.4 Procedures used to correct pouch-specific problems and their postoperative complications in 114 patients.

Category	Number of patients (%)			
	Anastomotic stricture (*n* = 42)	Perianal fistula/abscess (*n* = 30)	Intra-abdominal fistula/abscess (*n* = 29)	Unsatisfactory function (*n* = 13)
Ileostomy at presentation	13 (31)	10 (33)	15 (52)	3 (23)
Frequent procedures performed				
Dilatation of associated stricture	42 (100)	9 (30)		2 (15)
Fistulotomy/excision of fistula tract		17 (57)	4 (14)	
Primary closure of fistula		3 (10)	3 (10)	
Drainage of abscess		5 (17)	18 (62)	
Diverting ileostomy		3 (10)	6 (21)	
Redo ileal pouch anal anastomosis			5 (17)	4 (31)
Divide pouch septum				4 (31)
Shorten or excise efferent limb				2 (16)
Convert to different type pouch				3 (10)
Postoperative complications	25 (60)	23 (77)	18 (62)	4 (31)
Recurrent stricture	22 (52)	6 (2)		
Perianal fistula	2 (5)	16 (53)		
Perianal abscess	1 (2)	5 (17)		
Intra-abdominal fistula			5 (17)	1 (8)
Intra-abdominal abscess			9 (31)	1 (8)
Other				2 (16)
More than one operation for pouch-related complications	25 (60)	22 (73)	17 (59)	5 (38)

From Galandiuk *et al.* (1990) with permission.

Patients with anastomotic strictures were initially treated primarily by dilatation under anaesthesia. If strictures recurred, further operations were required, such as reconstruction of the ileal reservoir or, sometimes unfortunately, excision of the reservoir.

Patients with perianal abscess, fistula and sinus tracts were treated by local operations. After one operation the chance that there would be further complication was great. Ultimately, nearly 20% of patients who had a pouch-related complication after restorative proctocolectomy and who underwent a reoperation for it, needed to have their pouch excised.

Intra-abdominal abscess was probably the most serious complication. Drainage of such abscesses was required in all patients and all likewise were diverted. In some patients with a presacral abscess, percutaneous CT-guided drainage was performed, especially if the ileostomy had never been closed.

Reoperation was also required in patients with poor function. The different manifestations of poor function were: poor neorectal emptying due to a long efferent limb (S pouches), incontinence and obstruction caused by a J pouch septum, outlet obstruction due to mucosal prolapse, and recurrent pouchitis. Interestingly, even J pouches cannot empty efficiently if pulled through a long rectal muscular cuff which then subsequently fibroses; the result of such scarring is a tortuous outflow tract similar to that seen in some patients after S pouch anal anastomosis.

Some patients have had the efferent limb shortened. In others, the S shaped reservoir was excised and a J shaped reservoir constructed. We agree with Nicholls and Gilbert (1990) that a transabdominal approach nearly always is preferred to a transperineal approach in patients requiring pouch reconstruction.

Although the pouch excision rate was 20% for all patients with pouch-related complications requiring reoperation, it was even greater when the indication for reoperative surgery was a poor functional result (Fig. 4.7). Reoperation did, however, restore pouch function, in 67% of patients. Out of these, 70% had an excellent clinical outcome.

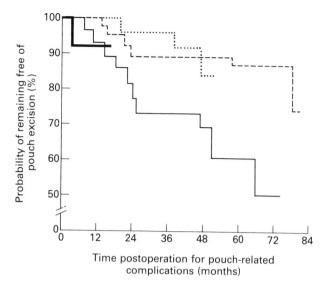

Fig. 4.7 Probability of pouch excision against time among groups of patients with pouch-related complications requiring reoperation after restorative proctocolectomy. ▬, functional; —, intra-abdominal abscess/fistula; . . . ., perianal abscess/fistula; ---, stricture. From Galandiuk *et al.* (1990) with permission.

As a final comment, it is reasonable to say that salvage procedures for pouch-specific complications are performed safely and will restore pouch function in many patients. However, the risk of subsequent complications and further reoperation, including pouch excision, is significantly high.

Pouchitis

Pouchitis is discussed in great detail in Chapter 8. Unfortunately, we also have considerable experience with this problem.

The incidence of pouchitis appears to be rising steadily at Mayo as the follow-up has lengthened. We reported in 1987 that the incidence of pouchitis was about 15% (Pemberton *et al.*, 1987). In our latest review of 734 patients in whom restorative proctocolectomy was performed between 1981 and 1988, the rate of pouchitis for all patients was 31% and for patients with familial adenomatous polyposis it was 7% (Lohmuller *et al.*, 1990). Whether pouchitis actually occurs after restorative proctocolectomy for familial adenomatous polyposis is debatable; it probably very rarely does, and is a variant of the type that occurs in patients with chronic ulcerative colitis.

We have chosen to define pouchitis clinically and not

endoscopically or histologically. The relationship of endoscopic appearance to clinical symptomatology is clouded. In addition, the major problem with histologic criteria alone are that biopsies from the pouch are heterogeneous; a biopsy from one part of the pouch may be read as 'normal colon', from another part as 'normal ileum', from another as 'chronic inflammation' and finally from another as chronic and acute inflammation. Although Shepherd *et al.* (1987) and Tytgat and Van Deventer (1988) suggested histologic criteria may be theoretically helpful, our experience has been that histologic changes may or may not be present in patients with classic signs and symptoms of pouchitis (O'Connell *et al.*, 1986) and vice versa. Indeed, acute and chronic inflammatory changes occur often in the pouch in the absence of clinical pouchitis (Kelly *et al.*, 1983; O'Connell *et al.*, 1986). We believe, therefore, that relying on endoscopic appearance and on biopsies to make a diagnosis of pouchitis is hazardous. Perhaps a combination of subjective and objective signs, organized into a 'pouchitis activity index' would be helpful.

At the Mayo Clinic, pouchitis is diagnosed if patients have abdominal cramps, frequency, watery diarrhoea (sometimes bloody), urgency, incontinence, malaise and fever. Although pouchitis is nearly always episodic in nature, it was reported to be a 'chronic problem' by 46% of the patients. The mean time between operation and first occurrence of pouchitis was 17 months. The earliest time to occurrence, however, was 2 days and the longest, 95 months. Therefore, patients after ileoanal anastomosis must always be considered at risk of pouchitis. Unfortunately, pouchitis *recurs* frequently; 61% of patients had at least one further episode.

We have documented that the incidence of pouchitis was not influenced significantly by the type of pouch constructed nor by the presence or absence of pelvic sepsis postoperatively. The age and sex of the patients also were not determinants of pouchitis.

We did identify one group of patients at increased risk. These patients were those who had extra-intestinal manifestations of inflammatory bowel disease before restorative proctocolectomy or at some time postoperatively. Among 671 chronic ulcerative colitis patients who underwent restorative proctocolectomy, extra-intestinal manifestations were present in 27%. They resolved in only 64% of the patients after operation. Extra-intestinal manifestations occurred *for the first time* postoperatively in 24 patients.

If extra-intestinal manifestations were present pre-

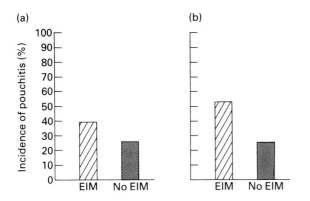

Fig. 4.8 Incidences of pouchitis in patients with and without extra-intestinal manifestations (EIM) of inflammatory bowel disease. (a) Preoperative, $p < 0.01$; (b) postoperative, $p < 0.001$.

operatively, pouchitis occurred in 39% of patients, while it occurred in only 26% if no preoperative extra-intestinal manifestations were present ($p < 0.001$) (Fig. 4.8). If *postoperative* extra-intestinal manifestations were present, 53% of patients developed pouchitis versus only 25% when no postoperative extra-intestinal manifestations were present ($p < 0.001$) (Fig. 4.8). Anecdotally, in seven patients, the extra-intestinal manifestations recurred when pouchitis occurred and abated when the pouchitis was treated.

The implications of this finding of an apparent association between pouchitis and extra-intestinal manifestations are that the pathophysiologic mechanisms underlying pouchitis may indeed provoke a systemic response similar to that which occurs in response to chronic ulcerative colitis itself.

The empiric treatment of pouchitis with metronidazole is largely successful and recurrent episodes have also been treated efficaciously with this medication. It is of interest that pouchitis is rare in polyposis patients in whom the occurrence of stagnation, overgrowth of bacteria, and ischaemia should not differ in degree from that present after operation in colitis patients. The rarity of pouchitis in polyposis patients, as opposed to those with colitis, would suggest that whatever causes colitis may predispose to pouchitis.

Homeostasis: the response to colectomy

The normal colon absorbs slightly more than 1000 ml of water and at least 100 mmol of NaCl/day (Phillips & Giller, 1973). Mineralocorticoids augment these salt retaining properties such that when salt depleted, the colon can reduce the faecal loss of NaCl to 1–2 mg/day. The small bowel cannot do this. Thus, after colectomy sodium is lost at the rate of 30–40 mmol/day from the small bowel (Kramer, 1966).

Ninety percent of enteric content is water (Kanaghinis *et al.*, 1963); the net weight can be increased by consuming food high in indigestible residue. After colectomy, if the intake of salt and water are adequate, patients with ileostomies are not salt or water depleted. But salt depletion occurs rapidly when patients get the flu, decrease their intake, vomit or perspire profusely (Gallagher *et al.*, 1962). Chronic oliguria is also common because patients lose about 500–700 ml of water in the enteric content per day compared to the 100 ml/day lost in the stool of patients with a colon. The composition of the urine changes causing stone formation in about 5% of patients after colectomy.

If the terminal ileum is resected together with the colon, bile acids and vitamin B_{12} malabsorption occurs. In addition, secondary bile acids disappear from bile (Morris *et al.*, 1973) after colectomy. Although no metabolic consequences have been identified, patients with ileostomies may be susceptible to gallstone formation. The primary homeostatic sequela of colectomy therefore is the potential for a salt losing state; patients must have a liberal salt and water intake.

Whether or not this precise situation occurs after restorative proctocolectomy was investigated by Christie *et al.* (1990). They could find no evidence that J pouch patients were chronically salt and water depleted. The amount of water and electrolytes lost in the enteric content was the same in patients after restorative proctocolectomy and in those after construction of a conventional ileostomy. Both patients with J pouches and those with conventional ileostomies did have increased fat stores compared with controls. Patients with conventional ileostomy as well as J pouch patients depend upon renal conservative mechanisms to compensate for the increased excretion of salt and water; the incidence of urinary calculi after restorative proctocolectomy, although not documented, should be similar to that reported after conventional ileostomy.

Complications in patients after restorative proctocolectomy for familial adenomatous polyposis

Out of 852 restorative proctocolectomy patients at the Mayo Clinic, 94 were operated upon for familial adenomatous polyposis. These patients appeared to

Table 4.5 Functional results after ileal pouch anal anastomosis: chronic ulcerative colitis vs. familial adenomatous polyposis.

Parameter	Colitis	Polyposis
Stools day/night-time (number)	6/1	5/1
Incontinent (% of patients), Spotting (day/night-time)	14/40	9/26*
Metamucil (% of patients)	31	20
Anti-diarrhoeal medication (% of patients)	26	17
Perianal irritation (% of patients)	33	31

*Differs from night-time spotting in colitis patients $p < 0.05$.

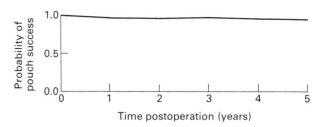

Fig. 4.9 The probability of successful outcome with functioning pouch against year after operation. No patient failed after 3 years. From Pemberton *et al.* (1987) with permission.

Table 4.6 Failure rates of ileal pouch anal anastomosis.

	Overall failure (% of patients)
Cohen *et al.* (1985)	2
Nicholls & Pezim (1985)	6
Becker & Raymond (1986)	10
Nasmyth *et al.* (1986)	12
Schoetz *et al.* (1986)	6
Morgan *et al.* (1987)	5
Pemberton *et al.* (1987)	6

tolerate the operation better, and had less *long-term* disability than did the colitis patients (Dozois *et al.*, 1989). However, the rate of postoperative complications appeared to be quite similar (26 and 29% of polyposis and colitis patients, respectively), and the need for reoperation for obstruction did not differ between the two groups. Pelvic sepsis requiring reoperation, on the other hand, was more common in colitis patients (6%) than in polyposis patients (0%). Furthermore, over the long term, polyposis patients had less night-time faecal spotting (13% of polyposis patients vs. 30% of colitis patients) (Table 4.5).

While it might be anticipated that polyposis patients would form desmoid tumours at a high rate postoperatively, mesenteric fibromatosis and/or desmoid tumours occurred in only one out of the 94 patients. Moreover, the overall incidence of small bowel obstruction was not different from that in colitis patients.

Failure

At the Mayo Clinic, 6% of patients after restorative proctocolectomy ultimately failed the operation and required excision of the pouch and/or construction of a permanent abdominal ileostomy. Ninety-four percent of the patients did well (Fig. 4.9). The most frequent causes of failure occurring alone or in combination were pelvic sepsis, gross faecal incontinence at night, multiple stools, and granulomatous colitis. Pouchitis by itself rarely led to failure of the operation (2% of all patients who failed). Of the patients who failed, 75% failed within one year, 12% within 2 years, and the final 12% within 3 years. All failures occurred in colitis patients; none occurred in patients with familial

adenomatous polyposis. For comparison, failure rates of other large series are listed in Table 4.6.

Complications of an alternative approach: the ileoanal pouch–distal rectal anastomosis

The major long-term functional complication after restorative proctocolectomy is faecal incontinence. This problem has prompted several authors to try another operation. This operation probably should be labelled ileal pouch distal rectal anastomosis (Kelly, 1991) for reasons explained here.

In this procedure, 1–3 cm of the full thickness of bowel above the dentate line, including the anal transitional mucosa (anal transition zone, ATZ) are left in situ. The ileal pouch is then sewn or stapled to this distal rectum or proximal anal canal at the level of the pelvic floor (Martin *et al.*, 1985; Johnston *et al.*, 1987; Kmiot & Keighley, 1989). The rationale is several fold: (i) this operation is easier to perform than standard restorative proctocolectomy, (ii) preservation of the transitional mucosa will maintain anal sensation, (iii) anal sphincter function and postoperative continence, especially at night, will be better achieved, and (iv) the transitional mucosa is not involved or is only minimally involved with colitis or polyposis and can, therefore, be safely left *in situ*.

Early results of uncontrolled series do indeed support several points of the rationale. The operation appears to be fast and easy to perform, and anal sensation and sphincter strength are usually well preserved, although not always (Nasymth *et al.*, 1986; Lavery *et al.*, 1990; Sagar *et al.*, 1991; Sugerman *et al.*, 1991.) As a result, faecal continence in these studies may be better than after standard restorative proctocolectomy, especially at night (Martin *et al.*, 1985; Johnston *et al.*, 1987; Lavery *et al.*, 1990.)

Importantly, in the only *prospective* trial conducted to date, no difference in function between conventional ileal pouch anal anastomosis and ileal pouch distal rectal anastomosis has been found (Seow-Choen *et al.*, 1991). Similar results have been reported from a non-randomized trial as well (Hallgren *et al.*, 1990).

The great concern with this operation is that it may leave diseased mucosa in situ. We recently examined 50 colitis specimens removed by conventional proctocolectomy and found that ulcerative colitis was present in the anal transition zone, within 1 cm of the dentate line, in 90% of the specimens (Ambrose *et al.*, 1991b). Preserving the anal transition zone, therefore, preserves disease in 90% of patients. This observation is supported by Sugerman *et al.* (1991) who observed that in 19 out of 20 ulcerative colitis patients, the distal doughnut of rectum after stapled ileal pouch distal rectal anastomosis harboured inflamed mucosa. Disease likewise may persist (Sugerman *et al.*, 1991; Tuckson *et al.*, 1991) and dysplasia and neoplasia can also be present or develop in this residual mucosa in patients with ulcerative colitis (Emblem *et al.*, 1988; King *et al.*, 1989; Tsunoda *et al.*, 1990) and in patients with familial adenomatous polyposis (Emblem *et al.*, 1988; Tsunoda *et al.*, 1990).

The role of this new operation thus remains unknown, particularly in younger patients. The results of this approach, reported anecdotally, *are* excellent and have prompted its rapid adoption by many. Although it *is* easier to perform, ileal pouch distal rectal anastomosis should probably be reserved for older patients who desire a restorative procedure, but because of age would not ordinarily be considered a candidate. The theoretic risk of leaving premalignant mucosa behind in older patients is minimal. Moreover, if there indeed is any improvement of sensation afforded by this approach, then the older patients will benefit the most. However, the sequelae of persistent and/or recurrent disease may be just as devastating in the older as in the younger patient.

Summary

Success after restorative proctocolectomy depends primarily upon two factors: preservation of the anal canal high pressure zone which acts as a barrier to outflow and restoration of adequate reservoir function. The anal sphincters and the pelvic floor are nearly always preserved, so a competent barricade to outflow is preserved. An adequate neorectal reservoir is restored if a J shaped ileal pouch is used. This kind of pouch anastomosed directly to the anal canal is as distensible, capacious and as readily evacuated as is the rectum of healthy people.

In patients in whom the internal or external anal sphincter had been damaged by the operation, incontinence is more likely. Likewise, in adults, straight ileoanal anastomosis without a pouch caused frequent stooling and poor faecal continence. Moreover, the use of S pouches or H pouches, those having efferent limbs between the pouch and the anal canal, sometimes lead to outflow obstruction and incomplete evacuation.

Furthermore, we have found that faecal continence does *not* depend upon the presence of intact rectal mucosa, intact rectal muscularis or the rectoanal inhibitory reflex; the operation destroys or alters all three, but patients are continent nonetheless.

There is little doubt, however, that patients after restorative proctocolectomy have an abnormal *pattern* of faecal continence. With distal enteric distention, frequent, large amplitude, propulsive contractions of the ileal pouch stress the anal sphincters more severely and more acutely than do either the infrequent, small amplitude, non-propulsive contractions or the clustered contractions present in healthy rectums. Moreover, patients must learn to recognize new signals heralding evacuation; the large pressure waves occurring in the ileal pouch at threshold volume trigger the sensation of urgency.

As a final insult, the consistency and the volume of stool are also changed; after operation, the stool volume increases to at least 600 ml/day, and becomes semi-solid, mushy, or even liquid in consistency. This doubtless places great strain on the anal sphincters; if the sphincters are damaged at all, or are not performing properly, faecal incontinence ensues invariably. Complications which might occur at any time after restorative proctocolectomy alter the balance between control and no control, reasonable stool frequency and unacceptable stool frequency and, therefore, ultimate success or failure. Clearly, the margin for error is small.

Among those who perform restorative proctocolectomy regularly, mortality is nearly non-existent and functional outcome predictably good. The rationale for performing the operation should not only include cure of the disease and preservation of anal continence, but also that the operation can be done safely. Clearly, this is the case. Just as clearly, however, restorative proctocolectomy is not a perfect operation, it is difficult to perform, not all patients are candidates (but ileal pouch distal *rectal* anastomosis may push the age envelop to 70 years), the complication rate remains moderate and the failure rate is 6%. However, among the alternatives to conventional ileostomy, ileal pouch anal anastomosis comes closest to restoring patients to some degree of normality than any other operation *without leaving disease in situ*.

At the Mayo Clinic, ileal J pouch anal anastomosis has been performed in 1218 patients since 1981. Satisfactory faecal continence was preserved in over 90% of the patients after operation. Some patients experienced intermittent leakage, particularly at night, but overall, results were excellent. A capacious reservoir and a well functioning anal sphincter, the central mechanisms of continence, were maintained by the operation. Other factors, however, were changed. These included an increased output of watery stool and the appearance of large amplitude waves in the ileal pouch upon distention. Better continence in patients after restorative proctocolectomy may be achieved by decreasing the volume of stool, increasing the stool consistency, and maximizing the threshold volume for pouch contractions. Perhaps the ileal pouch distal rectal anastomosis will resolve some of these concerns, but it is likely to do so only at the risk of leaving diseased mucosa behind.

There is little question that restorative proctocolectomy has had a profound impact upon surgery for ulcerative colitis and familial adenomatous polyposis. Several challenges lie ahead. The incidence of small bowel obstruction, fistulae and sphincter injury needs to be decreased, hopefully by improving surgical strategy and execution. Pouchitis remains an area of concern; although it rarely causes failure of the operation, it is bothersome. About 30% of our patients experienced at least one bout of clinically significant pouchitis. Importantly, acute, recurrent and chronic episodes are readily treated. However, an effective means of long-term prevention has yet to be devised. Finally, and perhaps most important, functional results will need to be monitored closely for signs of deterioration as the patients age.

References

Ambrose W, Beart R, Dozois R *et al.* (1991a) Treatment of fistulas following ileal pouch-anal anastomosis (abstract). *Dis Colon Rectum* **34**(4):20.

Ambrose WL, Pemberton JH, Dozois RR, Carpenter HA (1991b) Does retaining the anal transition zone (ATZ) fail to extirpate chronic ulcerative colitis (CUC) after ileal pouch-anal anastomosis (IPAA)? (abstract) *Dis Colon Rectum* **34**(4): 20.

Beart RW Jr, Dozois RR, Wolff BG, Pemberton JH (1985) Mechanisms of rectal continence: lessons from the ileoanal procedure. *Am J Surg* **149**:31–34.

Becker JM (1984) Anal sphincter function after coloectomy, mucosal proctectomy, and endorectal ileoanal pull-through. *Arch Surg* **119**:526–531.

Becker JM, Parodi JE (1989) Total colectomy with preservation of the anal sphincter. *Surg Annu* **21**:263–302.

Becker JM, Raymond JL (1986) Ileal-pouch anal anastomosis: a single surgeon's experience with 100 consecutive cases. *Ann Surg* **204**:375–381.

Cangemi JR, Wiesner RH, Beaver SJ *et al.* (1989) Effect of proctocolectomy for chronic ulcerative colitis on the natural history of primary sclerosing cholangitis. *Gastroenterology* **96**:790–794.

Chaussade S, Verduron A, Hautefeuille M *et al.* (1989) Proctocolectomy and ileoanal pouch anastomosis without conservation of a rectal muscular cuff. *Br J Surg* **76**:273–275.

Christie PM, Knight GS, Hill GL (1990) Metabolism of body water and electrolytes after surgery for ulcerative colitis: Conventional ileostomy versus J pouch. *Br J Surg* **77**: 149–151.

Cohen Z, McLeod RS, Stern H, Grant D, Nordgren S (1985) The pelvic pouch and ileoanal anastomosis procedure: Surgical technique and initial results. *Am J Surg* **150**: 601–607.

Deutsch A, McLeod RS, Cullen J, Cohen Z (1991) Results of the pelvic-pouch procedure in patients with Crohn's disease. *Dis Colon Rectum* **34**:475–477.

Dozois RR (1988) Pelvic and perianastomotic complications after ileoanal anastomosis. *Perspec Colon and Rectal Surg* **1**:113–121.

Dozois RR, Kelly KA, Welling DR *et al.* (1989) Ileal pouch-anal anastomosis: comparison of results in familiar adenomatous polyposis and chronic ulcerative colitis. *Ann Surg* **210**:268–273.

Emblem R, Bergan A, Larsen S (1988) Straight ileoanal anastomosis with preserved anal mucosa for ulcerative colitis and familial polyposis. *Scand J Gastroenterol* **23**: 493–500.

Everett WG, Pollard SG (1990) Restorative proctocolectomy without temporary ileostomy. *Br J Surg* **77**:621–622.

Francios Y, Dozois RR, Kelly KA, Beart RW Jr, Wolff BG, Pemberton JH, Ilstrup DM (1989) Small intestinal obstruction complicating ileal pouch anal anastomosis. *Ann Surg* **209**:46–50.

Galandiuk S, Scott NA, Dozois RR et al. (1990) Ileal pouch-anal anastomosis. Reoperation for pouch-related complications. *Ann Surg* **212**:446–454.

Gallagher ND, Harrison DD, Skyring AP (1962) Fluid and electrolyte disturbances in patients with long-established ileostomies. *Gut* **3**:219–223.

Hallgren T, Fasth S, Nordgren S, Öresland T, Hultén L (1990) The stapled ileal pouch-anal anastomosis. A randomized study comparing two different pouch designs. *Scand J Gastroenterol* **25**:1161–1168.

Harms BA, Hamilton JW, Yamamoto DT, Starling JR (1987) Quadruple-loop (W) ileal pouch reconstruction after proctocolectomy: analysis and function results. *Surgery* **102**:561–567.

Johnston D, Holdsworth PJ, Nasmyth DG, Neal DE, Primrose JN, Womack N, Axon AT (1987) Preservation of the entire anal canal in conservative proctocolectomy for ulcerative colitis: a pilot study comparing end-to-end ileo-anal anastomosis without mucosal resection with mucosal proctectomy and endo-anal anastomosis. *Br J Surg* **74**:940–944.

Kanaghinis T, Lubran M, Coghill NF (1963) The composition of ileostomy fluid. *Gut* **4**:322–338.

Kelly DG, Phillips SF, Kelly KA, Weinstein WM, Gilchrist MJ (1983) Dysfunction of the continent ileostomy: clinical features and bacteriology. *Gut* **24**:193–201.

Kelly KA (1992) Anal sphincter saving operation for chronic ulcerative colitis. *Am J Surg* **163**:5–11.

King DW, Lubowski DZ, Cook TA (1989) Anal mucosa in restorative proctocolectomy for ulcerative colitis. *Brit J Surg* **76**:970–972.

Kmiot WA, Keighley MRB (1989) Totally stapled abdominal restorative proctocolectomy. *Br J Surg* **76**:961–964.

Kramer P (1966) The effect of varying sodium loads on the ileal excreta of human ileostomized subjects. *J Clin Invest* **45**:1710–1718.

LaRusso NF, Wiesner RH, Ludwig J, MacCarty RL (1984) Current concepts. Primary sclerosing cholangitis. *N Engl J Med* **310**:899–903.

Lavery IC, Tuckson WB, Fazio VW, Oakley JR, Church JM, Milsom JW (1990) Pouch surgery – the importance of the transitional zone. *Can J Gastroenterol* **4**:428–431.

Lohmuller JL, Pemberton JH, Dozois RR, Ilstrup D, van Heerden J (1990) Pouchitis and extraintestinal manifestations of inflammatory bowel disease after ileal pouch-anal anastomosis. *Ann Surg* **211**:622–629.

McHugh SM, Diamant NE (1987) Effect of age, gender, and parity on anal canal pressures. Contribution of impaired anal sphincter function to fecal incontinence. *Dig Dis Sci* **32**:726–736.

McHugh SM, Diamant NE, McLeod R, Cohen Z (1987) S-pouches vs. J-pouches. A comparison of functional outcomes. *Dis Colon Rectum* **30**:671–677.

Martin LW, Torres AM, Fischer JE, Alexander F (1985) The critical level for preservation of continence in the ileoanal anastomosis. *J Pediatr Surg* **20**:664–667.

Metcalf AM, Dozois RR, Kelly KA (1986) Sexual function in women after proctocolectomy. *Ann Surg* **204**:624–627.

Morgan RA, Manning PB, Coran AG (1987) Experience with the straight endorectal pullthrough for the management of ulcerative colitis and familial polyposis in children and adults. *Ann Surg* **206**:595–599.

Morris JS, Low-Beer TS, Heaton KW (1973) Bile salt metabolism and the colon. *Scand J Gastroenterol* **8**:425–431.

Nasmyth DG, Williams NS, Johnston D (1986) Comparison of the function of triplicated and duplicated pelvic ileal reservoirs after mucosal proctectomy and ileoanal anastomosis for ulcerative colitis and adenomatous polyposis. *Br J Surg* **73**:361–366.

Nelson H, Dozois RR, Kelly KA, Malkasian GD, Wolff BG, Ilstrup DM (1989) The effect of pregnancy and delivery on the ileal pouch-anal anastomosis functions. *Dis Colon Rectum* **32**:384–388.

Nicholls RJ, Gilbert JM (1990) Surgical correction of the efferent limb for disordered defaecation following restorative proctocolectomy with the S ileal reservoir. *Br J Surg* **77**:152–154.

Nicholls RJ, Pezim ME (1985) Restorative proctocolectomy with ileal reservoir for ulcerative colitis and familial adenomatous polyposis: A comparison of three reservoir designs. *Br J Surg* **72**:470–474.

O'Connell PR, Pemberton JH, Weiland LH, Beart RWJ, Dozois RR, Wolff BG, Telander RL (1987) Does rectal mucosa regenerate after ileoanal anastomosis? *Dis Colon Rectum* **30**:1–5.

O'Connell PR, Rankin DR, Weiland LH, Kelly KA (1986) Enteric bacteriology, absorption, morphology and emptying after ileal pouch-anal anastomosis. *Br J Surg* **73**:909–914.

Peck DA (1988) Stapled ileal reservoir to anal anastomosis. *Surg Gynecol Obstet* **166**:562–564.

Pemberton JH (1992) Surgical approaches to proctocolectomy for inflammatory bowel disease. In Phillips SF, Pemberton JH, Shorter RG (ed) *The Large Intestine; Physiology, Pathophysiology and Disease*, New York, Raven Press.

Pemberton JH, Kelly KA, Beart RW, Jr, Dozois RR, Wolff BG, Ilstrup DM (1987) Ileal pouch-anal anastomosis for chronic ulcerative colitis: Long-term results. *Ann Surg* **206**:504–513.

Pemberton JH, Phillips SF, Dozois RR, Wendorf LJ (1985) Current clinical results of conventional ileostomy. In RR Dozois, (ed). *Alternatives to Conventional Ileostomy*, Chicago, Year Book Medical Publishers, pp. 40–50.

Pemberton JH, Phillips SF, Ready RR, Zinsmeister AR, Beahrs OH (1989) Quality of life after Brooke ileostomy and ileal pouch-anal anastomosis. Comparison of performance status. *Ann Surg* **209**:620–628.

Pezim ME, Pemberton JH, Beart RW, Jr et al. (1989) Outcome of 'indeterminant' colitis following ileal pouch-anal anastomosis. *Dis Colon Rectum* **32**:653–658.

Phillips RKS, Ritchie JK, Hawley PR (1989) Proctocolectomy and ileostomy for ulcerative colitis: the longer term story. *J R Soc Med* **82**:386–387.

Phillips SF, Giller J (1973) The contribution of the colon to electrolyte and water conservation in man. *J Lab Clin Med* **81**:733–746.

Roy PH, Sauer WG, Beahrs OH, Farrow GM (1970) Experience with ileostomies: evaluation of long-term rehabilitation in 497 patients. *Am J Surg* **119**:77–86.

Sagar PM, Holdsworth PJ, Johnston D (1991) Correlation between laboratory findings and clinical outcome after restorative proctocolectomy: serial studies in 20 patients after end to end pouch anal anastomosis. *Br J Surg* **78**:67–70.

Schoetz DJ, Jr, Coller JA, Veidenheimer MC (1986) Ileoanal reservoir for ulcerative colitis and familial polyposis. *Arch Surg* **121**:404–409.

Schoetz DJ, Coller JA, Veidenheimer MC (1988) Can the pouch be saved? *Dis Colon Rectum* **31**:671–675.

Scott NA, Dozois RR, Beart RW, Jr, Pemberton JH, Wolff BG, Ilstrup DM (1988) Postoperative intra-abdominal and pelvic sepsis complicating ileal pouch-anal anastomosis. *Int J Colorectal Dis* **3**:149–152.

Seow-Choen A, Tsunoda A, Nicholls RJ (1991) Prospective randomized trial comparing anal function after hand sewn ileoanal anastomosis with mucosectomy versus stapled ileoanal anastomosis with mucosectomy in restorative proctocolectomy. *Br J Surg* **78**:430–434.

Shepherd NA, Jass JR, Duval I, Moskowitz RL, Nicholls RJ, Morson BC (1987) Restorative proctocolectomy with ileal reservoir: pathological and histochemical study of mucosal biopsy specimens. *J Clin Pathol* **40**:601–607.

Stern H, Walfisch S, Mullen B, McLeod R, Cohen Z (1990) Cancer in an ileoanal reservoir: a new late complication. *Gut* **31**:473–475.

Sugerman HJ, Newsome HH, DeCosta G, Zfass AM (1991) Stapled ileoanal anastomosis for ulcerative colitis and familial polyposis without a temporary diverting ileostomy. *Ann Surg* **213**:606–619.

Taylor BM, Beart RW Jr, Dozois RR, Kelly KA, Phillips SF (1983) Straight ileoanal anastomosis versus ileal pouch-anal anastomosis and mucosal proctectomy. *Arch Surg* **118**:696–701.

Taylor BA, Wolff BG, Dozois RR, Kelly KA, Pemberton JH, Beart RW, Jr (1988) Ileal pouch-anal anastomosis for chronic ulcerative colitis and familial polyposis coli complicated by adenocarcinoma. *Dis Colon Rectum* **31**:358–362.

Tsao J, Galandiuk S, Pemberton J (1991) Pouchogram: a predictor of clinical outcome following ileal pouch-anal anastomosis (IPAA) (abstract). *Dis Colon Rectum* **34**(4):19.

Tsunoda A, Talbot IC, Nicholls RJ (1990) Incidence of dysplasia in the anorectal mucosa in patients having restorative proctocolectomy. *Br J Surg* **77**:506–508.

Tuckson WB, Lavery IC, Strong S, Fazio VW, Oakley JR, Church JM, Milsom JW (1991) Fate of preserved anal mucosa following TPC and stapled IPAA for MUC (abstract). *Dis Colon Rectum* **34**(4):19.

Tytgat GNJ, Van Deventer SJH (1988) Pouchitis. *Int J Colorectal Dis* **3**:226–228.

Utsunomiya J, Iwama T, Imajo M, Matsuo S, Sawai S, Yaegashi K, Hirayama R (1980) Total colectomy, mucosal protectomy and ileoanal anastomosis. *Dis Colon Rectum* **23**:459–466.

Watts J, DeDombal FT, Goligher JC (1966) Long-term complication and prognosis following major surgery for ulcerative colitis. *Br J Surg* **53**:1014–1023.

Wells AD, McMillan I, Price AB, Ritchie JK, Nicholls RJ (1991) Natural history of indeterminate colitis. *Br J Surg* **78**:179–181.

Wexner SD, James K, Jagelman DG (1991) The double-stabled ileal reservoir and ileoanal anastomosis. *Dis Colon Rectum* **34**:487–494.

Wiesner RH, LaRusso, NF, Dozois RR, Beaver SJ (1986) Peristomal varices after proctocolectomy in patients with primary sclerosing cholangitis. *Gastroenterology* **90**:316–322.

Williams NS, Johnston D (1985) The current state of mucosal proctectomy and ileo-anal anastomosis in the surgical treatment of ulcerative colitis and adenomatous polyposis. *Br J Surg* **72**:159–168.

Williams NS, Marzouk DEM, Hallan RI, Waldron DJ (1989) Function after ileal pouch and stapled pouch-anal anastomosis for ulcerative colitis. *Br J Surg* **76**:1168–1171.

Wong WD, Rothenberger DA, Goldberg SM (1985) Ileoanal pouch procedures. *Curr Probl Surg* **22**:1–78.

Chapter 5
Controversies and Practical Problem Solving

R. JOHN NICHOLLS

Introduction

Restorative proctocolectomy is in many ways an ideal operation for the colorectal surgeon. When surgery is necessary, the diseases in question involve specialist management. The procedure includes both abdominal and perineal phases which require training. Reconstruction is aimed to improve the quality of life by avoiding a permanent ileostomy which would not be achieved without ileoanal anastomosis. Furthermore, management of postoperative complications and special problems demand experience and sometimes improvization.

Since its introduction in the mid 1970s, the indications for restorative proctocolectomy have been expanded to include certain functional bowel diseases as well as ulcerative colitis and familial adenomatous polyposis. Almost every step of the operation as shown in Table 5.1, has become the subject of a degree of controversy. This has arisen partly to make the operation technically easier, partly to achieve the best function with a minimum of complications and partly from the natural desire of surgeons to be different in order to make a contribution.

However hard the surgeon tries, the procedure has a fairly high complication rate. Mortality, however, is low and despite complications which are sometimes serious, the large majority of patients ultimately have a satisfactory outcome. The sum total of experience puts operative mortality at below 1%. The complication rate taken from pooled data is anywhere from 20 to 50% (Dozois et al., 1986; Williams & Johnston, 1985). Many complications are minor but some may prejudice the success of the procedure or simply cause morbidity with extended treatment time with consequent suffering and financial cost. These more important complications include pelvic sepsis, usually associated with ileoanal anastomosis breakdown, intestinal obstruction and fistulation from the anastomosis or the reservoir itself to the exterior.

Technique and complications have been described in other chapters. It is clear that the operation itself can be accomplished by various different technical adaptations of a common theme. Some of these differences are controversial. In this chapter an attempt will be made to discuss those that are more important. Practical problems can be divided into intraoperative and postoperative. Postoperative problems may present in the immediate postoperative period while the patient is still in hospital, or they may be delayed.

Intraoperative phase

This has substantially been dealt with elsewhere. Attention to detail may be crucial for success.

Colonic dissection

Controversy

It has been suggested that during the colonic phase, division of blood vessels should be made proximally in order to achieve a radical regional lymphovascular clearance. This it is argued, would cover the eventuality of an unrecognized carcinoma. It is difficult to discuss this since there is as yet no information on how often this step would prove useful. However provided a patient with colitis has had a colonoscopy preoperatively by a competent practitioner, it is unlikely but not impossible that an invasive carcinoma or dysplasia would be missed. It would, therefore, seem common sense to widen the clearance where dysplasia is known to be present. In familial adenomatous polyposis this would apply to patients with large adenomas in which there might be a malignant focus.

Rectal dissection

Controversy: previous colectomy with ileostomy and preservation of the rectum

This operation is now the standard procedure for patients with severe colitis. It allows the patient's

Table 5.1 Restorative proctocolectomy: stages of the operation.

Colonic dissection
Rectal dissection
Level of division of the gut tube
Mobilization of the small bowel mesentery
Construction of reservoir
Mucosectomy ±
Ileoanal anastomosis
Temporary ileostomy

recovery of general health with the minimum of surgical interference. All future options are left open and the pathologist has an opportunity for making a precise diagnosis when this is in doubt.

Two controversies require comment. The first is whether the distal bowel should be exteriorized as a mucous fistula or closed and left within the abdomen. There are no objective data on the question. Thus the decision is made by the surgeon during the operation. A mucous fistula is difficult for the patient to manage and should be avoided if the surgeon considers it safe to close the distal large bowel. This will be determined by the general condition of the patient and the state of the bowel wall. It seems reasonable to close the stump if toxicity and malnutrition are minimal and there is no great oedema of the bowel. Otherwise a mucous fistula should be regarded as the safer method of managing the distal bowel. Alternatively the distal sigmoid can be closed and brought out through the rectus sheath subcutaneously with closure of the abdominal skin wound. This may be a satisfactory compromise.

The second question is the extent of distal bowel that should be removed. Some surgeons feel that the rectum either in whole or in part should be taken along with the colon. Alternatively the rectal mucosa can be removed by a mucosal proctectomy (Fallis & Barron, 1953; Fasth *et al.*, 1985). The aim of this approach is to remove as much disease as possible. Where bleeding is the indication for surgery, it often comes from ulceration in the rectum. Under this circumstance removal of the rectum is essential. However, bleeding is a rare reason for emergency surgery. For most patients severe inflammation is the indication and in these good recovery can be expected after a subtotal colectomy alone.

Although it is possible to carry out a subsequent ileoanal anastomosis after a previous proctocolectomy with distal mucosal proctectomy (Fasth *et al.*, 1986), the operation can be difficult risking damage to structures closely related to the rectum (see below). A long rectosigmoid stump as would occur where a mucous fistula has been created is easy to find and safely dissected to the pelvic floor (Fig. 5.1a). Where possible therefore a long stump should be left.

Problem: the short rectal stump

In cases previously treated by colectomy with ileostomy and preservation of the rectal stump where the rectum has been divided at the level of the pelvic peritoneum or below, it can be very difficult safely to identify and dissect the rectum. With a low division, the anterior structures tend to fall back posteriorly and scarring will make access to the rectal stump difficult. In males there is a danger of damaging the seminal vesicles and the autonomic nerves in the rectoprostatic septum, in females the vagina is at risk.

In dealing with this problem, the first step is to

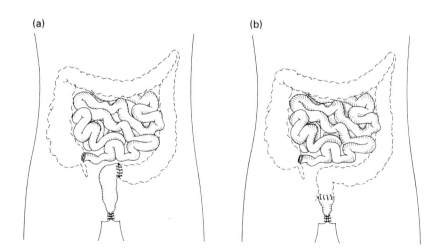

Fig. 5.1 Colectomy and ileostomy with (a) long and (b) short rectal stump.

identify the rectum and having done so, further dissection should be carried out close to the rectal wall. It is better to open the rectum, than damage surrounding structures. Because of the possible danger of opening the rectum during dissection, it is wise first to clean the rectal stump endoanally with an antiseptic solution, e.g. povidone iodine. On clearing the pelvis of small bowel loops, the rectum may be obvious. In other cases, all one may see is a healed-over pelvic peritoneum with some scarring at the site of the previous division of the rectum. In this circumstance, intraoperative digital examination via the anus may clearly demonstrate the rectal stump. In females it is often identified by simultaneous rectal and vaginal examination. In difficult cases, the surgeon should perform the digital examination, manipulating the rectum and vagina, to allow simultaneous scissor dissection using the other hand. With care and patience the longitudinal muscle fibres of the rectum will become apparent. Where there is tough scarring use of scalpel or heavy scissors is necessary.

There is a general tendency to dissect more anteriorly than is necessary. In females this error may be indicated by the occurrence of venous bleeding caused by damage to the postvaginal venous plexuses. In males the rectoprostatic plane is probably best entered in the following manner. A transverse incision is made on the peritoneum overlying the base of the bladder. The peritoneum is then elevated posteriorly and with gentle blunt dissection the seminal vesicles come into view. With further blunt dissection pushing the vesicles forward and the rectal stump backwards, the anatomical plane between rectum and prostate is entered. The surgeon will then be looking directly onto the Denonvilliers' fascia. In contrast with a rectal dissection for cancer, Denonvilliers' fascia should be divided transversely as soon as it is seen. This will minimize damage to the autonomic nerves on the base of the prostate, and allow entry into the immediate prerectal space which can then be developed down towards the pelvic floor. Thereafter the posterior and lateral aspects of the dissection follow easily on staying close to the rectal wall all the way down to the pelvic floor.

Identification and safe mobilization of a short rectal (Fig. 5.1b) stump can be extremely difficult and often requires all the surgeon's skill. As so often in surgery, care and patience will be rewarded. If the rectal stump is inadvertently opened the dissection may be easier but the additional factor of incomplete mucosal removal and contamination become important. The latter may be mitigated by a previous rectal antiseptic irrigation.

Controversy: perimuscular (close) rectal dissection

In patients with known rectal carcinoma or in those colitics with dysplasia, dissection should be carried out in the presacral space with full removal of the

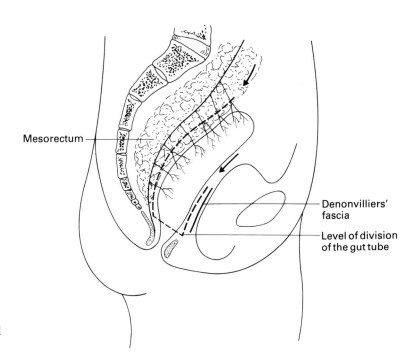

Mesorectum

Denonvilliers' fascia

Level of division of the gut tube

Fig. 5.2 Perimuscular (close) dissection of the rectum indicated by dashed lines. The level of division of the gut tube is at the level of the anorectal junction.

mesorectum. The presacral nerves should be routinely identified and safeguarded. They are easily seen entering the pelvis on the alae of the sacrum. As they pass downwards they become closely related to the lateral aspect of the rectum before ramifying within the pelvic autonomic plexus. They can be damaged at this point but this can be avoided by careful dissection sweeping the nerves laterally away from the rectum.

Where, however, there is no evidence of dysplasia or invasion, the question arises as to whether a close rectal or perimuscular dissection (Lee & Dowling, 1972) should be carried out. This technique involves division of all blood vessels lying between the superior and middle rectal vessels and the rectal wall. In addition Denonvilliers' fascia lies anterior to the anterior plane of dissection (Fig. 5.2). In conventional proctocolectomy with perimuscular dissection, Lyttle and Parks (1977) reported an incidence of sexual dysfunction in 7% and Lee did not have a single case out of a series of 115 patients operated on for ulcerative colitis or Crohn's disease (Berry 1987). With restorative proctocolectomy, the experience with close rectal dissection has been similar. Of the first 210 patients treated by Sir Alan Parks and the author, there were 97 males, out of these there was no single case of failure of ejaculation or orgasm. One patient had an incomplete erection but he was diagnosed to have Peyronie's disease. Subsequently there has been no case of sexual dysfunction in any male patient who has had a perimuscular rectal dissection. This is in contrast with the results after a conventional dissection of the rectum carried out in the anatomical plane between the mesorectum and the presacral fascia in which a retrograde ejaculation rate of nearly 10% has been reported (Taylor et al., 1988).

In females there is very little information on sexual function postoperatively. Thus it is difficult to be dogmatic on the necessity for a perimuscular dissection. Many surgeons carry out the mobilization in the anatomical plane with deliberate identification of the presacral nerves and a dissection in the lower pelvis close to the rectal wall.

Level of division of the gut tube

It was feared that a low division of the rectum might damage nerves or the pelvic floor muscles directly with the possibility of producing anal dysfunction. In the event it has been found that division of the gut tube at the level of the anorectal junction does not vitiate function (McHugh et al., 1987). Thus comparison be-

tween J and S reservoirs, each divided into two groups according to the length of the rectal cuff (long or short), did not show any significant difference between bowel frequency, night evacuation or soiling. A short cuff is associated with fewer postoperative complications (Cohen et al., 1985). There is general agreement that such a level of division is appropriate (Beart et al., 1985; Dozois et al., 1986). The operation is accelerated by division at this level owing to there being a shorter distal stump for mucosectomy (Fig. 5.2). In addition, complete removal of the rectum would reduce the possibility of leaving possibly dysplastic mucosa behind as was likely to have occurred in the case reported by Stern et al. (1990).

Mobilization of the small intestinal mesentery

The ability of the small intestine to descend to the anal level is the limiting factor for restorative proctocolectomy. The anatomy of the mesentery and the blood vessels within it just allow the terminal ileum to descend to the anal level. The most mobile part of the terminal ileum lies about 15 cm proximal to the ileocaecal junction.

In most cases there is no difficulty in achieving mobility. There is general agreement that the small intestinal mesentery should be freed up to the duodenum. In this, dissection should be continued up to the infraduodenal limit of the superior mesenteric vessels and the inferior pancreaticoduodenal artery must be recognized and avoided. Thereafter the mobility of small bowel to descend is determined chiefly by tension of the mesenteric vessels. In patients with a fatty mesentery or adhesions formed following a previous colectomy, mobility may be further reduced.

Problem: adequate mobility

In mobilizing the mesentery, there should be appropriate division of blood vessels combined with division of adhesions. It may also be useful to make several transverse cuts on the peritoneum of the mesentery. In assessing mobility, all surgeons are agreed that the most dependent point of the terminal ileum should be selected for the future ileoanal anastomosis, and that this should be stretched down over the pubis or directly down into the pelvis to the anal level before constructing the reservoir. There is a lot to recommend the latter of these two manoeuvres.

A trial descent before constructing the reservoir is

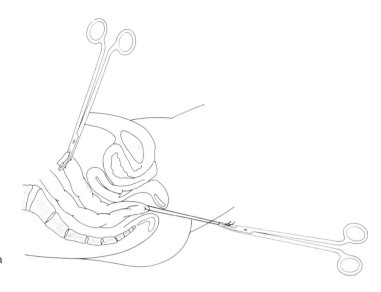

Fig. 5.3 Trial descent. The point on the terminal ileum chosen for the future ileoanal anastomosis is drawn down to the anal level before constructing the reservoir.

(a)　　　　　　　　　　　　　　　　(b)

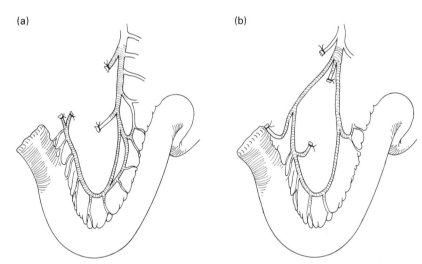

Fig. 5.4 Mobilization of the small intestinal mesentery with (a) division of the ileocolon artery, and (b) its preservation and division of arcades within the mesentery.

very helpful. The ultimate test of mobility is whether the loop of small bowel intended to form the ileal component of the ileoanal anastomosis goes down to the desired level. As suggested above, this can be most surely assessed by bringing the apex down through the pelvis to the level of the dentate line. In this manoeuvre a stay suture is placed on the apex of the intestinal loop. Following division of the gut at the anorectal junction, the surgical specimen is removed leaving the pelvis empty. A perineal operator then passes a long artery forceps through the anus to grasp the stay suture. The bowel is then drawn down through the pelvis to the anal canal level (Fig. 5.3). If it reaches the dentate line at this stage, it will do so after the reservoir is constructed. If it does not, more mobilization with division of mesenteric blood vessels is necessary.

Controversy

Some surgeons feel that the ileocolic artery should be preserved. If so mobility then has to be achieved by division of blood vessels within the arcade system (Schoetz *et al.*, 1986). This procedure can be time consuming and requires care not to devascularize the terminal ileum. Alternatively the ileocolic artery can be divided. This gives very considerable mobility and does not cause ischaemia (Fig. 5.4). Mesenteric thickening resulting from previous colectomy can almost always be resolved by appropriate mobilization of the mesentery and division of vessels and adhesions as necessary. Some surgeons have occasionally divided the superior mesenteric artery more proximal to achieve mobility. This must involve some increased risk of ischaemia and in the author's personal experience

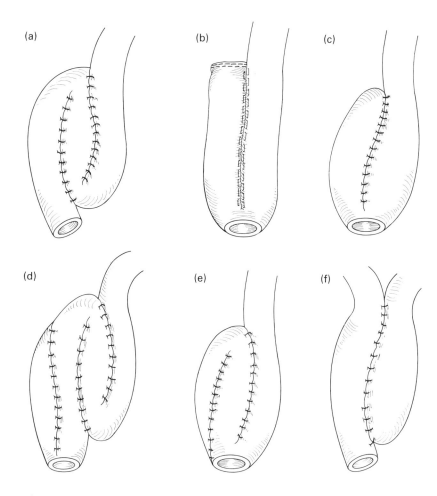

Fig. 5.5 Types of reservoir: (a) triple (S); (b) double (J) stapled; (c) double (J) hand-sutured, (d) quadruple (W), (e) modified triple (S), and (f) lateral isoperistaltic.

of 406 cases, it has never been necessary. On only two occasions has it proved impossible to obtain the necessary mobility of small bowel using the methods described above giving a failure rate, owing to immobility of two (0.5%) out of 408 attempts at the operation.

Controversy: construction of reservoir

Perhaps more has been written on the type of reservoir than on any other technical aspect of the restorative proctocolectomy (Fig. 5.5.) When restorative proctocolectomy with ileal reservoir was first described, it was asked whether a reservoir was necessary at all. The functional results of Ravitch's first two cases of proctocolectomy with straight ileoanal anastomosis were surprisingly good (Ravitch & Sabiston, 1947). However, subsequent experience with this operation showed that high frequency of defaecation including night evacuation especially and urgency, were very common. Indeed in a review in the mid 1950s by Valiente and Bacon (1955) it was concluded that function was unsatisfactory in 50% of cases. The same paper included the first mention of an ileal reservoir

constructed in dogs and speculated that this might be a possible way of improving function.

Martin *et al.* (1977) resurrected the straight restorative proctocolectomy procedure and gained good results although they did not itemize function in any detail. Nevertheless, a vogue was initiated. Not unexpectedly, however, it was found as before that frequency and urgency were significant problems (Telander & Perrault, 1981). So bad was function that balloon dilatation of the descended ileal segment was advocated to try to improve capacity, and therefore function.

The inferior performance of straight restorative proctocolectomy compared with reconstruction involving a reservoir was finally confirmed by the Mayo Clinic through an analysis of the outcome of each operation. Frequency, continence and patient acceptance were all better in the reservoir group (Taylor *et al.*, 1983). Subsequently, studies showing an inverse relationship between frequency and capacity (Nicholls & Pezim, 1985) confirmed that the reservoir served a useful physiological purpose.

More recently it has been suggested that capacity

may be improved by a longitudinal myotomy of a straight ileoanal reconstruction (Accarpio et al., 1983). While such a manoeuvre may reduce amplitude and frequency of ileal contraction in dogs (Sagar et al., 1990), there is little information as yet on the long-term results in humans (Aly & Fonkalsrud, 1988; Turnage et al., 1990). Whether there will be less morbidity and equivalent function as occurs after a formal ileal reservoir procedure remains to be seen.

In the original description of the reservoir procedure by Parks (Parks & Nicholls, 1978) a three loop or S reservoir was employed. Subsequently various modifications have been advocated. They differ in the number of loops of small bowel used and the nature of the outlet. The original S reservoir had a 5 cm length of terminal ileum projecting distally for the ileoanal anastomosis. This was found to give rise to failure of spontaneous evacuation requiring catheterization. Over 50% of such patients needed to catheterize (Nicholls et al., 1984) and a long distal ileal segment could be related to failure of spontaneous evacuation on dynamic radiological studies (Pescatori et al., 1983). In reports of function after construction of S reservoirs with a short or even absent distant ileal segment, the incidence of catheterization fell to less than 10% (Cohen et al., 1985; Vasilevsky et al., 1987). Furthermore secondary reconstructive surgery involving excision of the distal ileal segment and re-anastomosis of the reservoir itself to the anal canal resulted in a high incidence of conversion from catheterization to spontaneous evacuation (Nicholls & Gilbert, 1990). No one would dispute the necessity of avoiding such a distal ileal segment and with subsequent pouch designs, catheterization has become almost a thing of the past.

Another important consideration has been the ease of pouch construction. The two loop reservoir designed by Utsunomiya et al. (1980) is par excellence a simple pouch to make especially following the introduction of long-shafted stapling devices. When stapled, it is necessary to close the distal ileum leaving a short stump which may occasionally cause a complication. This is avoided when using a hand suture technique by incorporating the distal ileum end to side with the pouch (Fig. 5.5c). Other designs including the S and modified S (Pescatori, 1988), the four loop W (Nicholls & Lubowski, 1987) and the Kock reservoir used for restorative proctocolectomy without construction of a nipple value (Öresland et al., 1990b) are more involved reconstructions, although some may possibly yield a

better function (see below). The latero-lateral design of Fonkalsrud (1984) is, however, too involved for it to have attracted much of a following, as it requires a second laparotomy as part of the routine.

The J design is simple and quick to make, and is almost certainly the most widely used reconstruction. It was adopted by the Mayo Clinic, and within a short time during the late 1980s, a large experience with its use had been acquired. Its attraction was a spontaneous emptying that could be reliably expected. In this it had an obvious advantage over the S design, for which the modification to reduce the need for catheterization came too late to persuade general opinion in its favour. However, reported results of J reservoir function suggested fairly high frequency of defaecation particularly at night. Thus in an early report from the Mayo Clinic mean frequency of defaecation per 24 hours was 7.2 in a series of 186 patients (Metcalf et al., 1984). This included a mean frequency of evacuation at night of 1.2 times. Reporting a comparison of frequency of defaecation of S, J and four loop (W) reservoirs, Nicholls and Pezim (1985) observed an inverse relationship between frequency of defaecation and maximal tolerated volume of the reservoir measured by inflation of a balloon introduced into the pouch per anum. A similar regression had been established for straight ileoanal reconstruction (Heppel et al., 1982) and for coloanal colic pouches (Lazorthes et al., 1986). Thus capacity is a factor determining frequency. It was largely to obtain a reservoir more capacious that the W and modified S designs were introduced.

Factors besides capacity which influence frequency of defaecation include mucosal inflammation (Moskowitz et al., 1986), possibly completeness of evacuation (O'Connell et al., 1987) and small intestinal motility (Levitt et al., 1990). None of these can reliably be influenced by the surgeon. Only capacity can be.

Function can be divided into components which include frequency, urgency, continence and the need for anti-diarrhoeal medication. An important aspect of frequency is the occurrence of night-time evacuation. Diurnal frequency may well be affected by various factors including micturition, habit and consciousness of bowel function. At night these do not apply. For example a patient may not need to defaecate for many hours while occupied at work, but then may go several times in quick succession on getting home in the evening. Nobody would willingly get up at night unless forced to do so; thus night evacuation may well be a more sensitive guide of function than overall 24-hour frequency. The need for anti-diarrhoeal medication may also be a sensitive guide to function.

In this regard, Nicholls and Pezim (1985) found significant differences in 24-hour frequency between S and W reservoirs on the one hand and J reservoirs on the other. Mean frequency of defaecation in the former two groups were from 3.6 and 3.7 times per 24 hours in contrast with 5.5 in the latter. Night evacuation was defined as the need to get up at night to defaecate at least one or more times per week. In this regard, over 50% of patients required to do so, compared with less than 30% in the S and W groups. The need for anti-diarrhoeal medication in the J, S and W groups was 58, 26 and 22% respectively.

In a similar non-randomized study, Nasmyth *et al.* (1986) reported on nine patients having an S reservoir and 12 with a J reservoir. While frequency was not much different, urgency of defaecation was significantly better in the S than the J group. More recently Tuckson and Fazio (1991) studied function and physiological variables in 35 patients operated on by one surgeon. Of these, 17 had a J and 18 an S reservoir. With patients followed for more than 6 months, there were significant differences in favour of the S reconstruction. Results of S and J reservoirs respectively were as follows: 24-hour frequency 4 vs. 6, night frequency 0 vs. 1, compliance 14.1 vs. 7.6 ml/mmHg, and night leakage 25 vs. 53%. These data show that capacity and compliance are important physiological variables affecting function. Generally large reservoirs lead to less frequency of defaecation. In support of the study of Nicholls and Pezim (1985), O'Connell *et al.* (1987) and Öresland *et al.* (1990a) also demonstrated that capacity and frequency were inversely related in 23 and 67 J reservoirs respectively. Öresland *et al.* (1990b) found in addition that good compliance correlates with satisfactory overall function. In another study comparing function of S ($n = 19$) with J ($n = 51$) reservoirs there was also no significant difference (McHugh *et al.*, 1987), although S pouch frequency was 1 time per 24 hours less than in the J group. Uncontrolled data from reports of function after four loop (W) reservoir construction support the view that this larger type is likely to yield lower frequency of defaecation. Nicholls and Lubowski (1987) and Everett (1989) reported a mean frequency of defaecation of 3.3 and 3.8 per 24 hours respectively.

However, probably it does not matter what form of pouch is used provided it is large enough. There is an

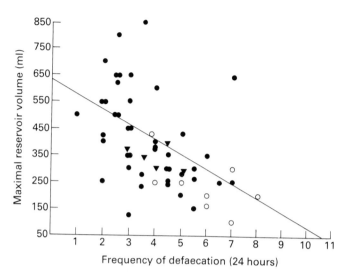

Fig. 5.6 The relationship between pouch capacity (maximal tolerated volume) and frequency of defaecation. (○), double loop reservoir; (▼), quadruple loop reservoir; (•), triple loop reservoir.

increase in pouch volume following ileostomy closure with the passage of time. This occurs up to about 6 months from ileostomy closure (Öresland *et al.*, 1990a). From the regression shown in Fig. 5.6 it would seem that a pouch volume of about 400 ml corresponds with a frequency of 4 or so per 24 hours. An S or a W construction reasonably reliably achieves this volume. It could well be the case that a large J reservoir using 20 cm of loop length could be equivalent but further study is necessary to show this. In a prospective trial of J vs. W reservoirs, 18 and 15 patients respectively were randomized to each group. No difference was found in the frequency of defaecation or any other functional parameter (Keighley *et al.*, 1988). However, three patients from the J group were excluded from analysis and the numbers were small. Further trials are necessary. Mathematical considerations concerning volume achieved per unit length of intestine used, favour a more 'spherical' reservoir, as occurs with the W or S compared with the J construction (Thomson *et al.*, 1987).

Mucosectomy: yes or no?

Controversy

The term mucosectomy refers to the removal of the epithelial lining of the gut tube down to the level of the dentate line. The mucosa in question is referred to as

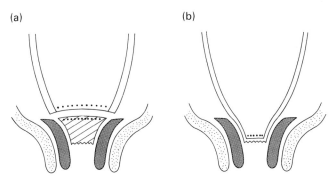

(a)   (b)

Fig. 5.7 Ileoanal anastomosis with (a) and without (b) preservation of the anal transitional zone mucosa.

the transitional zone. It contains sensory receptors and its presence has been shown in man to contribute to the defaecation sampling reflex (Miller *et al.*, 1988).

The issue concerning mucosectomy is linked to the method of anastomosis. The original description of restorative proctocolectomy included a mucosectomy down to the dentate line with a manual endoanal anastomosis. Advocates of preservation of the transitional zone have carried out the anastomosis at the level of the anorectal junction using stapling techniques (Fig. 5.7). Until recently it has been impossible to separate the physiological question of preservation of the mucosa with the possible stretching effects on the anal sphincter of a hand-sutured versus a stapled anastomosis.

Johnston *et al.* (1987) in a pilot study of 12 patients having a stapled ileoanal anastomosis at the anorectal junction (therefore without mucosectomy) compared the results achieved with a retrospective series of 24 patients who had had a mucosectomy with a manual anastomosis made a few millimetres above the dentate line. Postoperative anal resting pressures were significantly higher in the former group (70 vs. 40 cm water) and anal canal length was greater (4 vs. 2 cm). Non-mucosectomy patients had better continence. It was normal in 11 out of the 12 compared with 14 out of the 24 following mucosectomy. The conclusion was that preservation of the rectal mucosa was responsible for the difference in function.

However, this difference might well have simply been due to technical factors which include the learning curve phenomenon and the duration of anal dilatation necessary to carry out a manual anastomosis. It would not be possible from this result to state that preservation of sensory receptors was the factor responsible. Keighley *et al.* (1987) measured anal

canal sensation in 15 patients who had had an anal mucosectomy and six who had not. The results were compared with 14 patients with colitis and an intact rectum and also with 14 normal controls. Although a significant increase in the minimum current perceived after mucosectomy was found, discrimination between faeces and flatus as well as nocturnal leakage was no different in any of the groups. Subsequently, Holdsworth and Johnston (1988) reported on 14 and 13 patients having no mucosectomy and mucosectomy respectively. There was a significant difference in the ability of patients in each group to discriminate flatus from faeces but this was not correlated with function including continence.

In a prospective trial in which patients were randomized to having a mucosectomy with hand-sutured ileoanal anastomosis at the level of the dentate line and a stapled anastomosis at the ileoanal rectal junction without mucosectomy, there was no significant difference in complications in 15 and 17 patients respectively entering each group. Out of these, 14 in each group were assessed at a median of 12 months (range 5 to 17 months) from closure of the ileostomy. In these there was no significant difference in any clinical functional variable. Thus frequency, urgency, night evacuation and continence were similar. Continence was normal in 11 and 12 patients respectively. Mucous leakage occurred in three and two patients respectively, of which one in each group used a pad. There was no incidence of faecal leakage. Furthermore eight out of 14 and 10 out of 14 were able to discriminate flatus from faeces. There was, however, a significantly greater fall of resting anal pressure in the patients who had had a manual anastomosis (Seow-Choen *et al.*, 1991). This reflected a previous report of Neale *et al.* (1982) who had demonstrated that a manual anastomosis causes longstanding resting anal hypotonia. Whether this physiological observation will become clinically significant with the passage of time remains to be seen. As far as can be judged at present, a manual is no more likely to incur functional disturbances than a stapled anastomosis provided the anal sphincters are not too greatly stretched.

If this is true, then the important question centres around the completeness of excision of the disease itself. In this regard there is now some information on the incidence of dysplasia in the mucosa within the anal canal in patients suffering from both colitis and polyposis. King *et al.* (1989) reported the findings in 16 consecutive patients with colitis. Out of these, four had moderate dysplasia in the anal mucosa and in one case there was a poorly differentiated carcinoma. This demonstrates that the anal canal is not free of risk of malignant transformation. Tsunoda *et al.* (1990) reviewed a larger group of 118 patients with colitis. Out of these, three (3%) had dysplasia within the anal strippings as judged by the criteria internationally accepted (Riddell *et al.*, 1983). Although a low incidence, two of the three patients were in the subgroup of eight patients who had an established carcinoma in the large bowel. It may therefore be that the presence of carcinoma in colitis can pose a greater risk on the anal mucosa. Further work is necessary to confirm this result, which is not a surprising finding. With regard to polyposis, out of the 14 patients in the same study, 12 had dysplasia in the anal mucosa. This observation would also be expected from a basic knowledge of the pathology of familial adenomatous polyposis. If these observations are true, it implies that a mucosectomy ought to be carried out in patients with colitis who have a carcinoma and also in all patients with polyposis. The functional results so far do not suggest that removal of this area will vitiate function.

There is, to date, little information in the literature to suggest that preservation of the anal mucosa increases the chance of cancer developing in that segment. However, Stern *et al.* (1990) have reported a patient who developed an adenocarcinoma in the rectal cuff 4 years after the operation. The presence of severe dysplasia was the indication for surgery and after removal of the proximal rectum, a mucosectomy of the distal rectum was performed. It is likely that the carcinoma was already established at the time of surgery or resulted from dysplastic epithelium remaining after mucosectomy.

There is no doubt that stapled anastomosis speeds up the procedure and it also avoids the need for a perineal phase of the operation. These technical and economic advantages have to be set against the cost of stapling and other advantages. For example, there is a small but significant incidence of technical failure. When this occurs, salvage will only be possible by means of a manual suture. Thus it is incumbent upon surgeons to be competent at both techniques of anastomosis if they are to offer a comprehensive service to the patient. It is a paradox that manual anastomosis when required under these circumstances will be more testing than when used in a routine manner. Thus a surgeon who routinely staples may not be getting sufficient practice at manual anastomosis to be in a

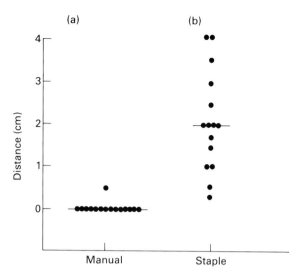

Fig. 5.8 Distance (cm) of the ileoanal anastomosis from the dentate line (a) after manual suture with mucosectomy, and (b) stapled anastomosis without mucosectomy. Bars represent median values.

competent position to use it under the difficult conditions following failure of a stapled.

When the double staple technique is used, it may be difficult precisely to achieve an anastomosis at the anorectal junction. There is some evidence that this can lead to a longer stump than desired. For example, Fig. 5.8 shows the distance of the ileoanal anastomosis from the anal verge in a group of patients randomized to (a) hand suture versus (b) stapled (Seow-Choen *et al.*, 1991). It can be seen that a few of the patients in the stapled group had an anastomosis significantly above the anorectal junction. When using the double staple technique, it may be difficult to get the transverse stapler down to the appropriate level and this explains the observation shown. Other methods of stapling, including the placement of a purse-string suture per anum via an endoanal approach or after eversion of the mobilized rectal stump (Brough & Schofield, 1989) may overcome this problem.

A further disadvantage of stapling concerns stenosis which seems to occur more often than after manual anastomosis. In a retrospective review of 266 patients undergoing restorative proctocolectomy, 218 had a handsewn and 48 a stapled anastomosis. There were 50 cases who developed stenosis at the ileoanal anastomosis. Out of these 38 persisted and required repeated dilatations. The incidence of stenosis after manual (31/218; 14%) was significantly less than after stapled anastomosis (19/48; 40%).

The question of mucosectomy and the relative merits of hand-sutured anastomosis will only become fully appreciated with the passage of time. So far the evidence with regard to clearance of disease-prone tissue and cost weighs in favour of mucosectomy. With regard to function, there seems to be no present significant difference between a stapled or a hand-sutured anastomosis. Further follow-up is, however, necessary.

Manual ileoanal anastomosis

Problem: sphincter stretching

There is no doubt that a manual anastomosis using an endoanal technique can lead to damage to the anal sphincter. While this may be subclinical in most cases, there is ample information to show that resting anal tone after a manual anastomosis is reduced and is likely to remain so indefinitely (Neale *et al.*, 1982; Öresland *et al.*, 1989; Seow-Choen *et al.*, 1991). It follows, therefore, that all efforts should be made to minimize dilatation of the sphincter in doing the anastomosis. The Gelpi retractor works by stretching the perianal skin to bring the anal canal more distal. This may cause some stretch on the lower part of the sphincter only. Using a true endoanal technique, it is necessary to expose the entire anal canal when placing sutures and here greater care should be taken not to overstretch. The Eisenhammer retractor (Fig. 5.9a) is an excellent instrument for this purpose. It can be inserted and withdrawn with great ease and the rigidity of the blades allows a reasonable adjustment of stretch to allow exposure. The stretch can be minimized by using the retractor only for the time taken to put in each individual stitch. It can be removed on each occasion. Using this strategy, the average period of anal dilatation including a mucosectomy (if this is to be carried out) is of the order of 20 minutes. This also is minimized by opening the blade just sufficiently to obtain access. The mucosectomy is of course easier and quicker if the gut tube has been divided at the level of the pelvic floor.

Problem: orientation

A manual ileoanal anastomosis has the advantage of precision in the level of placement of sutures and in achieving a complete circumferential union without any defect. The type of needle used for the anastomosis is important. It should be strong and small. A 25-mm

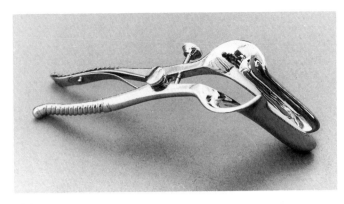

(a)

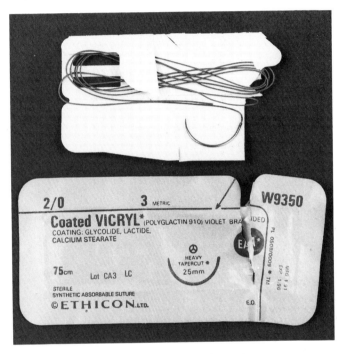

(b)

Fig. 5.9 (a) Eisenhammer's anal speculum. (b) Taper cut (25 mm) needle with 2/0 polyglactin suture.

taper cut needle on a 2/0 suture (Ethicon) is ideal (Fig. 5.9b). It can be easily manipulated within the anal canal and does not bend or break.

However, problems can be encountered. The reservoir may be brought down twisted on its mesenteric axis. This can be avoided by the manoeuvre shown in Fig. 5.10. Two sutures are placed during the abdominal phase, one on the left, the other on the right side of the enterotomy in the reservoir after orientation of the mesentery such that its free edge lies on the right side of the patient. Each is then grasped by a long artery forceps passed through the anus and the pouch is brought down into the pelvis by gentle traction on the

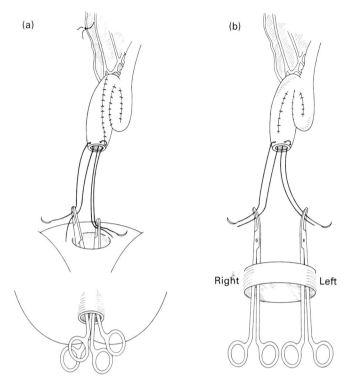

Fig. 5.10 Method of achieving correct orientation of the reservoir on descent to the anal level for the ileoanal anastomosis. (a) Stay sutures grasped by artery forceps introduced per anum. (b) Pouch drawn down with correct right-left orientation.

sutures. The perineal operator then takes each needle and places a suture taking a deep bite of the tissue at the dentate line on the left and the right aspect of the anal canal. When these are tied, the reservoir is approximated to the anal canal with the correct orientation. Two further sutures are placed, one anteriorly the other posteriorly, and with fixation of the ileoanal anastomosis at these cardinal points, it is then an easy matter to place further sutures into each quadrant. Clearly there are other ways of approximating the

reservoir to the anal canal in doing a manual anastomosis but the method described simplifies the technique and avoids the problem of twisting.

Problem: tearing

Using the manual method, there is a danger of tearing the small bowel in the reservoir just above the anastomosis when the retractor is opened. This can be a very difficult situation to handle. It can best be avoided by first leaving an adequate diameter of enterotomy on the pouch for the anastomosis. When the pouch is being constructed, leaving an enterotomy which comfortably takes two fingers, seems to be about right. Such a diameter will accommodate the anal retractor with a minimal chance of splitting. If splitting does occur, then it may be possible to repair the defect if its longitudinal length is short, i.e. no more than about 2 cm. This is shown in Fig. 5.11, the defect being repaired transversely by interrupted sutures. If the defect is longer, or access and poor vision prevent a clear definition of the damage, the safest course of action is to take down the anastomosis and deliver the pouch back to the abdomen. Here the damage can be repaired and another attempt at the ileoanal anastomosis made using the same descent technique as before.

Stapled ileoanal anastomosis

Problem: level of division

Surgeons who prefer stapled anastomosis do so for two main reasons: (i) the anal transitional zone is preserved, and (ii) the anastomosis is carried out without stretching the anal sphincter. The aim is to achieve an anastomosis at the level of the anorectal junction.

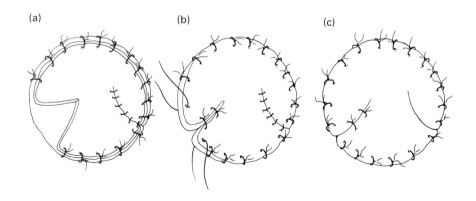

Fig. 5.11 Repair of split in reservoir during the ileoanal anastomosis. Interrupted transverse sutures should be used. (a) Tear in pouch; (b) transverse sutures placed; (c) anastomosis complete.

However, it is important to judge this accurately in order to avoid leaving a significant rectal stump. While it is too early to say whether inadvertent preservation of the rectal stump might lead to the subsequent development of cancer later, there is already some evidence that residual inflamed mucosa may be symptomatic (Keighley *et al.*, 1989).

If a purse-string suture technique is to be used, the level of division of the gut tube can be directly assessed in the following manner. With the rectum completely dissected down to the pelvic floor, an assistant passes an anal speculum and identifies the dentate line. A point on the anterior rectal wall about 2 cm above this level is then indicated to the abdominal surgeon by the perineal surgeon using an instrument introduced through the anus to expose the mucosa. Alternatively the level of division can be gauged by digital examination per anum. A suitable level corresponds to the length of the two distal phalanges of the adult index finger. The abdominal surgeon then divides the mucosa at that point. A similar manoeuvre can be employed to place a transverse row of staples at the same level when using the double staple technique. Alternatively the eversion method described by Brough and Schofield (1989) allows direct visualization of the point of division of the gut tube as seen from the mucosal side.

Problem: reservoir suture

If a stapled ileoanal anastomosis is to be used with a reservoir made by hand-suture, the surgeon should be aware not to use a continuous suture down to the point on the pouch to be used for the anastomosis. Inevitably the suture will be cut by the knife of the circular stapler. A continuous suture should be taken down to a point on the reservoir safely above the zone that will be incorporated into the stapling device. This latter portion should be completed using interrupted sutures (Fig. 5.12). Since a stapled anastomosis seems more likely to result in stenosis than a manual suture the largest instrument should be used.

Ileostomy

Problem

A loop ileostomy even with the Turnbull modification is a difficult stoma for the patient to handle. Despite the eversion of the proximal limb, many retract in the

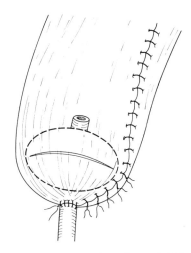

Fig. 5.12 Hand-sutured pouch with stapled ileoanal anastomosis. Interrupted sutures should be used on the distal reservoir which will be drawn over the anvil of the stapler.

postoperative period. It can be difficult to maintain an appliance satisfactorily in place, and leakage with consequent skin damage is common. Excessive tension in the mesentery can occasionally lead to such serious retraction in the postoperative period that revision may be necessary. Very occasionally this has to be done as an emergency procedure if peritoneal contamination occurs.

As with any stoma, it is important to site its position preoperatively. A loop ileostomy can be brought out on either side of the abdomen and there is no special merit of having it on the right. Thus the area of skin with the best contour in the iliac fossa on either side should be selected and marked preoperatively. Excessive tension can be avoided by carefully selecting the loop to be exteriorized at a point closest to the reservoir proximally which does not result in tension within the mesentery. A retracted ileostomy may not defunction properly. It is difficult to know whether this matters particularly, although incomplete defunctioning clearly defeats the purpose of doing an ileostomy in the first place. It may well be that faecal contamination around a disrupting ileoanal anastomosis could be an important factor in determining the outcome for the patient. Wong and Goldberg (1987) recommend division of the small bowel, closure of the distal limb and exteriorization of the proximal as an everted end ileostomy. Besides completely defunctioning the patient, this stoma has the advantage of being easier for the patient to manage enabling him or her to appreciate an ileostomy under optimal conditions. Closure is still readily possible.

Controversy

The use of a temporary ileostomy has been a routine procedure. It is argued that it mitigates the effects of anastomotic breakdown. However *per se* it may lead to complications and it also extends the total treatment time and cost.

The need for a temporary ileostomy was questioned initially by Thow (1985) who drew attention to the potential complications and costs of this stage of the procedure. He described a series of 21 patients operated on over a 4-year period to whom no covering ileostomy was given. His technique required a somewhat involved system of intubation of the small bowel itself as well as of the reservoir. The former was cannulated by a double lumen gastrointestinal tube passed via a gastrostomy to enter the reservoir *ab oram* where it was retained by a balloon. The latter was intubated by a drain placed per anum. A sump suction drain was then placed in the space between the reservoir and denuded rectal cuff. While early postoperative complications were fairly high (including nine patients with fever, obstruction, haemorrhage and subphrenic abscess) only one patient required a subsequent temporary ileostomy for these. There were, however, late complications which included abscess from ileoanal fistulae (one case), rectovaginal fistula (one case), pelvic inflammation (one case) and diarrhoea (one case). Three of these required a subsequent permanent ileostomy. It is of course impossible to know whether these failures would have been avoided by the use of an initial temporary ileostomy.

At about the same time there was a general consensus among a group of surgeons who had had considerable experience with the operation that a covering ileostomy was desirable (Dozois *et al.*, 1986). In particular Dozois *et al.* (1986) reported that five out of six patients in whom no ileostomy had been carried out developed a septic complication. They had clearly been discouraged by the experience.

Thow (1985) had emphasized the need for careful patient selection in performing a one stage procedure. Subsequently Everett and Pollard (1990) in reporting their experience of 60 cases, discussed the advantages and disadvantages of a single stage procedure. Twenty of the patients had had no ileostomy, these included 15 with ulcerative colitis and five with familial adenomatous polyposis. Of these, four developed a significant complication, which required subsequent defunctioning in two. The majority however, made a good recovery and had a significantly shorter hospital stay when compared with the two stage procedure. Thus in the 16 uncomplicated cases this amounted to a mean of 11.7 days compared with a mean of 27.9 days for the two stage patients when hospital stay for both procedures was combined. Even when the few one stage patients with complications were added to the 16 uncomplicated, total hospital stay was 17.8 days. Everett feels however that cases should be selected for no ileostomy on the basis of simple criteria including ease of construction of the anastomosis, vascularity, tension and a patient in good general condition as judged by the absence of 'high dose' steroid medication. However valid these may be, the important point to recognize is that patients should be selected on individual merit for avoidance of a temporary ileostomy.

In a report of 16 patients having no ileostomy, Kmiot and Keighley (1989) commended this approach on the basis that 13 had no major complications. In these the median hospital stay was 14 days (range 11–17 days). However, three patients experienced severe septic postoperative complications requiring a subsequent ileostomy, permanent in at least one. Whether these might have been less serious had a covering ileostomy been performed cannot be said.

There is no doubt that an ileostomy carries its own morbidity. Furthermore, a loop ileostomy may not entirely defunction the distal intestine. In this regard Winslet *et al.* (1987) showed that failure to defunction was likely in cases with stomal retraction. There is furthermore a suggestion from a retrospective study of 982 patients that inadequate defunctioning by an ileostomy may be associated with an increased incidence of pelvic sepsis (Galandiuk *et al.*, 1990). There is now some information on ileostomy-related morbidity. Winslet *et al.* (1991) reported a series of 34 patients with an ileostomy-related complication rate in formation and closure of 41 and 30% respectively. The complications were divided into minor and major, only the latter category requiring hospital admission. Of the 34 patients only two had major complications, including excessive output (one case) and retraction (one case). With regard to closure, eight patients had complications requiring hospitalization. These included enterocutaneous fistula (nine (19%) cases) and intestinal obstruction (two (6%) cases). Further surgery was required in five of these. In the light of such morbidity, the authors had discontinued the routine use of loop ileostomy reserving defunctioning for cases of technical difficulty in construction. The incidence of nearly 20% of enterocutaneous fistula was high in this series.

In a larger series of 296 patients, 17 (5.7%) had complications related to the formation of the ileostomy. These included: small bowel obstruction requiring laparotomy (seven (2.4%) cases), retraction needing revision (three (1%) cases) and eight (2.7%) with minor complications. Following closure in 263 patients, major complications occurred in 21 (8%). These included small bowel obstruction requiring laparotomy (11 (4.2%) cases), laparotomy to close the ileostomy (five (1.9%) cases), enterocutaneous fistula (two (0.9%) cases) and peritonitis requiring laparotomy (three (1.1%) cases) (Senapati *et al.*, 1992). These results reveal that intestinal obstruction related to the ileostomy is a significant complication, however the experience also shows that leakage rates on closure (2%) can be very low.

The arguments for and against a defunctioning ileostomy include on the one hand avoidance of the morbidity associated with the procedure, and on the other, the cost of another operation and a shorter treatment time. In favour is the contention that an ileostomy minimizes the consequence of anastomotic leakage and pelvic sepsis when it occurs. There is another factor in support of an ileostomy albeit difficult to quantify. Patients who are advised to have a restorative proctocolectomy may be disappointed with the functional result. In particular, those with normal function preoperatively such as many with familial adenomatous polyposis and some with ulcerative colitis for whom the indication is dysplasia are unlikely to have the same or better function postoperatively. Patients having a one-stage restorative proctocolectomy will never have experienced an ileostomy, however temporary, and will therefore not be in as good a position to accept any functional difficulty, as if they had. Thus it might be more difficult for them to accept what they perceive to be poor function compared with those who have lived with the alternative, namely an ileostomy. The author has found having patients with experience of an ileostomy to be invaluable.

The obvious response to settling this controversy is a prospective randomized clinical trial. While this is simple in theory, it is likely to be difficult in practice. The first question involves case selection. It would not be ethical to randomize without taking the circumstances of the individual case into account. Thus technical difficulty and pathological differences would need to be standardized to create a group that could justifiably be randomized. To set such criteria would be difficult and they may themselves not be appropriate, involving as they do subjective decisions in the 'difficulty' of the operation or any other significant step in the procedure. There is general agreement that there should be a degree of case selection when deciding when or not to do an ileostomy. The question is, how does one decide objectively? As with low anterior resection, in all probability the answer will come by gradual evolution through general experience.

Postoperative phase

Complications are common after the procedure (see Chapter 4), occurring in anywhere from 20 to 50% of patients. However, provided two aspects of the postoperative course remain satisfactory, all is likely to be well with the minimum of inconvenience to the patient. These include return of intestinal function and absence of septic complications.

Normal postoperative course

In-patient course

As with any other major abdominal operation, satisfactory progress in the first 24 hours will be indicated by stable vital signs and only a small amount of blood loss from the abdominal drain. This is usually no more than 200 ml and occurs chiefly during the first 6 hours or so postoperatively, after which it usually stops. As a result, there is usually no good reason to keep the drain in for longer than 12–24 hours postoperatively. The ileostomy begins functioning within around 2–5 days. There may be a considerable output from it initially and it is wise to keep the intravenous infusion in place for a day or two after the ileostomy has begun to act. With resumption of oral intake, it is very important to emphasize to the patient the need to maintain an adequate sodium intake. The patient should also be warned to expect a discharge of bloody mucus per anum. Initially this may leak out without control but the patient should be reassured that this will settle. Some surgeons leave a drain through the anus in the pouch. This might be advisable in cases defunctioned by an end ileostomy with a closed distal stump or perhaps in those who have had no ileostomy at all. In those with a loop ileostomy, however, there is the opportunity for the pouch to decompress proximally through the distal limb of the ileostomy. An anal catheter can alert the surgeon to haemorrhage from the pouch. It is usually well tolerated by the patient although not always. There is the theoretical possibility that it can cause damage to the anastomosis by local pressure. However there is no published evidence that it has any advantage over not using a drain.

Unless there is a particular indication for example, the suspicion of an ileo anastomotic complication, it is unnecessary to carry out a digital examination before the patient leaves hospital. It is only likely to cause damage.

In the uncomplicated case, patients who have had a previous ileostomy can usually be discharged between 8 and 10 days postoperatively. For those who have not, a few more days may be necessary for them to become confident with the appliance. Time spent at this stage on stoma care with expert advice may avoid unnecessary skin complications later. If there is a fairly high ileostomy output (>1 litre/24 hours) it is advisable to prescribe an electrolyte mixture to continue after leaving hospital and to re-emphasize the need for an adequate sodium intake in the diet.

Out-patient course

The patient should be seen at about a month from discharge. Appetite, weight, return of wellbeing and ileostomy function (including evidence of sodium depletion), should all be assessed. The ability of the anus to hold secretion should be determined. The ileostomy and the abdominal wound should be inspected and a digital examination per anum then carried out. The finger should slide easily into the pouch and the circumference of the anastomosis should be palpated. Signs of induration should be felt for. A thin, mobile suture line without induration is evidence of satisfactory healing. Some induration at this stage is not uncommon. If it is associated with tenderness or a pit or obvious defect in the anastomosis, then incomplete healing should be inferred. Under this circumstance, the patient should be seen a month or so later, by which time there is a good chance that healing will have occurred. Not infrequently a narrowing is felt by the finger. This can be real or 'apparent'. In the former case there is a true stenosis from fibrosis around the suture line due to reaction to the sutures (more common after a stapled anastomosis), localized sepsis with subsequent scar formation, or some degree of

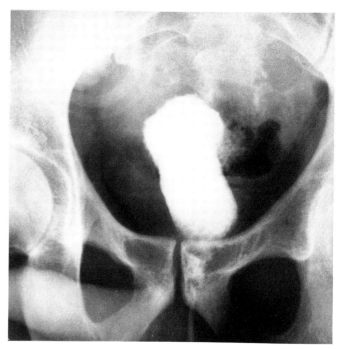

(a)

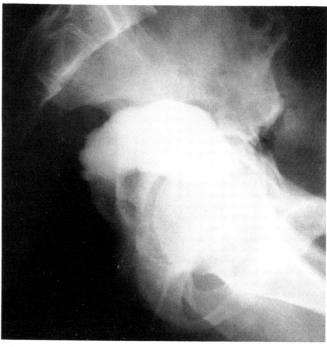

(b)

Fig. 5.13 Normal pouchogram. No leakage of contrast from the reservoir or restorative proctocolectomy. (a) AP view, (b) lateral view.

separation of the suture line with proximal retraction of the reservoir. An 'apparent' stenosis gives way on gentle finger pressure to leave a lumen of adequate diameter. In this situation, one has the impression that there has been adhesion formation in the transverse plane across the suture line where points on the circumference of the suture line have come into contact with each other. The finger is simply breaking down these adhesions and there is no true stenosis.

In the absence of any signs suggesting incomplete healing, a decision to close the ileostomy can then be taken. It is desirable to have a contrast radiograph (pouchogram) (Fig. 5.13), this should include views of the ileum up to the level of the ileostomy to look for evidence of obstruction. The pouchogram may sometimes reveal a track from the lumen and an excessively wide presacral space might suggest a collection behind the reservoir. Certainly the combination of a satisfactory digital examination with a normal pouchogram is an indication that the ileostomy can be closed.

On restoration of anal function, frequency of defaecation including evacuation at night, may be initially high. There may be episodes of leakage per anum, soreness of the perianal skin is very common and a suitable barrier cream should be prescribed at this stage. All these disturbances tend to improve spontaneously with time even up to as long as 12–18 months after closure of the ileostomy.

Complications of postoperative phase

Problems: bleeding

Bleeding may be reactionary or secondary. It must be distinguished from the normal bloody discharge from the pouch. In the latter case, the blood is altered and obviously diluted by mucus. The patient and nurses are however, likely to be concerned and the discharged material should be inspected. No action is necessary other than reassurance.

Reactionary haemorrhage

Reactionary haemorrhage occurs within the first few hours after operation. It is detected by the usual alteration in vital signs. Bleeding may be intraperitoneal or within the reservoir. In the former case there may well be an increased output of blood from the abdominal drain (if used) of several hundred millilitres during the first few hours. In the latter, there will be bleeding per anum.

The surgeon naturally hopes the bleeding will stop without the need for further intervention. When bleeding is coming from the reservoir, this is usually easy to judge. Occasionally the sphincter can retain blood in the pouch obscuring the haemorrhage. However, when it is intraperitoneal, assessment is much more difficult. Restoration of vital signs with the diminution of output from the drain might lead to a decision not to reoperate. However, if on clinical assessment, there is a reasonable suspicion that a significant intra-abdominal haematoma has formed, it is probably preferable to re-explore. A haematoma particularly in the pelvis can lead to serious postoperative infective complications and is an easy matter to resolve in the immediate postoperative period. Where bleeding continues, surgery will obviously be necessary.

The patient should be taken back to the operating theatre and anaesthetized. If bleeding is from the pouch, then there is every good prospect of stopping it by endoscopic means. The pouch is irrigated and the bleeding point identified. Diathermy coagulation or under-running with a suture if the bleeding point is accessible, should be employed. Very occasionally there may be so much blood in the pouch that the ileoanal anastomosis has been disrupted by its distension. At this early stage the anastomosis can readily be revised after stopping the bleeding. Where bleeding is inaccessible via an endoanal approach, the abdomen will need to be reopened.

In cases where there is intraperitoneal bleeding, the abdomen should be reopened and blood clot evacuated. There are three likely sites of bleeding, the colonic or rectal bed, the lateral pelvic wall in the region of the middle rectal vessels and the divided anorectal stump. It may well be possible to identify and stop a bleeding point without undue traction on the reservoir. However, bleeding from the divided anorectal stump can be inaccessible to vision with the pouch in place. In this rare circumstance, it is a feasible manoeuvre to detach the ileoanal anastomosis and bring the pouch up into the abdomen to gain vision in the pelvis. The bleeding point can then be dealt with and the anastomosis refashioned.

Secondary haemorrhage

Secondary haemorrhage is rare and when it occurs is usually from the reservoir or ileoanal anastomosis. It is associated with pelvic sepsis. Where minor, observation only is required. If significant and where it shows no sign of stopping, an examination under anaesthetic should be carried out. An anal retractor is

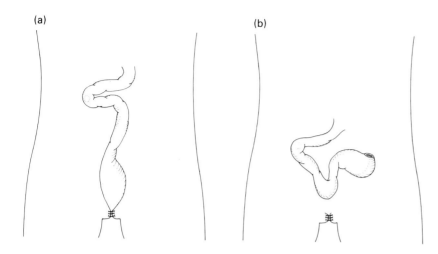

Fig. 5.14 Method of salvage for secondary haemorrhage or chronic sepsis in the pelvis showing detachment of restorative proctocolectomy and exteriorization of the reservoir. This method should only be used in highly selected cases. (a) Initial situation; (b) ileoanal anastomosis detached and pouch exteriorized as a mucosal fistula.

inserted through the anastomosis and the situation assessed. A defect in the anastomosis is likely to be found and secondary haemorrhage is most likely to be coming from a vessel (or vessels) on the edge of the reservoir at the point of disruption. It may be possible by diathermy or underrunning to stop this. No attempt should be made to close the gap in the disrupted anastomosis.

Occasionally a secondary haemorrhage may be coming from within the pelvis, again associated with sepsis. In this circumstance a laparotomy will be necessary. The surgeon might be tempted to excise the pouch and stop the haemorrhage, but salvage should be aimed for. The author has been in this position on two occasions and on each salvage has ultimately been achieved by the following manoeuvre. The ileoanal anastomosis is completely detached and the pouch delivered to the abdomen. With the pelvis exposed, the bleeding point is then dealt with. The pelvis is then filled with small bowel loops and any residual omentum and the pouch itself exteriorized as a mucous fistula in the iliac fossa on the opposite side to the defunctioning ileostomy (Fig. 5.14). With recovery of the patient, subsequent operation is carried out some weeks to months later. In this the mucous fistula and pouch are mobilized, the abdomen is opened, the small bowel cleared from the pelvis and the ileoanal anastomosis is refashioned. All being well it will then be possible to close the ileostomy subsequently.

Sepsis

Sepsis includes abscess formation within the abdomen and the pelvis. There may be differences in reporting the incidence based on definitions. Some surgeons consider a minor defect of the ileoanal anastomosis to be included within the general heading of pelvic sepsis. Others would only include cases in whom pelvic sepsis has posed a significant clinical problem. They would thus exclude cases with a minor anastomotic defect. It is important to remember that fever in the postoperative period can be due simply to the presence of infected mucus within the reservoir.

Early sepsis

Pelvic sepsis usually presents during the in-patient postoperative course. Early features tend to occur around the 5th postoperative day. They include the symptoms of pain or pressure in the perineum associated with a desire to expel material per anum. Signs include tachycardia, pyrexia and leukocytosis. The differential diagnosis includes any cause of postoperative pyrexia but in addition retained infected mucus within the reservoir can be the reason for the fever. Urinary infection is uncommon, and if the abdominal wound is satisfactory and there are no obvious sites of tenderness or masses within the abdomen, a septic complication in the pelvis is extremely likely. The pelvic sepsis itself will be due to an abscess around the reservoir, usually posteriorly, with or without the presence of a defect in the ileoanal anastomosis or the reservoir itself. Reservoir defects are very much less common than anastomotic.

Diagnosis is made by anal examination. First, however, an attempt is made to exclude an abdominal collection by clinical and ultrasound examination. If negative, then a digital examination should be performed. This can usually be done at the bedside but if too painful, an examination under anaesthetic will be necessary, any obvious defect may then be felt.

Alternatively, there may be an indurated or fluctuant fullness outside the reservoir which when present is usually posterior. A proctoscope should be introduced. This will drain any retained infected mucus and will resolve the problem if this is the cause for the pyrexia.

Patients with an abscess outside the reservoir will need drainage under anaesthetic. Needle aspiration of a presacral abscess via the intestinal lumen may well be worth trying although in the author's experience this is unlikely to lead to permanent resolution. It may be better to effect drainage through the ileoanal anastomosis by incising it over a controlled distance of 1–2 cm. Antibiotics should be given. Only in about one in 20 cases with abscess formation does this treatment fail.

Where an abscess is not found but suspicion remains, a water soluble contrast enema and a CT scan of the abdomen and pelvis may help to identify the focus. This may allow a CT-guided drainage of pus.

A leak from the reservoir is uncommon. It may close spontaneously or fistulate or remain associated with a chronic abscess. When a fistula forms, it is usually through the lower part of the abdominal wound. Management will depend on the degree of acuteness of this complication. Formation of an abscess will require drainage. A persisting fistula may require formal surgical closure after the acute phase has passed.

Delayed sepsis

Induration or the presence of a track may be discovered on out-patient assessment after discharge from hospital by clinical or radiological examination (Fig. 5.15). Where minor, there is a good chance that healing will occur providing drainage is satisfactory. It may be necessary to perform an examination under anaesthetic and to widen any sinus communication into the gut tube from an abscess cavity outside the reservoir.

Where resolution does not occur despite such measures, there are two possibilities in management. First the reservoir can be removed and a permanent ileostomy established. Alternatively a salvage procedure can be attempted. The indications for each will depend upon a general assessment of the severity of the sepsis and the condition of the patient. The patient's own personal feelings should be taken into account. A salvage procedure has a limited chance of

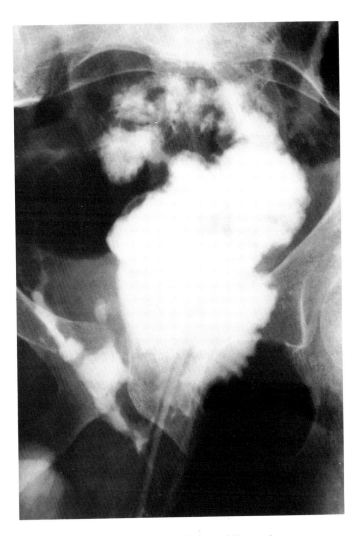

Fig. 5.15 Pouchogram showing defect of ileoanal anastomosis and associated extramural cavity.

success, and the patient should be allowed to decide whether such a chance is worth taking.

The operation will involve an abdominal approach. The source of the sepsis should be identified and the extent of chronic abscess formation assessed. It may be possible to close a defect and to drain the cavity. If this is not feasible then detachment of the pouch from the anus and its exteriorization as described above for secondary haemorrhage, should be considered. The abscess cavity is curetted and filled with loops of small bowel. If the infection resolves, then it may subsequently be possible to refashion the ileoanal anastomosis. The disadvantages of such surgery include the risks of further major surgery with a limited chance of success coupled with hospitalization and consequent disruption of the patient's life. The patient should certainly not be encouraged and the surgeon must also be realistic about the chances of success and must also have made a reasonable assessment of the patient's psychological state. For example, the patient can become obsessed with the desire to lose the ileostomy at all costs.

Ischaemia

Ischaemia in the reservoir is rare. A combination of too much surgical division of mesenteric vessels with stretch due to tension on bringing the pouch down to the anus can lead to arterial or venous insufficiency within the mesentery. The condition presents early in the postoperative period. There is considerable loss of dark blood stained mucus from the anus associated with a tachycardia and a markedly raised white cell count (usually $30\,000/mm^3$ or more). The patient may feel a pressure and heaviness in the perineum. If the ischaemia is severe, toxicity will develop. If it affects the full thickness of the bowel wall, perforation with peritonitis will follow. The diagnosis is confirmed by inspection of the reservoir using a small sigmoidoscope. It may be very difficult to see the mucosa clearly owing to the volume of exudate, and it may be necessary to carry out the inspection with the patient under general anaesthetic. Where complete necrosis is taking place, there will be a characteristic odour and the mucosa will look grey. In incomplete ischaemia, there will be oedematous elevated areas of mucosa with intervening ulceration oozing blood.

Where the pouch is thought to be non-viable, it should be removed and an end ileostomy established. Where oedema and ulceration are seen, the patient should be treated expectantly. There is a reasonable possibility that recovery will occur. Management should also include maintaining the circulation by the necessary measures.

In the author's personal experience of 406 cases, recognized ischaemia has occurred in one case only. Although the condition resolved spontaneously, the patient was left with a severe stricture at the ileoanal anastomosis. This subsequently required a major revision involving excision of the stricture via an abdominal approach and re-anastomosis.

Water and sodium loss

This common complication results from excessive output from the defunctioning ileostomy. It is one of the more important complications of an ileostomy and occasionally it can be severe. It can occur either as a result of a high output stoma or the failure to replace sodium lost from a stoma that is not producing excessively, or a combination of both.

High output ileostomy

During the early postoperative period the effluent from the ileostomy may be excessive in some patients. A 24-hour output of 2 or more litres can occur. This may be due to the stoma being placed too proximally but in most cases a functional cause is presumed. There is a tendency for the output to settle with time.

It is important to measure the ileostomy output during the in-patient period and the general condition of the patient should be monitored to anticipate features of sodium depletion which causes a contraction of the intravascular compartment. The symptoms include weakness, postural hypotension, anorexia, and nausea. A tachycardia will be present and in severe cases there will be peripheral vasoconstriction. Urinary output will fall and there is reduced tissue turgor. The serum sodium concentration may not necessarily be low if the concurrent loss of water has not been replaced. Often it is, however, and in advanced cases, there will be biochemical evidence of prerenal failure. Thus the serum creatinine, urea and potassium levels may be raised. There may be acidosis.

In patients on steroids or in those who have recently been taking them, sodium loss through the kidney may be an additional factor leading to sodium depletion. Steroid suppression combined with sodium depletion can precipitate Addisonian crisis. In these, steroids should be given along with intravenous infusion of normal saline which should apply to all cases. The patient's progress should be monitored with the measurement of ileostomy and urine output and serum electrolyte levels. Usually an initially high ileostomy output settles over a period of 1–2 weeks. However, if it persists, then the most effective treatment is to close the ileostomy, albeit earlier than anticipated.

Failure to replace sodium loss

Even in patients without an excessive ileostomy output, sodium depletion can occur if the patient does not maintain an adequate intake of sodium. Sodium concentration in ileostomy effluent is around 100 mmol per litre. While water loss from the body tends to be replaced through the stimulus of thirst, there is no such mechanism for sodium in man. On leaving hospital the patient's appetite and general wellbeing may not be particularly good in any case, and there is therefore a real danger of failing to replace sodium loss. A daily deficit of for example 50 mmol by the end of a week or two will have amounted to a significant fraction of the total exchangeable body sodium of around 2500 mmol. With the occurrence of sodium depletion, strength and appetite can be depressed leading to a vicious circle of worsening negative sodium balance.

The possibility of sodium depletion should be explained to all patients at the time of discharge from hospital, and if there is any doubt as to the patient's competence to add salt to food, an electrolyte mixture should be prescribed. When the patient attends for the out-patient follow-up visit signs of sodium loss should be looked for. If present, management will proceed as described above. If possible the condition should be treated by increasing oral intake but sometimes admission to hospital for intravenous sodium replacement will be necessary.

Obstruction

Obstruction is common occurring in 10% or more of cases. It can take place in the immediate postoperative period or after closure of a temporary ileostomy. Chronic obstructive symptoms can persist for weeks or months thereafter. The diagnosis and management are basically the same as described in standard textbooks on abdominal surgery. However, there are certain points worth emphasizing.

Obstruction before ileostomy closure

Causes of obstruction include not only simple adhesion formation, but also a hypertrophic peritoneal reaction encasing the small bowel. In addition, torsion of the ileostomy may occur. In this situation the obstruction may be intermittent and the plain abdominal X-ray may demonstrate dilated loops of small bowel down to the site of the ileostomy (Fig. 5.16). The author has tried to relieve obstruction due to stomal torsion by placing a catheter through the proximal limb of the ileostomy. While this may temporarily relieve the obstruction, the manoeuvre has failed to avoid an operation in the end.

Strangulation must be extremely rare and there has been no case in the author's series. Thus when

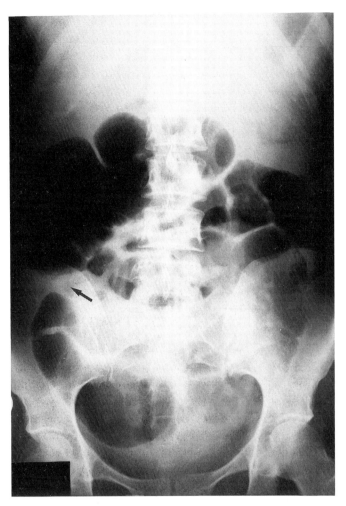

Fig. 5.16 Obstruction at the site of the ileostomy (arrow). Plain X-ray shows dilated loops down to the site of the stoma.

obstruction occurs, it is well worth persisting with conservative management with or without intravenous alimentation depending on the nutritional state of the patient. Where the condition does not resolve depending upon the clinical assessment, surgery will be necessary. It is then seriously worth considering closing the ileostomy at the same time as dealing with the obstruction provided the ileoanal anastomosis is satisfactory.

Obstruction after ileostomy closure

Since the ileostomy had been functioning satisfactory preoperatively, obstruction following closure is usually due to occlusion more distal. The location is likely to be at three possible points, including the ileostomy closure site itself, the distal small bowel between the ileostomy site and the pouch, and thirdly at the anal level. When obstruction occurs, the first step is to examine the ileoanal anastomosis and insert a sigmoidoscope or catheter into the pouch. This may immediately make the diagnosis of an outlet obstruction, which can be caused either by a physical stenosis of the ileoanal anastomosis, or a functional outlet problem. If no obstruction is revealed at the anal level, it is possible that there is impedance to flow at the site of the ileostomy closure by oedema at the suture line. This should settle over a few days and it is thus worth waiting. If the obstruction does not settle then a laparotomy will be necessary.

Chronic obstruction

Sometimes patients develop symptoms of chronic obstruction with colicky pains, episodes of abdominal distension and borborygmi. These may be associated with functional disturbances including frequency and urgency of defaecation. A small bowel contrast enema may identify the site of obstruction. The condition may improve spontaneously but if it does not then surgery will be necessary. While the pains and distension may improve, the surgeon should not expect frequency to diminish. In cases with no obvious local site of obstruction, it is worth placing an enteric tube from the jejunum through the small bowel to the pouch. This can be removed 10 or so days postoperatively.

Dysfunction

In reporting functional results the following should be stated: frequency of defaecation per 24 hours, number of defaecations at night, urgency (less or equal to 5 minutes, less or equal to 15 minutes, less or equal to 30 minutes), mode of evacuation (spontaneous or assisted), the need for anti-diarrhoeal medication and continence.

Continence is reported by different surgeons in various ways, but the following system is simple and satisfactory.

Normal	Complete continence for faeces and flatus
Abnormal	
Minor	⎫ Faecal or mucoid
Major	⎬ Day or night or both
	⎭ Pad or no pad

The presence or absence of anal soreness should be recorded. Function tends to improve spontaneously with the passage of time.

Abnormal frequency

While mean frequency of defaecation in large series of patients is about 4–6 times per 24 hours, there is a natural variance with a standard deviation of 1–2 (see Chapters 6 & 7). Abnormal frequency may be inferred if there is a rise in the number of stools per 24 hours from a previously stable figure or if the figure exceeds 7 or 8 times per 24 hours, i.e. more than two standard deviations above the mean.

Differential diagnosis

There are several reasons for abnormal frequency. First it may be time-related occurring in the early period following resumption of anal function. This form of frequency tends to improve with time. However, it should show signs of doing so within a few weeks, with reduction in frequency continuing over 6–12 months or more. Treatment is by anti-diarrhoeal agents and reassurance. Frequency may be an idiosyncratic feature determined presumably by the intrinsic motility of the intestine in that person. Sometimes such 'functional' frequency is phasic. For example the patient may go infrequently during the working day but several times in quick succession during the evening or at night. It is diagnosed when investigation (see below) has failed to identify a mechanical or inflammatory cause for the frequency. Little can be done to help it other than offering symptomatic treatment in the form of medicaments to reduce intestinal motility, for example loperamide, diphenoxylate, or codeine phosphate. It may be that certain elements of the diet affect frequency. If these can be genuinely identified, then avoiding them may help. Patients, however, tend to ascribe frequency too readily to diet.

Night evacuation occurs in 20–50% of patients depending on the series (Dozois et al., 1986). It is probably the most sensitive symptomatic guide to function. While the need to get up at night diminishes gradually with time in most patients, some are still left with troublesome night-time frequency. This may be associated with nocturnal leakage and sometimes major incontinence with the expulsion of a full faecal bolus.

Patients with night evacuation should be advised to eat early in the evening and to defaecate just before going to bed. Some of these may need to use a catheter to do so (see below). In addition an anti-diarrhoeal agent should be taken in maximum dose just before retiring.

Table 5.2 Assessment of frequency of defaecation.

	History	Examination	Histopathology (biopsy)	Radiology	Pouch Volume	Pouch Pressure
Pouchitis	Liquid stool ± Blood ± Urgency Anorexia	Proctoscopy Inflammation	Diagnostic	NC	NC	NC
Chronic intestinal obstruction	Abdominal pain Distension ± Failure to thrive	Abdominal distension Proctoscopy Pouch not distended	NC	Plain film Dilated loops Contrast X-ray possible site of obstruction	NC	NC
Evacuation disorder *Ileoanal stenosis*	Frequent small volume stool	Catheter test Stenosis at IAA	Excludes pouchitis	Pouchogram: (i) Dilatation of pouch, (ii) Poor emptying, (iii) ± Long distal segment	High MTV High compliance	Low High compliance
Long distal segment		Seen on proctoscopy N	Excludes pouchitis	(i) As above (ii) As above (iii) Long distal segment		
'Functional'						
Low capacitance reservoir	Frequent small volume stool ± Urgency	No stenosis Urgency on distension with air	Excludes pouchitis	Pouchogram: (i) Small reservoir, (ii) ↑ Motility on distension	Low MTV Low sensory threshold Low compliance	↑ Pressure Wave activity on distension Low compliance
'Functional' frequency	Frequency often phasic (see text)	N	Excludes pouchitis	N	N	Ambulant pressure monitoring ↑ activity of tonic waves

IAA, ileoanal anastomosis; MTV, maximal tolerated volume; N, normal; NC, non-contributory.

There are four circumstances causing frequency which the clinician may be able to improve. These include chronic intestinal obstruction, an evacuation disorder, inflammation of the reservoir (pouchitis) and a low capacitance pouch. Obstruction and pouchitis have been dealt with elsewhere.

Investigation

The assessment of the patient includes clinical examination and special investigations. It is helpful to follow a protocol as outlined in Table 5.2. From the history it may be possible to distinguish frequency with the passage of small volume e.g. evacuation disorder from a larger volume e.g. pouchitis stool. The history will also reveal systemic symptoms more suggestive of intestinal obstruction and pouchitis than a local mechanical problem. Digital examination of the ileo-anal anastomosis will detect stricture formation. Proctoscopy will demonstrate a long distal ileal segment and mucosal inflammation. A biopsy should be taken. There must be evidence of severe acute inflammation to diagnose pouchitis. If there is not, frequency is due to another cause.

The catheter test and contrast radiology of the pouch are essential to diagnose an evacuation disorder. A small capacity reservoir can be seen on contrast radiology but volumetric and manometric studies are the mainstay of diagnosis. With the introduction of ambulant pressure monitoring will come a greater understanding of so-called 'functional' frequency where there is no obvious mechanical or anatomical cause.

Evacuation disorder

In this condition there is the frequent passage of a small volume of stool often associated with a feeling of fullness and discomfort in the perineum or lower abdomen. It can be due to a stenosis at the ileoanal anastomosis, the presence of a significant distal ileal segment between the pouch and the anus as often occurred with the triplicated design or a functional incomplete emptying in the absence of a physical narrowing or persisting segment.

The diagnosis of incomplete evacuation is made by anorectal examination. A stricture or a long ileal segment will be identified in cases with a mechanical cause. Dilatation of the pouch may be obvious on proctoscopy. There is almost always a residual volume after defaecation which can be demonstrated on proctoscopy or by passing a catheter (the catheter test) into the reservoir. A pouchogram is essential, it will usually show dilatation of the reservoir and an ileoanal stricture if present (Fig. 5.17). If facilities for video proctography are available, a qualitative assessment of the effectiveness of emptying can be made.

Stenosis

Some degree of stenosis of the ileoanal anastomosis requiring treatment occurs in 20–30% of cases (Dozois *et al.*, 1986). It should only be treated if judged to be producing symptoms and the first line of management is a dilatation. If the stenosis is mild, this can be done as an out-patient. If not, a general anaesthetic will be needed. About 25% of stenoses will respond to one dilatation and more than one will be required in a further 75% and in a small but important minority (about 5%) a surgical revision will be necessary. As indicated above, there appears to be a greater likelihood of stenosis occurring after a stapled rather than a handsewn anastomosis. Revision is a major under-

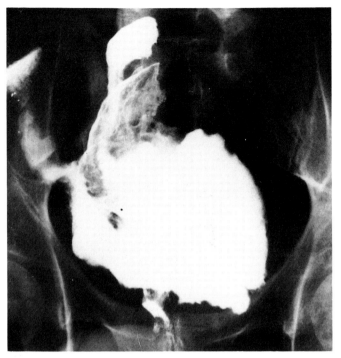

(a)

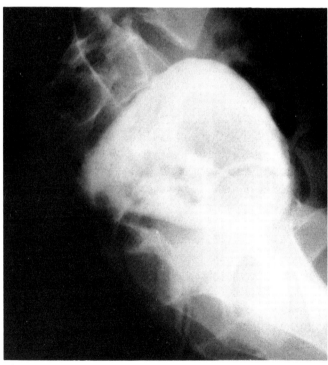

(b)

Fig. 5.17 Pouchogram of reservoir obstructed at the ileoanal level by stricture. (a) AP view, (b) lateral view.

taking, since it will require almost certainly an abdominal approach covered by a defunctioning ileostomy. The operation should aim to excise the stenosed segment and refashion the ileoanal anastomosis under the minimum of tension.

Distal ileal segment

The improvement in function with a reduction in the need to catheterization following surgical excision of the distal ileal segment has already been dealt with in Chapter 4. This again is major surgery and should not be offered to the patient if he or she is happy with intermittent catheterization. In any event, with modern reservoir designs, this particular problem has become rare.

Functional evacuation disorder

If after a normal clinical examination the proctogram shows poor evacuation with no stenosis or angulation of the reservoir at the ileoanal level then a 'functional' obstruction is inferred. It is likely that the condition is due to a gradual increasing distension of the reservoir with resulting reduction in propulsive power due to the cumulative effect over several weeks of incomplete evacuation. All that can be offered the patient is catheterization. Some surgeons regard this as 'failure'. While no one would pretend that catheterization is an ideal solution, patients who have to use the method do so usually without regarding it as particularly inconvenient. The reason is clear. A frequency of 8 or more times per 24 hours can be reduced by catheterization to a very acceptable level. Catheterization often seems to be required indefinitely in these patients. However in some it can be dispensed with after several weeks to months. Here perhaps, catheterization has allowed return of muscle tone following relief of over-distension with the establishment of adequate emptying.

Small capacity

Given the inverse relationship between capacity and frequency, the size of reservoir may be the critical factor causing poor function. A contracted reservoir may occur as the result of persisting unremitting pouchitis, but a low volume can also be due to the construction, the most extreme example being a straight ileal segment.

Small capacity is inferred from contrast radiology and volumetric studies. Balloon volumetry carried out with the patient at rest in the left lateral position can establish three parameters. These include sensory threshold, the volume producing the desire to defaecate and the maximum tolerated volume, and are compared with median and range values for the normal rectum. An example is shown in Fig. 5.18.

Treatment in the first instance should be medical including anti-diarrhoeal agents and dietary modification to reduce stool volume. If unacceptable frequency persists the patient has two options. Either the pouch should be removed and a permanent ileostomy established, or an attempt at revision of the reservoir should be considered. In cases with a straight ileoanal anastomosis, the procedure is well worth attempting by replacing the straight segment with a reservoir. The reservoir is mobilized via an abdominal approach and the ileoanal anastomosis detached. Its volume is augmented by incorporating a loop of ileum immediately proximal and the ileoanal anastomosis is then refashioned. The author has performed an operation of

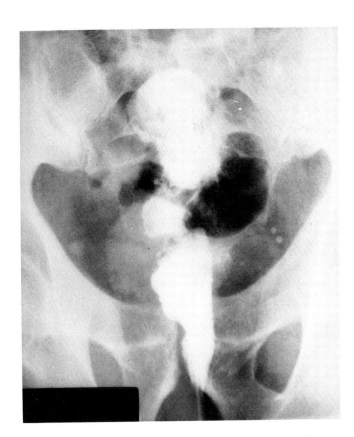

Fig. 5.18 Small capacity reservoir with frequency. Small reservoir on pouchogram with reduced sensory threshold, urge and maximal tolerated volumes.

this type on two occasions, resulting in each case in a marked and sustained diminution of frequency to an acceptable level.

Incontinence

In patients with minor disturbances of continence, treatment should be expectant hoping that matters will improve with time. There is almost always coexistent anal soreness and it will be necessary to advise the patient on anal skin care (see below). Anti-diarrhoeal agents should be prescribed to reduce frequency and thicken the stool.

Where continence disturbances are more severe, then further investigation is necessary. There are two basic factors leading to incontinence including an incompetent anal sphincter mechanism and an increased propulsive force from above. The latter may be due to increased irritability of the pouch as with pouchitis, or reduced capacitance. Soiling also occurs in cases with an evacuation disorder. It can also be 'functional' due to some undefined motility disturbance.

The investigation of incontinence is therefore similar to that outlined above in the assessment of abnormal frequency with the addition of clinical and physiological study of the anal sphincter. Physiological tests formalize in figures the clinical findings on digital examination. They may be useful in establishing the presence or absence of a diffuse pelvic floor weakness with changes suggesting neuropathy. Some fall in resting tone should be expected especially after a manual ileoanal anastomosis, but a reduction in voluntary contraction pressure associated with the symptom of incontinence is significant, indicating sphincter weakness to be the important factor. Under this circumstance there may be an indication to attempt a repair. The nature of this will depend on the nature of the injury. If a localized disruption is present a direct sphincter repair is indicated. If on the other hand there is a diffuse weakness in the presence of an intact sphincter ring, some form of pelvic floor repair, e.g. a post-anal repair should be offered. There is little information from the literature or personal experience, as to how effective sphincter reconstruction after restorative proctocolectomy is. It may, however, be the only treatment available before resorting to excision and a permanent ileostomy.

In cases shown to have poor capacity or an evacuation disorder associated with incontinence, treatment should follow the lines described above for the management of abnormal frequency.

'Functional' incontinence in which there is a precipitant evacuation often at night is rare, occurring in the author's series in less than 2%. Treatment should be the same as for nocturnal frequency (see above). In addition it may be helpful for the patient to be woken by an alarm clock at a time set to precede that when incontinence usually occurs.

Problem

Anal irritation

Some degree of irritation of the perianal skin occurs in 20–50% of patients after restoration of anal function. In most cases it resolves spontaneously although it may take some weeks to months to do so. In some patients, however, sometimes severe anal ulceration and fissure formation occur. These lesions may closely resemble those occurring in anal Crohn's disease but review of the original histological sections usually still shows the features of ulcerative colitis. The cause is unknown but it is possibly due to the proteolytic enzyme activity of the faeces combined with the general irritation of high volume frequent defaecations in the early days to weeks after ileostomy closure. Frequency of defaecation is often associated with soreness presumably due to the increased contact of irritant liquid stools with the perianal skin.

Management

Management includes local skin care and reduction in the frequency of defaecation using anti-diarrhoeal agents. There is improvement with the passage of time in most cases. Even in severe cases with widespread ulceration, there is every good chance that healing will occur provided the true diagnosis is not Crohn's disease. Local skin care involves gently washing and drying the anal skin after defaecation followed by the application of a barrier cream. Those used to protect the skin around an abdominal stoma have been disappointing in the author's experience. However, tincture of benzene spray can be extremely effective. In severe cases it may be necessary to admit the patient to hospital for intensive nursing of deep painful ulceration. Here it is worth trying to reduce contact of faeces with skin. This can be achieved by placing an indwelling wide bore balloon catheter (28F) in the reservoir for 1–2 weeks. If tolerated, the skin then has a chance to recover. Other than the occasional case of ulceration due to Crohn's disease, there has been no single case in the author's series of failure as defined by removal of the pouch and establishment of a permanent ileostomy due to anal ulceration. There is every good reason therefore for the clinician to encourage and reassure the patient that with time and skin care, ulceration and irritation will resolve.

Pouch–vaginal fistula

Fistulation from the reservoir to the vagina or directly to the perineum is becoming one of the major problems following restorative proctocolectomy. It is difficult to manage and with few exceptions some active treatment is obligatory. Diagnosis is necessary. Some females complain of the passage of flatus per vaginam without there being any demonstrable fistula on clinical or radiological examination. In cases where digital examination per anum and per vaginam do not show a fistula, it may be helpful to carry out proctoscopy. Air insufflated into the pouch may be seen to emerge through the vagina. This finding is diagnostic.

In a review of 304 patients operated on in 11 centres, Wexner *et al.* (1989) reported 21 (6.4%) cases of pouch–vaginal fistulae. In a series of 345 patients operated on at St Mark's Hospital there were 15 (9.7%) instances among 155 females. Overall, 20 cases have been treated at St Mark's including five additional patients referred. The fistulous opening into the pouch occurred at the ileoanal anastomosis in all cases. In only one patient was Crohn's disease found to be present after review of all available histological material. It may be that use of a stapled technique increases the possibility of a pouch–vaginal fistula developing. Thus in the St Mark's series of 155 females, there were nine (7.8%) out of 114 having a manual and six (15%) out of 41 having a stapled anastomosis. Larger numbers of cases need to be accrued to be sure on this point. Pelvic abscess formation or an anastomotic defect is undoubtedly a very common precursor. Of the 20 St Mark's cases this was a certain association in 12 (60%) of cases. Intraoperative vaginal injury accounted for three, and the fistula were associated with pouchitis in two cases. There may also have been a surgeon-related factor (Groom *et al.*, in press). Crohn's disease was rarely responsible.

Pouch–vaginal fistula can present either before or after closure of the ileostomy. If the St Mark's data are representative, this appears to be an important prognostic factor. In six out of the 20 patients the fistula occurred in the immediate postoperative period before closure of the ileostomy. Of these closure was achieved in five (82%) and only one patient (18%) required excision of the reservoir. Of the five closures, four occurred spontaneously and one following surgical repair. In contrast there were only five (35%) healed cases among the 14 patients presenting after closure of the ileostomy. The appearance of the fistula was often delayed and indeed it occurred at a median time of 28 weeks following closure. Of the 14, three (21%) patients had to have the pouch excised and a permanent ileostomy established. Of the five healed cases, two occurred spontaneously, the remaining three only closed after surgical intervention. In this series, nine patients underwent 11 surgical attempts of closure, including fistulotomy ($n = 3$, success $= 1$), direct repair ($n = 4$, success $= 1$), pouch advancement flap ($n = 2$, success $= 1$), and complete detachment of the ileoanal anastomosis with a more distal re-anastomosis ($n = 2$, success $= 0$). Overall therefore closure was achieved in only three out of 11 surgical attempts. Failure seems to be likely where there is significant persisting sepsis. Failure is also certain where the repair is under tension as it was in both the author's cases of distal revision of the ileoanal anastomosis which cannot therefore be recommended for pouch–vaginal fistula.

Fleshman *et al.* (1988) reported 24 (12.8%) out of a series of 188 patients who developed significant complications at the ileoanal anastomosis. These were divided into 19 who suffered a disruption owing to failure of the anastomosis to heal and five in whom a fistula developed late after a prolonged period of healing. There were five pouch–vaginal fistulae overall. The remaining cases were composed of those with blind tracks from the anastomosis and tracks emerging through the perineum. Forty-four operations were carried out in the 24 patients. These can be grouped into: (i) resuturing of the anastomosis and drainage of abscess (seven patients were treated by 12 procedures with healing achieved in three); and (ii) pouch advancement flap with drainage of abscess (nine patients were treated by 10 procedures with healing occurring in six). The results were not specifically reported for pouch–vaginal fistula but overall healing was achieved in 12 out of the 24 patients. Simple drainage or defunctioning was not successful as judged by one case of healing among the 16 patients in whom it was tried. Results of treatment in the 19 patients (11 healed) with early presentation seemed better than in the five (one healed) who presented late.

From the information currently available it is reasonable to draw the following tentative conclusions relating to pouch–vaginal fistulae. Prognosis is better if the onset is pre- rather than postoperative. If occurring preoperatively, spontaneous closure is reasonably likely and therefore it is worth adopting an expectant policy. Any local sepsis with abscess formation should be treated by drainage. Defunctioning by ileostomy is essential in all but the mildest cases and certainly whenever a surgical attempt at closure is to be made. Of the operations tried, closure with an advancement flap seems to have been the least unsuccessful procedure. Laying open to allow sepsis to settle followed by a subsequent sphincter repair procedure is another possibility. Refashioning of the ileoanal anastomosis distal to the origin of the fistula fails owing to proximal retraction of the pouch due to tension. The condition is difficult to treat.

References

Accarpio G, Scardamalgia R, Mignon D, Pizoatti A, Accarpio V (1983) Total colectomy and ileoanal anastomosis and myotomy in the treatment of patients with colonic diseases. *Coloproctology* 5:263–285.

Aly A, Fonkalsrud EW (1988) Construction of ileal reservoir with longitudinal ileal myotomy. *Am Surg* 54:475–478.

Beart RW, Metcalf AM, Dozois RR, Kelly KA (1985) The J ileal pouch-anal anastomosis: the Mayo Clinic experience. In Alternatives to Conventional Ileostomy, RR Dozois (ed). Chicago, Year Book Medical Publishers, pp. 384–401.

Berry AR (1987) Conservative techniques during rectal dissection. In *Surgery of Inflammatory Bowel Disorders*, ECG Lee (ed). Edinburgh, Churchill Livingstone, pp. 59–64.

Brough WA, Schofield PF (1989) An improved technique of J-pouch construction and ileoanal anastomosis. *Br J Surg* 76:350–351.

Cohen Z, McLeod RS, Stern H, Grant D, Nordgren S (1985) The pelvic pouch and ileo-anal anastomosis procedure. Surgical technique and initial results. *Am J Surg* 150:601–607.

Dozois RR, Goldberg SM, Rothenberger DA, *et al.* (1986) Restorative proctocolectomy with ileal reservoir. *Int J Colorectal Dis* 1:2–19.

Everett WG (1989) Experience of restorative proctocolectomy with ileal reservoir. *Br J Surg* 76:77–81.

Everett WG, Pollard SG (1990) Restorative proctocolectomy without temporary ileostomy. *Br J Surg* 77:621–622.

Fallis LS, Barron J (1953) Modified technique for total colectomy in ulcerative colitis. *Arch Surg* 67:363–369.

Fasth S, Öresland T, Ahren C, Hulten L (1985) Mucosal proctectomy and ileostomy as an alternative to conventional proctectomy. *Dis Colon Rectum* 28:31–34.

Fasth S, Scaglia M, Nordgren S, Öresland T, Hultén L (1986) Restoration of intestinal continuity (pelvic pouch) after previous proctocolectomy with distal mucosal protectomy. *Int J Colorectal Dis* 1:256–258.

Fleshman JW, McLeod RS, Cohen Z, Stern H (1988) Improved results following use of an advancement technique in the treatment of ileoanal anastomotic complications. *Int J Colorectal Dis* 3:161–165.

Fonkalsrud EW (1984) Endorectal ileoanal anastomosis with isoperistaltic ileal reservoir after colectomy and mucosal proctectomy. *Ann Surg* 199:151–157.

Galandiuk S, Scott NA, Dozois RR *et al.* (1990) Ileal pouch-anal anastomosis. Reoperation for pouch-related complications. *Ann Surg* 212:446–454.

Groom J, Nicholls RJ, Harley PR, Phillips RKS (1993) Pouch vaginal fistula. *British J Surg.* (in press).

Heppel J, Kelly KA, Phillips SF, Beart RW, Telander RL, Perrault J (1982) Physiologic aspects of continence after colectomy, mucosal proctocolectomy and endorectal ileo-anal anstomosis. *Ann Surg* 195:435–443.

Holdsworth PJ, Johnston D (1988) Anal sensation after restorative proctocolectomy for ulcerative colitis. *Br J Surg* 75:993–996.

Johnston D, Holsworth PJ, Nasmyth DG, Neal DE, Primrose JN, Womack N, Axon ATR (1987) Preservation of the entire anal canal in conservative proctocolectomy for ulcerative colitis: a pilot study. *Br J Surg* 74:940–944.

Keighley MRB, Winslet MC, Flinn R, Kmiot W (1989) Multivariate analysis of factors influencing the results of restorative proctocolectomy. *Br J Surg* 76:740–744.

Keighley MRB, Winslet MC, Yoshioka K, Lightwood R (1987) Discrimination is not impaired by excision of the anal transitional zone after restorative proctocolectomy. *Br J Surg* 74:1118–1121.

Keighley MRB, Yoshioka K, Kmiot W (1988) Prospective randomised trial to compare the stapled double lumen pouch and the sutured quadruple pouch for restorative proctocolectomy. *Br J Surg* 75:1009–1011.

King DW, Lubowski DZ, Cook TA (1989) Anal canal mucosa in restorative proctocolectomy for ulcerative colitis. *Br J Surg* 76:970–972.

Kmiot WA, Keighley MRB (1989) Totally stapled abdominal restorative proctocolectomy. *Br J Surg* 76:961–964.

Lazorthes F, Fages P, Chiotasso P, Lemozy J, Bloom E (1986) Resection of the rectum with construction of colonic reservoir and coloanal anastomosis for carcinoma of the rectum. *Br J Surg* 73:136–138.

Lee ECG, Dowling BL (1972) Perimuscular excision of the rectum for Crohn's disease and ulcerative colitis. *Br J Surg* 59:29–43.

Levitt MD, van der Sijp JRM, Kamm MA, Nicholls RJ (1990) Prospective pouch and anal ambulatory motility to characterise good and bad function. *Gut* 31:A1169.

Lyttle JA, Parks AG (1977) Intersphincteric excision of the rectum. *Br J Surg* 64:413–416.

McHugh SM, Diamant NE, McLeod R, Cohen Z (1987) S-pouches vs. J-pouches. A comparison of functional outcome. *Dis Colon Rectum* 30:671–677.

Martin LW, LeCoultre C, Schubert WK (1977) Total colectomy

and mucosal proctectomy with preservation of continence in ulcerative colitis. *Ann of Surg* **188**:245–248.

Metcalf AM, Beart RW, Dozois RR, Kelly KA, Rochester MN (1984) *Ileal-Pouch Anal Anastomosis: The Procedure of Choice?* Proceeding of the 83rd Annual Meeting of the American Society of Colon and Rectal Surgeons, New Orleans.

Miller K, Bartolo DCC, Roe AM, Mortensen NJMcC (1988) Anorectal sampling: a comparison of normal and incontinent patients. *Br J Surg* **75**:44–46.

Moskowitz RL, Shepherd NA, Nicholls RJ (1986) Inflammation in the reservoir after restorative proctocolectomy with ileal reservoir. *Int J Colorectal Dis* **1**:167–174.

Nasmyth DG, Johnston D, Godwin PGR, Dixon MF, Smith A, Williams NS (1986) Factors influencing bowel function after ileal pouch-anal anastomosis. *Br J Surg* **73**:469–473.

Neale DE, Williams NW, Johnston D (1982) Rectal, bladder and sexual function after mucosal proctectomy with and without a pelvic ileal reservoir for colitis and polyposis. *Br J Surg* **69**:599–604.

Nicholls RJ, Gilbert J (1990) Surgical correction of the afferent ileal limb for disordered defaecation following restorative proctocolectomy with the S ileal reservoir. *Br J Surg* **77**:152–154.

Nicholls RJ, Lubowski DZ (1987) Restorative proctocolectomy: the four loop (W) reservoir. *Br J Surg* **4**:564–566.

Nicholls RJ, Pezim ME (1985) Restorative proctocolectomy with ileal reservoir for ulcerative colitis and familial adenomatous polyposis: a comparison of three reservoir designs. *Br J Surg* **72**:470–474.

Nicholls RJ, Pescatori M, Motson RW, Pezim ME (1984) Restorative proctocolectomy with a three loop ileal reservoir for ulcerative colitis and familial adenomatous polyposis: clinical results in 66 patients followed for up to 6 years. *Ann Surg* **199**:383–388.

O'Connell PR, Pemberton JH, Brown ML, Kelly KA (1987) Determinants of stool frequency after ileal pouch-anal anastomosis. *Am J Surg* **153**:157–164.

Öresland T, Fasth S, Nordgren S, Hultén L (1989) The clinical and functional outcome after restorative proctocolectomy. A prospective study in 100 patients. *Int J Colorectal Dis* **4**:50–56.

Öresland T, Fasth S, Nordgren S, Akervall S, Hultén L (1990a) Pouch size: the important functional determinant after restorative proctocolectomy. *Br J Surg* **77**:265–269.

Öresland T, Fasth S, Nordgren S, Hallgren T, Hultén L (1990b) A prospective randomised comparison of two different pouch designs. *Scand J Gastroenterol* **25**:986–996.

Parks AG, Nicholls RJ (1978) Proctocolectomy without ileostomy for ulcerative colitis. *Br Med J* **2**:85–88.

Pescatori M (1988) A modified three loop ileoanal reservoir. *Dis Colon Rectum* **31**:823–824.

Pescatori M, Manhire A, Bartram CI (1983) Evacuation pouchography in the evaluation of ileo-anal reservoir function. *Dis Colon Rectum* **26**:365–368.

Ravitch MM, Sabiston DC (1947) Anal ileostomy with preservation of the sphincter. *Surg Gynecol Obstet* **84**:1095–1099.

Riddell RH, Goldman H, Rausohoff DF *et al.* (1983) Dysplasia in inflammatory bowel disease. Standard classification with provisional clinical applications. *Hum Pathol* **14**:931–968.

Sagar PM, Roldsworth PJ, King RFGJ, Salter G, Johnston D (1990) Single lumen ileum with myectomy: a possible alternative to the pelvic reservoir in restorative proctocolectomy. *Br J Surg* **77**:1030–1035.

Seow-Choen A, Tsunoda A, Nicholls RJ (1991) Prospective randomised trial comparing anal function after hand sewn ileoanal anastomosis with mucosectomy versus stapled ileoanal anastomosis without mucosectomy in restorative proctocolectomy. *Br J Surg* **78**:430–434.

Schoetz DJ, Coker JA, Veidenheimer MC (1986) Ileoanal reservoir for ulcerative coitis and familial polyposis. *Arch Surg* **121**:404–409.

Senapati A, Tibbs C, Nicholls RJ, Hawley PR (1992) Complications of defunctioning ileostomy in restorative proctocolectomy. (in press).

Stern H, Walfisch S, Mullen B, McLeod R, Cohen Z (1990) Cancer in an ileoanal reservoir: a new late complication? *Gut* **31**:473–475.

Taylor BM, Beart RW, Dozois RR, Kelly KA, Phillips SF (1983) Straight ileoanal anastomosis vs. ileal pouch-anal anastomosis after colectomy and mucosal proctectomy. *Arch Surg* **118**:696–701.

Taylor BA, Wolff BG, Dozois RR, Kelly KA, Pemberton JH, Beart RW (1988) Ileal pouch-anal anastomosis for chonic ulcerative colitis and familial polyposis coli complicated by adenocarcinoma. *Dis Colon Rectum* **31**:358–362.

Telander RL, Perrault J (1981) Colectomy with rectal mucosectomy and ileoanal anastomosis in young patients. *Arch Surg* **16**:623–629.

Thompson WHF, Simpson AHRW, Wheeler JL (1987) Mathematical prediction of ileal pouch capacity. *Br J Surg* **74**:567–568.

Thow GB (1985) Single-stage colectomy and mucosal proctectomy with stapled antiperistaltic ileoanal reservoir. In *Alternatives to Conventional Ileostomy*, RR Dozois (ed). Chicago, Year Book Medical Publishers, pp. 420–432.

Tsunoda A, Talbot IC, Nicholls RJ (1990) Incidence of dysplasia in the anorectal mucosa in patients having restorative proctocolectomy. *Br J Surg* **77**:506–509.

Tuckson WB, Fazio VW (1991) Functional comparison between double and triple ileal loop pouches. *Dis Colon Rectum* **34**:17–21.

Turnage RH, Coran AG, Drongowski RA (1990) The value of intestinal myotomy and myectomy in improving the reservoir capacity of the endorectal pull-through. *Ann Surg* **221**:463–469.

Utsunomiya AJJ, Iwama T, Imajo M, Matsuo S, Saurai S, Yaegashi K, Hirayama R (1980) Total colectomy, mucosal proctectomy and ileoanal anastomosis. *Dis Colon Rectum* **23**:459–466.

Valiente MA, Bacon HE (1955) Construction of pouch using 'pantaloon' technique for pull-through of ileum following colectomy. *Am J Surg* **90**:742–750.

Vasilevsky CA, Rothenberger DA, Goldberg SM (1987) The S ileal pouch anal anastomosis. *World J Surg* **11**:742–750.

Wexner SD, Rothenberger DA, Jensen L (1989) Ileal pouch vaginal fistulas: incidence, etiology and management. *Dis Colon Rectum* **32**:460–465.

Williams NS, Johnston D (1985) The current status of mucosal proctectomy and ileoanal anastomosis in the surgical treatment of ulcerative colitis and adenomatous polyposis. *Br J Surg* **72**:159–168.

Winslet MC, Drac Z, Allan A, Keighley MRB (1987) The aetiology of continued defaecation in the presence of a loop ileostomy. *Br J Surg* **74**:1157.

Winslet MC, Barsoum G, Pringle W, Fox K, Keighley MRB (1991) Loop ileostomy after ileal pouch-anal anastomosis – is it necessary? *Dis Colon Rectum* **34**:267–270.

Wong WD, Goldberg SM (1987) The S pouch. In *Surgery of Inflammatory Bowel Disease.* Lee ECG, (ed). Edinburgh, Churchill Livingstone, pp. 87–88.

Chapter 6
Physiological Studies following Restorative Proctocolectomy

DAVID C.C. BARTOLO AND GRAEME S. DUTHIE

Introduction

Restorative proctocolectomy is now the established treatment of choice for most patients with ulcerative colitis and a significant proportion with familial adenomatous polyposis. Most patients obtain good function, but the results vary. Physiological tests provide an objective means of auditing the results based on age, sex, pouch design, construction and type of anastomosis.

In this chapter, we will discuss the routine and research investigations we have used to study 60 patients who have undergone physiological assessment before and after surgery.

Patient assessment of pouch function

Many studies have been undertaken to assess pouch function. Very few however use similar techniques for this assessment which makes interpretation between studies quite difficult. In addition assessment by the surgeon may induce bias, since most patients are considerably improved simply because they no longer have a disease, indeed patient satisfaction is normally high after proctocolectomy and ileostomy (Pemberton et al., 1989). For this reason, we compared three questionnaires, one from the case records where the patients were interviewed by the surgeon, a second following interview by a research fellow and a third, the result of a survey by the stoma therapist. Table 6.1 depicts these results. All the pouch procedures reported here have been undertaken, or directly supervised by one of the authors (D.C.C.B.).

The results for both surveys were similar with two exceptions. More patients reported leakage on the nursing questionnaire. This question asked whether the patients had experienced leakage at any time, and therefore included early function, and these data are in agreement with those from other surveys. In a report from the Mayo Clinic, 36% of patients experienced minor soiling during the early stages, and 4%

reported incontinence. By 5 years, 23% still had minor soiling (Pemberton et al., 1987). In our series, more patients reported complete satisfaction with their functional outcome in response to the stoma therapist's inquiry than to those of the medical attendants.

Questions on subjective variables had the answers rated on a four point scale. 'Always' reflected a feature occurring on greater than 75% of occasions, and 'usually', 'occasionally' and 'rarely' reflect the other optional quartiles, 75, 50 and 25% respectively. While it is possible to divide the options further to improve the accuracy of the assessment we felt simplicity rather than confusion would achieve a better response.

Physiological assessment

There are several methods for measuring anal pressures, sensitivity, and function. We have used standard techniques throughout. Anal pressures were measured using a closed air-filled microballoon system (Miller et al., 1988b), a station pull-through technique.

Anal canal sensitivity was assessed using the method described by Roe et al. (1986). Pouch sensitivity was assessed using a compliance balloon which measured the volume of first sensation, sensation of fullness, and maximum tolerable volume. The slope of the inflation volume–pressure relationship allowed the compliance to be calculated (Duthie & Bartolo, 1991).

We used an ambulatory system to study patients in their home environment. This gave us the opportunity to carry out night-time motility studies, when most episodes of minor seepage occur. This method allowed us to analyse the dynamics of motility changes that cause episodes of minor incontinence. Moreover we were able to compare early and later investigations to determine what leads to improvement of pouch function.

We were particularly interested in the analysis of those patients who experienced nocturnal leakage. Most of these recovered over the first 6 months following ileostomy closure.

Table 6.1 An analysis of the functional results following restorative proctocolectomy comparing three independent assessments.

	Operator	Researcher	Stoma nurse
24-hour frequency*	5 (3–12)	5 (2–11)	6 (3–13)
Night frequency*	0 (0–6)	1 (0–3)	1 (0–3)
Delay emptying (> 1 hour)	61%	71%	76%
Differentiate flatus/ solids	42%	58%	63%
Pass flatus	18%	23%	33%
Seepage			
Daytime	5%	5%	27%
Night-time	10%	15%	45%
Anti-diarrhoeal drugs	20%	18%	33%
Satisfaction with result			
Very happy			
5	/	46%	61%
4	/	37%	29%
3	/	6%	8%
2	/	11%	2%
1	/	0%	0%
Very unhappy			
Prefer pouch to ileostomy†	100%	100%	100%

*Numbers in brackets are range of frequency medians.
†All patients had a temporary ileostomy.

We used the ambulatory Gaeltec system which featured a four channel pressure catheter with microtransducer pressure sensors (Gaeltec, Dun Bheagan, Scotland). Investigation of electrical events in the internal sphincter after the pouch procedure was undertaken with an improved system using the four pressure channels and in addition there were three EMG channels. One measured low frequency electrical activity from the internal anal sphincter (IES EMG), while the other two high frequency EMG channels measured electrical activity in the external anal sphincter (EAS EMG) and puborectalis respectively. These were stored on a portable computer, and subsequently off-loaded onto a desk top computer for subsequent analysis.

We have not undertaken routine radiological investigations of pouch function in our patients.

Functional assessment of outcome

Most of the patients undergoing restorative proctocolectomy had ulcerative colitis. The predominant anorectal symptom during the preoperative period, particularly during acute exacerbations was urgency and stool frequency. Anal canal pressures were normal, and leakage occurred as a consequence of high pressure waves in the diseased rectum. The neorectum following pouch construction is normally compliant, and this allows patients to defer pouch emptying until it is socially convenient without experiencing urgency or leakage.

Reduced anal canal resting pressures were the most common abnormality seen in the postoperative patient (Nasmyth et al., 1986a; Primrose et al., 1987; O'Connell et al., 1988; Scott et al., 1989). This has been attributed to the sphincter dilatation that is necessary to carry out a mucosectomy and construct an endoanal anastomosis (Keighley et al., 1987; Lavery et al., 1989). It has been reported that stapling the pouch to the anus prevents this reduction in resting anal canal pressures, (Holdsworth & Johnston, 1988) but Seow-Choen et al. (1991) in a randomized controlled study were unable to confirm these findings. They compared pouches which were stapled at the level of the anorectal junction with conventional endoanal anastomosis following mucosectomy carried out at the dentate line. No differences in functional outcome were found.

Attempts to prevent reductions in anal pressures have led to increasing use of stapled pouch anal anastomosis. However, other authors have also reported similar falls in resting sphincter pressures using this technique (Williams et al., 1989). Johnston and his co-workers have reported improved function when compared to historical controls, and maintain that anal function does not deteriorate following stapled ileoanal anastomosis (Landi et al., 1991; Sagar et al., 1991). In these cases function may be better preserved because the authors are undertaking pouch-rectal rather than pouch anal anastomosis (q.v.). In spite of the reductions in pressure regularly seen, continence is satisfactory in most groups, and Levitt and Lewis (1991) suggest incontinence reflects poor case selection especially with regard to patients with previous sphincter injury or decreased function due to age. It is possible that because pouch anal anastomosis is simpler to construct using the stapled technique, that there are fewer septic sequelae, and this in turn accounts for improved function.

Interestingly there may be significant recovery of sphincter function with time (Kmiot *et al.*, 1989), although this is not a universal finding.

Many authors relate emptying frequency to pouch volume and certainly the larger pouches of some series reflect this (Nicholls & Pezim, 1985; Keighley *et al.*, 1988). Stool frequency and efficiency of pouch emptying are also related (O'Connell *et al.*, 1987; Pemberton *et al.*, 1987). Pouch size increases with time (Becker *et al.*, 1985) and accounts for the reduction of stool frequency. This all suggests these factors are interrelated, but increases in pouch volume will only translate into reduced stool frequency if pouch emptying is efficient. A large volume pouch may still have a relatively small functional capacity and a high emptying frequency if it empties only 50% of contents at any given time. Inefficient emptying may also account for both the urgency and leakage experienced by some patients.

Our patients had a median emptying frequency of 5 per 24 hours with a range varying between three and eight times daily. The median nocturnal frequency was one ranging between zero and two. Only five patients could not defer evacuation for less than 1 hour after first awareness of pouch fullness. No patients experienced such urgency that they could not delay pouch emptying for less than 15 minutes. Sixty-eight percent of our patients can differentiate flatus but less than 20% report passing flatus, or indeed the need to do so apart from during defaecation.

The results of Holdsworth and Johnston (1988) are better in this respect, but we believe this may reflect the higher anastomoses, and possibly the retention of an integral rectoanal reflex in their patients. Only one of our patients had a rectoanal reflex postoperatively, and in this case, the anastomosis was 2 cm above the dentate line.

As most patients achieve acceptable continence, it may be argued that retention of the rectoanal inhibitory reflex is not important. Despite the lack of reflex sampling, awareness of the need to evacuate and discrimination are retained and not determined by the presence or absence of sensory upper anal canal epithelium (Beart *et al.*, 1985; Keighley *et al.*, 1987; Pemberton *et al.*, 1987).

From our survey, all our patients are usually or always aware of the need to empty their pouches and few suffer any real urgency. Four of the 60 patients could only defer for between 30 and 60 minutes, the remainder could defer for at least 1 hour. The majority do not have to strain to defaecate and most feel the

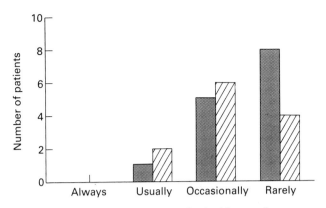

Fig. 6.1 There was little change in the incidence of urgency with time over 12 months. ■, 12 months after ileostomy closure; ▨, 25–36 months after ileostomy closure.

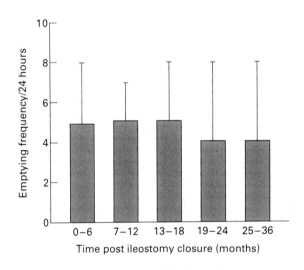

Fig. 6.2 Emptying frequency/24 h. Emptying frequency is constant although there is a trend to decrease with time.

pouch is emptying completely. Only three patients reported a sensation of incomplete evacuation. Forty percent use drugs to reduce emptying frequency. In a more long-term view, comparing patients in the first 6 months after surgery with those 2–3 years after surgery there is little alteration in the incidence of urgency (Fig. 6.1) but in our study neither nocturnal frequency nor overall 24-hour emptying frequency changes with time (Fig. 6.2) in contrast to the improvement reported by Becker *et al.* (1985).

Table 6.2 Pre- and postoperative anorectal physiological measurements.

	Preoperative	Postoperative
24-hour frequency		5 (3–8)
Day frequency		4 (2–7)
Night frequency		1 (0–2)
Sphincter length (cm)	3 (2–4.5)	3 (2–4)
Maximum resting pressure (cmH$_2$O)	110 (35–250)	75 (30–175)*
Maximum voluntary contraction pressure (cmH$_2$O)	240 (90–650)	242.5 (50–450)
Electrosensitivity (mV)		
Lower anal canal	5 (2–15)	5 (2–11)
Mid anal canal	5 (2–15)	6.7 (3–13)*
Upper anal canal	7 (3–26)	12 (5–26)*
First appreciation of reservoir filling (ml)	30 (10–190)	55 (10–255)*
Maximum tolerable reservoir volume (ml)	90 (25–425)	320 (100–700)*
Maximum tolerable reservoir pressure (cmH$_2$O)	80 (25–140)	110 (30–225)*
Reservoir compliance (ml/cmH$_2$O)	1.3 (0.2–4.5)	4 (1.25–16)*

All numbers in brackets are range of medians.
* $p < 0.05$, Wilcoxon signed rank test.

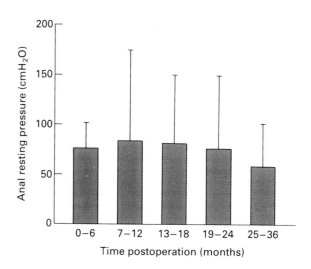

Fig. 6.4 Relationship of anal resting pressure with time. Our figures suggest there is no significant alteration of the resting pressures with increasing postoperative time. All figures were in the normal range.

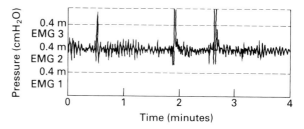

Fig. 6.5 Normal internal anal sphincter electromyogram. EMG 3 is low frequency electromyogram (0.01–10 Hz) showing the normal wave form of anal smooth muscle. (Full scale deflection 0.4 mV.)

Physiological changes with restorative proctocolectomy

Anal canal manometry (Table 6.2)

Pescatori and Parks (1984), Hatakeyama *et al.* (1989), Scott *et al.* (1989) and Lindquist (1990) all report a significant drop in resting sphincter pressures postoperatively although Stryker *et al.* (1986) found pre- and postoperative values did not change significantly. Our patients showed a significant drop after surgery (Fig. 6.3) and studying patients at intervals after surgery reveals no evidence of resting pressure recovery (Fig. 6.4). Indeed, there is in fact a tendency in our studies for resting pressures to drop slightly with time. It is however interesting to look at the electrical activity of the internal anal sphincter after surgery.

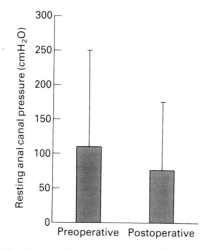

Fig. 6.3 Resting anal canal pressure. There is a significant fall in anal pressures postoperatively. Preoperative pressures were significantly above the normal range and postoperative values were still within the normal range.

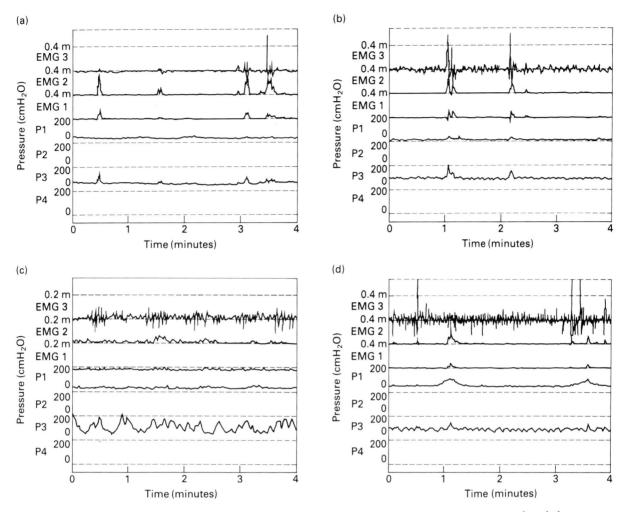

Fig. 6.6 Recovery of internal and sphincter electromyogram with time. (a) Patient 3 months post pouch, (b) patient 12 months post pouch, (c) patient 18 months post pouch, (d) patient 24 months post pouch. These progressive recordings confirm normal function of the somatic sphincters throughout. Recovery of the internal anal sphincter electrical activity is associated with recovery of anal slow pressure waves. There is good recruitment of somatic muscles in response to rises in pouch pressure. EMG 1, integrated puborectalis electromyogram; EMG 2, integrated external anal sphincter; EMG 3, raw internal anal sphincter; P1, pouch pressure; P3, anal canal pressure.

Normal internal anal sphincter electrical activity is shown in Fig. 6.5. Figure 6.6 shows the effect of surgery which almost abolishes electrical activity in the immediate postoperative period. Over the ensuing months there is a stepwise recovery towards more normal activity as the patients are followed up. Recovery of internal sphincter electrical activity can take 12 months or more to occur. In addition, anal slow pressure wave activity is not seen without this recovery of normal internal sphincter EMG activity (Fig. 6.6). Whether or not this electrical recovery represents the slow integration of internal sphincter and ileal neural plexuses remains speculative at present but to date, only one of our patients has a postoperative rectoanal inhibitory reflex. This is the patient described above who had a stapled anastomosis 2 cm above the dentate line. Studies of this patient showed an almost immediate return to normal anal function after closure of the ileostomy with a normal internal sphincter EMG with typical anal slow pressure wave activity (Fig. 6.7). The comparison of this result with the rest of our pouch studies suggests the importance of the distal 1–2 cm of rectum in normal integrated anorectal function. This immediate recovery may also explain the excellent results of Sagar *et al.* (1991) who intentionally leave a short cuff of rectum behind.

The resting pressures recorded preoperatively are in fact higher than our normal control group but this may be related in some way to the colitic activity preoperatively (Loening-Baucke *et al.*, 1989). Disruption

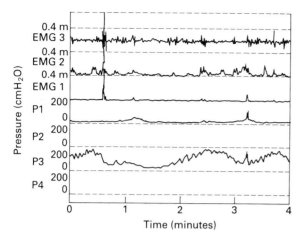

Fig. 6.7 Early function following stapled restorative proctocolectomy, 2 cm above the dentate line. The mark is an awareness of presence of flatus. The pressure recordings show a typical sampling reflex with equilibration of anal and rectal pressures and relaxation of the internal anal sphincter electromyogram. EMG 1, integrated puborectalis electromyogram; EMG 2, integrated external anal sphincter electromyogram; EMG 3, raw internal anal sphincter electromyogram; P1, pouch pressure; P3, anal canal pressure.

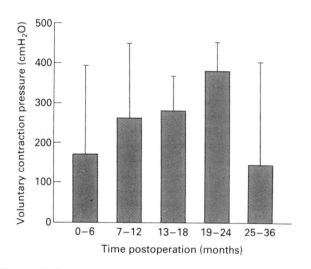

Fig. 6.8 Voluntary contraction pressure. This remains unaffected by surgery and lies within the normal range. There is no difference with postoperative time.

of the excitatory rectal neural connections leaves the internal anal sphincter with predominantly myogenic activity. Restoration of electrical activity may well reflect the recovery of a neurogenic element to the resting anal pressure and hence be responsible for the rise in pressure seen with time by some authors.

Rectal excision as carried out for restorative proctocolectomy does not interfere with somatic sphincter function. Thus like others, we did not find any reduc-

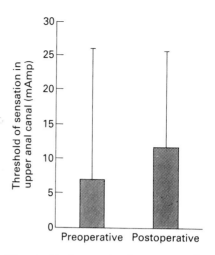

Fig. 6.9 Threshold of sensation in upper anal canal. Typical increase in threshold levels for anal sensitivity to electrical stimuli. Similar changes are found in the mid anal canal, though the increase is less marked.

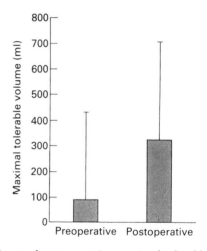

Fig. 6.10 Pre- and postoperative maximal tolerable volume. This confirms the significant increase in capacity between the diseased rectum and the pouch.

tions in measurements of postoperative sphincter voluntary contraction pressures. Longitudinal studies were carried on our patients, these did not alter with time (Fig. 6.8).

Anal canal sensitivity

The results of mucosectomy are discussed in detail below. In brief while lower anal canal sensation did not change postoperatively, the threshold of sensitivity rises after surgery in the mid and upper canal, this change being most pronounced in the upper canal (Fig. 6.9).

Pouch variables

The rectum and pelvic floor are responsible for appreciation of filling in normal individuals (Winckler, 1958; Öresland *et al.*, 1990). While most have emphasized the importance of the pelvic floor, the small volumes of stool in the diseased rectum that cause severe urgency in many colitic patients suggest the rectal component may be very important, since the colitis is not likely to affect the deep seated pelvic floor proprioceptors. It should not be expected that ileal and rectal walls would have similar sensations mediated by stretch receptors. The increase in volume seen for simple awareness of filling, and the change in the maximum tolerable volume (Fig. 6.10) from less than 100 ml preoperatively to a capacity of over 300 ml after pouch construction underline the importance of neorectal capacity in relation to the functional outcome. The pouch is better able to cope with higher filling pressures and this volume–pressure relationship is reflected in the high compliance of the reservoir. Although Becker *et al.* (1985), and Dozois *et al.* (1986) suggest capacity and compliance rise with time, in our patients maximum pouch volume and compliance are reached rapidly after operation, certainly within the first 3 months, and the long-term results show that these values are maintained but not improved upon (Fig. 6.11).

Overall we feel function after surgery is related to both anal and pouch variables. Indubitably anal pressures and the somatic sphincter response to challenge are important, but probably of more importance is the pouch capacity and compliance as previously discussed. There are still some interesting unanswered questions about pouch physiology and we will attempt to address these below.

Does pouch configuration affect functional outcome?

Since functional outcome seems to be related to the volume of the pouch, many studies have concentrated on pouch design. The initial S configuration with the long efferent limb described by Parks *et al.* (1980) has fallen into disrepute because of the associated emptying difficulties. Our series contains two S pouches, both done for purely technical reasons, one of which needs to catheterize to evacuate efficiently. Because of the tendency of the efferent limb to elongate, and lead to problems with evacuation, we normally avoid S pouches, since it is normally possible to obtain adequate length with a J or W configuration. If length is a problem, then, it is normally straightforward to staple the ileoanal anastomosis since length is far less critical with this technique.

The more ileum used to construct the pouch, the larger its volume. Overall four-limb W pouches are larger than three-limbed S pouches and two-limbed Js (Nicholls & Pezim, 1985; Nasmyth *et al.*, 1986b, Nicholls & Lubowski, 1987; Everett, 1989). The main difficulty in assessing the various designs has been the variable amount of ileum used for the pouch limbs. We have endeavoured to use approximately 40 cm of ileum for both the J and W configured pouches and believe that the pouch volume is often limited by the available pelvic space rather than by the configuration. A W

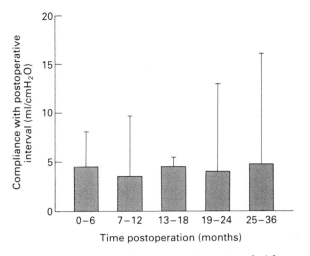

Fig. 6.11 Compliance with postoperative interval. After a very rapid adaption in the first week the compliance of pouches remains constant.

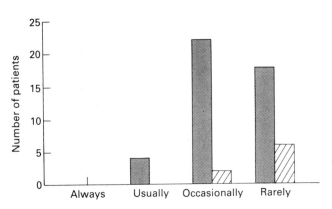

Fig. 6.12 Urgency of emptying J and W pouches. There are similar proportions in both groups. The J pouch is not associated with increased urgency. ■, J pouch; ▨, W pouch.

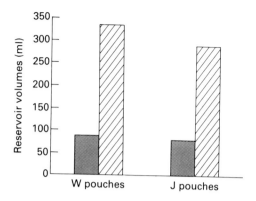

Fig. 6.13 Pre- and postoperative reservoir volumes in J and W pouches. Both J and W pouches have similar final volumes that reflects their similar functional state. ▩, preoperative; ▨, postoperative.

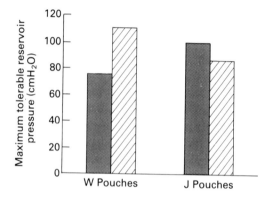

Fig. 6.14 Maximum tolerable reservoir pressure in J and W pouches. W pouches tolerate significantly higher post-operative pressures. ▩, preoperative; ▨, postoperative.

pouch in a small male pelvis will have a different final capacity compared to one in a wide female pelvis.

Our own studies show a daily emptying frequency of five (range 3–8) for W pouches and five (3 to 6) for J pouches. Similar proportions in both groups can defer emptying for greater than 1 hour, and can differentiate and pass flatus. Three of our W pouch patients require to catheterize for complete emptying compared to none in the J group. There are similar proportions in both groups who are aware of the need to evacuate and few in either group experience any urgency (Fig. 6.12).

Routine manometric and sensory assessment of the anal canal is identical in both groups, nor should they be different. The maximum filling volume for both pouch types is similar (Fig. 6.13) although W pouches tolerated significantly higher filling pressure before urgency occurred (Fig. 6.14). Pouch compliance was similar for both designs. Keighley *et al.* (1988) reported

similar findings and like our own unit, used similar lengths of bowel for the formation of both pouch types. This simply confirms the difficulty in comparing pouch designs between units. We believe that using our technique, functional results of W and J pouches are similar and this leaves the surgeon in a position to choose the configuration to suit each patient without the worry of inferior results from one or other pouch design.

Does a stapled anastomosis improve the functional result?

Normal continence is a complex phenomenon but we know that one of the major factors is the resting pressure of the anal canal and the pressure response of the muscles to challenge (Bartolo *et al.*, 1986). Anal stretching reduces anal pressure partly by disrupting the internal sphincter fibres and we recognize that a small proportion of patients experience seepage of pouch contents in the early postoperative period. Nasmyth *et al.* (1986a) considered anal resting pressure one of the most important determinants of functional outcome. Keighley *et al.* (1988) reported that patients with less than perfect continence have lower pressures. Similar postoperative drops in pressures have been recorded by most other authors.

To undertake a mucosectomy and endoanal anastomosis requires at least some dilatation of the anal canal, and it has been suggested this trauma may be minimized by the use of a stapled as opposed to handsewn anastomosis. Williams *et al.* (1989) have shown that even stapled anastomosis, while in their hands being superior to a handsewn anastomosis, are

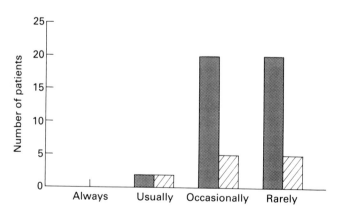

Fig. 6.15 Comparison of urgency of emptying, between stapled and sewn anastomoses. The proportions in both groups were similar. ▩, sewn; ▨, stapled.

associated with significant sphincter impairment. This is not therefore due to prolonged anal retraction; Seow-Choen *et al.* (1991) have shown no difference in functional outcome comparing a stapled and sutured anastomosis. The drop in pressure seen after either procedure may therefore be due to the impairment of the electrical activity of the sphincter caused by removal of the neural connections from the distal rectum. In addition to this drop in pressure there is of course the potential for sphincter injury if prolonged anal retraction is required for the mucosectomy and endoanal anastomosis. We attempt to reduce this risk by the use of Gelpi retractors rather than the more conventional bladed retractors. We believe these allow adequate access for safe surgery with minimal retraction.

In our hands, the functional results following endoanal and stapled anastomoses were similar. The emptying frequency was 5/24 hours and there was no difference in the proportion of patients suffering anal seepage, nor in the ability to discriminate and pass flatus successfully. Urgency to evacuate and the awareness of the need to evacuate were similar in both groups (Fig. 6.15).

The use of the Gelpi retractors has resulted in no additional reduction in anal pressure in the handsewn group (Fig. 6.16) although there was still a significant drop in pressure compared to preoperative values. The excellent results reported by the Leeds group (Sagar *et al.*, 1991) require more careful interpretation since they indubitably do pouch–rectal anastomoses pre-

serving 1–2 cm of rectum and therefore do not disturb the neural input to the same extent as when the anastomosis is close to the dentate line. Landi *et al.* (1990) reported a series of patients in whom stapled anastomoses were constructed above the transitional zone. They showed no significant fall in resting pressure using a stapling technique. It is difficult to ascertain the precise level of the anastomotic line in this series.

Overall we conclude that careful anal retraction does not itself damage the sphincter more than the rectal dissection and transection itself. There seems no good evidence to support the view that stapled anastomosis should be undertaken for functional reasons. Moreover, introduction of the circular stapler dilates the anus, and reductions in anal pressure were reported by Kirwan *et al.* (1989) following low rectal anastomoses using this technique, so it is difficult to understand why the same factors should not prevail following ileoanal anastomosis.

What remains to be seen is whether in the long term, patients develop cancers in the small distal rectal remnant. If function is better, then there may be a good case for adopting the Leeds policy so long as the long-term cost does not outweigh this. There is no doubt that it is much easier to staple the pouch to the top of the anus or distal rectum. Clearly patients with dysplasia should have a complete mucosectomy if possible, but even then, islands of colitic mucosa are preserved. It is too early to answer many of these questions, and what is important, is for the major centres carefully to audit the outcome, in order to try and answer these important questions.

Is preservation of the anal transitional zone important?

The importance of the anal sampling reflex in sensory discrimination of rectal contents is well known. Duthie and Gairns (1960) first described the sensory supply of the anal canal and postulated the importance of sampling in continence (Duthie & Bennett, 1963). We have shown defective sampling in incontinent individuals (Miller *et al.*, 1988a) and it seems logical to assume that pouch patients undergoing mucosectomy, in whom the upper anal canal lining is stripped off to remove all potentially diseased mucosa, will have impaired sensation. It may also be implicit that retained awareness might allow improved functional results.

In our series approximately half of the patients have had a complete mucosectomy to the dentate line.

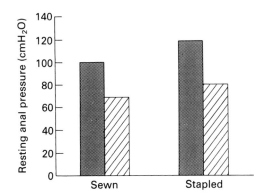

Fig. 6.16 Pre- and postoperative resting anal pressures in the handsewn and stapled ileoanal anastomosis groups. Postoperative pressures were significantly below preoperative values, but were similar for both groups. The results do not suggest an advantage for stapled anastomoses. ▨, preoperative; ▨, postoperative.

The remainder had a variable amount of transitional mucosa retained above this level. This has made no significant difference to emptying frequency either during the day or night. In addition continence did not differ between the two groups. Thus retention of the transitional zone did not translate into improved function. Five patients had anal seepage after mucosectomy, and four patients experienced similar symptoms in the group where the mucosa was left intact. These results are similar to those reported by Keighley *et al.* (1987). Holdsworth and Johnston (1988) record improved ability to discriminate and pass flatus successfully in patients where the anal transitional zone was retained but our own results suggest there is no difference between these groups. The Leeds group noted a large proportion of patients with recovery of the rectoanal reflex in the patients who did not undergo mucosectomy. This suggests 1–2 cm of rectum and normal rectal mucosa is being retained in this group since these local reflexes appear to be dependent on rectal input. It is conceivable that retention of a longer rectal cuff aids this even after mucosectomy.

It could be postulated that safe passage of flatus depends on the integrity of this reflex rather than intact sensation. In fact Read and Read (1982) found no deterioration in continence during rectal infusion of saline when anal canal sensation was reduced by the use of topical anaesthetics, although in this study, no measurements of anal sensation were carried out, so it really was not clear how much sensation was abolished during their studies. It appears that although anal sensation may have a role to play in fine tuning, it is not a major determinant of continence.

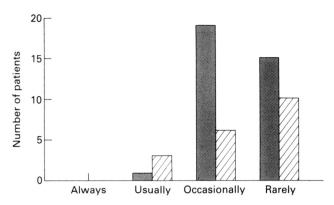

Fig. 6.18 Urgency of emptying is not increased with excision of the anal transitional zone. Neither group suffers urgency of emptying with any regularity and the proportions in the groups are not significantly different. ■, excised; ▨, retained.

Functionally we found no difference in the awareness of the need to evacuate (Fig. 6.17), nor did we have any evidence that reduced sensation leads to greater urgency (Fig. 6.18). Seow-Choen *et al.* (1991) similarly report no detrimental effects on function as a result of a formal mucosectomy. It may be that function depends more on the pelvic floor stretch receptors, although Öresland *et al.* (1990) have shown that the rectal wall itself has some role to play in detecting the need to empty.

Overall, our results and those of other authors (Keighley *et al.*, 1987, Seow-Choen *et al.*, 1991) suggest the anal transitional zone may be removed without affecting continence adversely. Since this area has potentially colitic mucosa, and therefore the potential for malignancy we believe this zone should be excised where practicable.

Continence and ileoanal pouch function

One of the main dilemmas with regard to pouch function is the incidence of incontinence. The majority of patients are continent preoperatively, although urgency due to acute colitis is known to overwhelm normal sphincters in otherwise normal individuals. For restorative proctocolectomy to be acceptable, it is essential that continence is maintained in this young group of patients. Incontinence rates vary from 47 to 0% (Martin & Fischer 1982; Williams & Johnston, 1984; Nicholls 1984; Rothenberger *et al.*, 1985; King *et al.*, 1987; Seow-Choen *et al.*, 1991), but the degree of incontinence varies from minor soiling to serious incontinence. The investigation and minimization of this

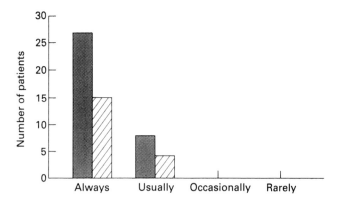

Fig. 6.17 Awareness of emptying is independent of the anal transitional zone. The presence or absence of the anal transitional zone does not affect patients' ability to perceive the need to empty their pouches. ■, excised transitional zone; ▨, retained transitional zone.

problem is imperative if continence is to be improved in this procedure.

It has been suggested that incontinence may be due to excessive anal sphincter stretching during ileo-anal anastomosis (Becker 1984; Keighley *et al.*, 1988; Luukkonen 1988 and Lavery *et al.*, 1989). However Williams *et al.* (1989) suggest that a stapled anastomosis will still result in sphincter pressure reduction despite the lack of anal stretch, and this reduction in pressure was confirmed by Johnston *et al.* (1987) and Seow-Choen *et al.* (1991). Pemberton (1991) related continence mainly to pouch reservoir function and compliance. This is the most plausible theory. High pressure pouch waves are associated with a desire to empty and a degree of urgency (Heppel *et al.*, 1987; Stryker *et al.*, 1986; O'Connell *et al.*, 1987). The abolition of these waves after pouch emptying, and the increased frequency of these waves during pouch filling all confirm their relevance to pouch function. During nocturnal studies, we have shown that high pressure waves exceed anal canal pressures. This suggests pouch filling, compliance and the anal pressure response to pressure waves are important in continence and leakage.

Our own experience relates to nine patients with pouch leakage. We have been fortunate not to have any patient with frank incontinence and only three of these patients routinely use pads emphasizing the minor nature of their problems. Only three out of nine have recorded leaks during the day and this occurs only on about 1 day per week. Only one of the patients reporting anal seepage used pads during the day. Interestingly, a further three continent patients use pads diurnally mainly because of anxiety that leakage might occur, and report lack of confidence as the principle reason. We have demonstrated that in our hands, postoperative anal pressures after endoanal sutured and stapled anastomoses are similar. This has been discussed, on p. 91. The ratio of patients reporting seepage following sewn or stapled anastomoses was 7:2 which was not a significant difference. This suggests a carefully constructed endo-anal anastomosis is not inferior with respect to function. A similar picture was seen when we compared the ratios of patients with excised and retained anal transitional zones, in whom there was no significant difference in upper and mid anal canal sensitivity. There was a trend for patients with seepage to have poorer sensation (Fig. 6.19). A similar trend was also found with respect to awareness of pouch filling. There were no differences in maximum

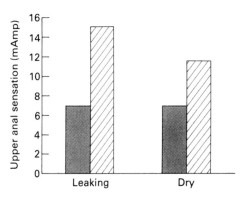

Fig. 6.19 Upper anal sensation in patients with seepage and in those with perfect continence. This is impaired more in seeping patients in the postoperative period although the change is not significant. ■, preoperative; ▨, postoperative.

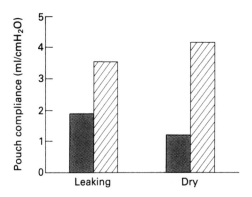

Fig. 6.20 Pouch compliance in leaking and dry patients. Pouch compliance is significantly higher postoperatively in those with perfect continence. ■, preoperative; ▨, postoperative.

pouch volumes in these patients (incontinent = 320-ml median, continent = 315 ml), but the pouch compliance was higher in the continent group (Fig. 6.20). This suggests pouch filling, volume and sensitivity to filling are closely related to the functional outcome.

Emptying frequencies in our two groups were similar (median five per 24 hours, 1 per night). Three patients initially experienced troublesome leakage which was abolished by catheterization. This suggests that emptying was inefficient as one would not expect catheterization to prevent leakage in the presence of impaired sphincter function. One elderly patient was normally continent during the daytime, but leaked at night. She had a large pouch which was not emptying efficiently. Her leakage was abolished by emptying her pouch with a catheter before retiring. In a further patient, leakage was almost abolished by division of a pouch

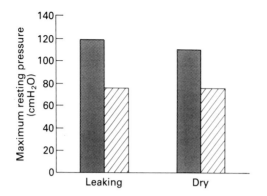

Fig. 6.21 Pre- and postoperative maximum resting pressures comparing leaking and dry patients. Both groups show a significant drop postoperatively but there is no difference between the groups. ■, preoperative; ▨, postoperative.

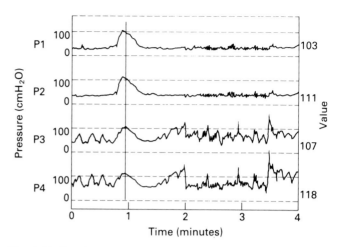

Fig. 6.22 Pouch pressure waves during daytime recording. P1 and P2, pouch pressure; P3, upper anal canal pressure; P4, mid anal canal pressure. The pouch pressure wave seen in P1 and P2 is covered by the anal canal pressure response in channels 3 and 4 resulting in a continent pressure gradient.

anal anastomosic stricture. All these patients were failing to empty their pouches adequately, supporting the conclusion that leakage was the result of poor emptying although this has only been deduced in most instances by clinical assessment including endoscopy following pouch evacuation. One patient with frequency (21/day), suffering urgency and leakage gained excellent function once his pouch was emptied with regular catheterization. Here once more, impaired emptying explained his dysfunction. Pemberton (1991) suggests patients with poor evacuation have increased frequency as they have less filling reserve and O'Connell *et al.* (1988) has directly related stool frequency with output volume. Our patients with seepage have significantly greater urgency of emptying than our continent group tending to confirm this thesis.

Resting anal canal pressures surprisingly, do not appear to correlate with continence. Patients who experience seepage, compared to those with perfect continence had similar anal sphincter pressures. Moreover, preoperative values did not discriminate between them or predict which patients would have less than perfect control (Fig. 6.21).

We attempted to elucidate the pathophysiology of nocturnal seepage in a study in which we compared the findings in 10 normal controls, 10 patients with perfect continence following restorative proctocolectomy, and five patients who experienced nocturnal seepage, and wore pads (Duthie & Bartolo, 1990). The patients were studied using the ambulatory system described on p. 87, which allowed recordings to be made during sleep in the patients' homes. Average ambulatory daytime anal pressures were similar in all three groups. At night, anal pressures fell in normal subjects and

following restorative proctocolectomy. However, anal pressures were significantly lower in the pouch patients compared to the normal controls. Despite this, anal pressure measurements did not discriminate *per se* between those with seepage and those with perfect continence. Although pressures were lower in those with leakage, this difference was not significant.

High pressure pouch waves were detected in 80% of the patients with impaired continence during prolonged ambulatory manometry, with an average frequency of 5 per hour. During the daytime, none of the patients reported leakage of pouch contents. Pouch pressures during reservoir contractions tended to approach anal pressures, but no episodes of leakage were reported despite this, and continence was maintained. During these instances, the anal canal pressure response was sufficient to maintain a continent pressure gradient (Fig. 6.22). The same scenario was perpetuated at night, except that during a quarter of the recorded high pressure pouch contractions, pouch pressures exceeded the anal canal pressure response. We concluded that these pouch contractions which were not compensated for by an adequate sphincter response caused leakage. Similar inversion of the pouch anal pressure gradient was not observed at night-time during recordings from the patients with perfect continence (Fig. 6.23).

These studies indicate that function is determined primarily by pouch variables. We cannot from these

(a)

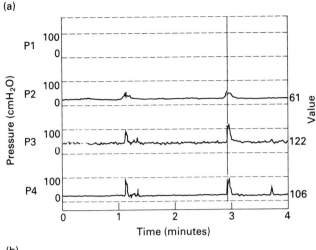

(b)

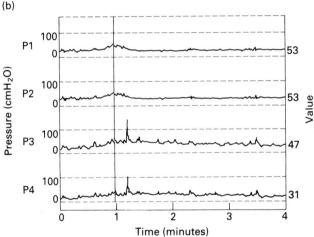

Fig. 6.23 Pouch pressure waves during nocturnal recording. P1 and P2, pouch pressure channels; P3, upper anal canal pressure; P4, mid anal canal pressure. (a) Upper figure 04.57 h pouch pressure waves are well covered by the anal sphincter response. (b) Lower figure at 00.28 h shows a pressure wave that elicits a poor anal pressure response with a pressure gradient in favour of incontinence, and a delayed external sphincter response.

studies prove that pouch design was the cause of high pressure contractions, but we suspect they might be prevented in larger pouches. Against this hypothesis were our findings in an earlier study of ambulant pouch motility (Miller *et al.*, 1990). High pressure pouch waves were seen in a patient with nocturnal leakage who had a very large pouch which emptied inefficiently (see above). This however, may simply reflect a reduced functional capacity due to a large residual stool volume. Thus increasing pouch volume will only translate into better function when emptying is efficient.

Pouch motility is clearly important, and hypermotility

appears to be the prime cause of nocturnal leakage. It may be possible to prevent these high pressure phenomena by pharmacological manipulation, but to date no studies have been carried out to try and modify pouch motility. We could not ascribe these waves to pouchitis, since none of the patients studied had significant pouch inflammation. Pelvic sepsis may cause fibrosis and lead to impairment of function, but again, none of the patients had sepsis to account for impaired function.

Resting anal pressures are not directly related to leakage, except during these waves, and when they are due to poor emptying, then catheterization will improve pouch emptying and give the patient an acceptably functioning pouch.

Patients presenting with incontinence require investigation of pouch emptying as a priority but it may be appropriate simply to assess residual volume after emptying rather than embark on more complex radiological investigations. Simple catheterization or correction of outflow obstruction, for example due to a pouch-anal stricture may restore continence or certainly limit the disability associated with this problem.

Is restorative proctocolectomy an appropriate procedure in older patients?

The majority of series report on pouch function in patients who are aged under 50, in whom function is normally expected to be satisfactory. There has been a tendency to exclude older patients, and recommend total proctocolectomy and ileostomy because of fears about the functional outcome. There is good evidence that anal function deteriorates with age (McHugh & Diament, 1987; Laurberg & Swash, 1989) and the reluctance to perform pouch procedures in older patients appears to be based on this. Attitudes are, however, changing. Keighley and Kmiot (1990) and Lewis *et al.* (1991) report that they are prepared to restore intestinal continuity in patients up to 65 years of age providing anal function is satisfactory preoperatively.

We have adopted a liberal selection policy in our unit and have been prepared, after fully counselling older patients, to carry out restorative pouch procedures on any older patients who are fit enough. Indeed in many ways, the operative procedure is simpler, as a perineal wound can be avoided, and we do not find the operative procedure is any more traumatic than a total proctocolectomy and end ileostomy.

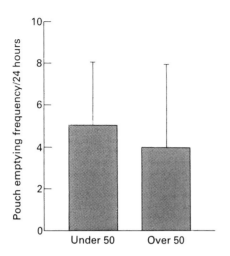

Fig. 6.24 Pouch emptying frequency comparing patients under and over 50 years old. There is no difference between the groups.

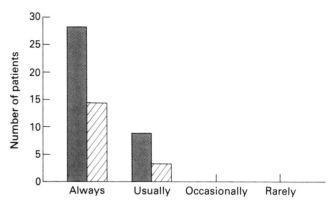

Fig. 6.25 Awareness of need to evacuate. In both younger and older patients there was satisfactory awareness of the need to empty the pouch. ▓, under 50 years; ▨, over 50 years.

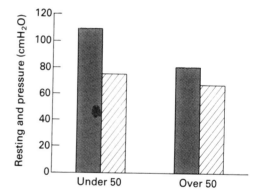

Fig. 6.26 Pre- and postoperative resting anal pressures in young and older patients. Both groups fall significantly in the postoperative period but older patients had significantly lower pressures preoperatively. ▓, preoperative; ▨, postoperative.

We compared the outcome in patients who were older than 50, with the younger ones, and assessed the functional outcome. Forty-two patients (median age 35.5, range 17–47) in the younger group were compared with seventeen older patients (median age 60, range 50–71). The cut off for the groups was 50 years of age.

More of the younger group had a three-staged procedure (17 vs. 5) and this simply reflected the more acute presentation of colitis in this group. The sex ratios were similar for the two groups.

There were 10 stapled anastomoses in young patients, and four in the group aged 50 or greater. Three of the former, and one in the latter group used a catheter to empty their pouches because of inefficient emptying. The overall pouch emptying frequency was not significantly different (Fig. 6.24) with ranges of 3–8 per 24-hour period in both groups. The median nocturnal frequency of once a night was again similar. Minimal soiling of underclothes was seen in seven younger and two older patients but was not considered by the patients to be significant and in fact only five out of these nine wore pads as protection emphasizing the minor nature of the problem. Poorer anal function might have been expected to result in a higher incidence of urgency in the older group, but only one patient compared with four in the younger group complained of any significant urgency of defaecation. This was not a major problem, as they simply reported they could not defer for an hour when an urge to defaecate was felt. In addition, the ability to discri-

minate between gas and stool, was similar for old and young patients. In the under 50s group, 27 patients accurately discriminated flatus, and seven were secure enough to pass it, while in the older group, the numbers were 14 and three respectively. It was noted that both groups rarely felt the need to pass flatus, and most were only confident to pass it while lying on their side in bed.

Older patients appeared to complain less of abdominal colic. Both groups were similar in appreciating awareness of the need to empty their pouches (Fig. 6.25) and rarely had urgency.

Physiologically older patients had significantly worse baseline sphincter function compared to the younger group but both results fell within our normal range (median 85, range 50–140 cmH$_2$O). Interestingly in

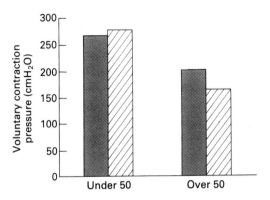

Fig. 6.27 Pre- and postoperative voluntary contraction pressures in young and older patients. Although older patients had significantly poorer anal function, in neither group was the contraction pressure significantly affected by surgery. ▓ , preoperative; ▨ , postoperative.

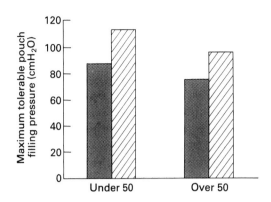

Fig. 6.28 Maximum tolerable pre- and postoperative pouch-filling pressures. A significant improvement was seen in both groups in keeping with removal of the non-compliant rectum. ▓ , preoperative; ▨ , postoperative.

both groups, pressures fell postoperatively to similar levels (Fig. 6.26). This might be in keeping with our previous hypothesis that rectal excision affects the modulation of sphincter pressures by removal of the intrinsic neural connections thereby leaving pressures in the postoperative period that reflect the intrinsic myogenic tone alone.

A similar picture was seen in the results of pre-operative voluntary contraction sphincter pressures (Fig. 6.27), the older had significantly poorer function (Table 6.3) but as expected the surgery itself had little effect on this, since the pelvic nerves remained undisturbed.

The anal transition zone was excised in 16 out of 42 younger patients and in 5 out of 12 older. This is reflected in the almost identical lower anal canal sensa-tion of both groups and the progressive widening of the pre- and postoperative sensory thresholds in the mid and upper anal canals, although none of these results (Table 6.3) attained significance within the groups as a whole. This related well to the awareness of emptying and lack of urgency previously recorded. Rectal sensation seems less acute after surgery and although the majority of this sensory input is reputed to come from pelvic floor muscle spindles, the loss of sensitivity does suggest some input comes from the

Table 6.3 Older vs. younger (<50 years) patients: a comparison of manometric and sensory data.

	Under 50 Years		Over 50 Years	
	Preoperative	Postoperative	Preoperative	Postoperative
Sphincter length (cm)	3 (2–4.5)	3 (2–4)	3.5 (2–4)	3 (2–4)
Maximum resting pressure (cmH$_2$O)	110 (70–250)[†]	75 (30–175)*	80 (35–125)	68 (35–150)*
Maximum voluntary contraction (cmH$_2$O)	270 (90–650)[†]	280 (100–450)	200 (100–275)	163 (50–400)
Electrosensitivity (mV)				
Mid anal canal	5 (2–15)	6 (3–13)	5 (3–10)	7 (4–13)
Upper anal canal	7 (3–26)	11 (5–26)*	9 (3–26)	13 (5–26)*
Threshold of first reservoir sensation (ml)	30 (10–130)	53 (10–250)*	30 (10–190)	60 (25–120)
Maximum tolerable reservoir volume (ml)	80 (40–425)	305 (100–700)*	110 (25–280)	340 (150–550)*
Reservoir compliance (ml/cmH$_2$O)	1.1 (0.3–4.5)	3.9 (1.3–16)*	1.6 (0.2–3.5)	5.2 (2.3–13)*

Numbers in brackets are range of frequency medians.
* Significant preoperative vs. postoperative: $p < 0.05$.
[†] Significant >50 vs. <50: $p < 0.05$.

rectum itself in keeping with the findings of Öresland *et al.* (1990). In addition the argument of this perceived change being due to the removal of the uncompliant diseased rectum still holds and the increased tolerance to higher filling pressures (Fig. 6.28) and increased compliance in both groups lends support to this argument.

Overall there seems no good evidence to suggest these procedures constitute a greater risk in more elderly patients despite the significantly poorer anal sphincter function. We would suggest that restorative proctocolectomy should be considered whenever a proctocolectomy is being carried out. Our only contraindication to such surgery would be severely impaired sphincter function prior to surgery.

Summary

Physiological testing has allowed us to carefully audit the effects of restorative proctocolectomy. We have been able to understand the pathophysiology of nocturnal anal seepage and objectively assess function. It does not predict function. We firmly believe that no patient should be denied reconstructive surgery on the basis of physiology testing. We could not correlate preoperative resting or squeeze pressures with outcome. Moreover, incontinence before surgery is usually the result of a rigid non-compliant rectum. Clearly a patient with obstetric trauma, or one who has had his sphincters divided for fistulae will be expected to have incontinence following restorative proctocolectomy. This is a clinical assessment which is different from finding that pressures are rather low and advising the patient against reconstructive surgery.

Restorative proctocolectomy is clearly the procedure of choice for the vast majority of patients with ulcerative colitis irrespective of age, so long as the patients are fit enough to cope with the procedure and its implications. Our data suggest that age *per se* should not preclude reconstructive surgery. If patients are to have an endo-anal anastomosis, then a mucosectomy can be carried out to the dentate line without anxieties about compromising ultimate function. Although there is evidence of improved anal sensitivity when the anal columns are preserved, this does not in our experience translate into better function. We do believe anal retraction should be kept to a minimum. Clearly if the internal anal sphincter is damaged by over zealous retraction, low pressures will ensue, and this is likely to be associated with impaired function. Pouch design does not appear to be important, so long as the pouch is of adequate volume. In this respect we are in agreement with Hultén (see Chapter 7). His group has shown that smaller pouches give rise to poorer function, and this is in agreement with the details outlined by Nicholls (see Chapter 5). We do not favour the S pouch design since it does tend to be associated with outlet obstruction even if the efferent limb is kept short.

The two areas which are currently causing the most debate are whether the ileoanal anastomosis should be stapled or sutured. If the anastomosis is stapled to the dentate line there does not appear to be any advantage for either method. The improved results reported by Johnston and his co-workers are most interesting, and clearly need to be taken on board. If function is indeed better with preservation of the most distal rectum, and there are both anatomic and physiologic advantages for believing this, then their approach may be the correct one. The disadvantage is the potential for recurrent symptoms and the risk of carcinoma. This is obviously small, but is a real one that should not be ignored. There is clearly a functional advantage compared to ileorectal anastomosis where the rectal reservoir is non-compliant, and urgency is a major disadvantage. The principal gain with restorative proctocolectomy is that most patients achieve socially acceptable defaecation without urgency. The majority of patients with colitis severe enough to warrant surgery will have urgency that interferes with everyday activity, to the extent that it stops them pursuing activities or employment where the lack of proximity to a toilet would risk embarrassing incontinence. If in addition, the operation carried out in this fashion does not require an ileostomy, then it has even more to commend it. Ileorectal anastomosis fell into disrepute because of late cancer development. To some extent we may be following the same paths with what can be described as near total proctocolectomy. The purist will argue that the disease should be eradicated, and the results in the majority justify this approach. For the minority with poor function, the price is too high. On the other hand, patients with polyposis, and those who are having surgery either because of dysplasia or carcinoma must surely have the whole of their diseased mucosa excised.

It is clearly important for the surgeon to be conversant with all the available options and be able to tailor the surgery to the disease. A rigid approach is counterproductive and as in all other branches of surgery, treatment should complement the patient's requirements.

References

Bartolo DCC, Roe AM, Locke-Edmunds JC, Virjee J, Mortensen NJMCC (1986) Flap valve theory of anorectal incontinence. *Br J Surg* **73**:1012–1014.

Beart RW, Dozois RR, Wolff BG, Pemberton JH (1985) Mechanisms of rectal continence: lessons from the ileoanal procedure. *Am J Surg* **149**:31–34.

Becker JM (1984) Anal sphincter function after colectomy, mucosal proctectomy and endorectal ileoanal pull-through. *Arch Surg* **119**:526–531.

Becker JM, Hillard AE, Mann FA, Kestenberg A, Nelson JA (1985) Functional assessment after colectomy, mucosal proctectomy, and endorectal pullthrough. *World J Surg* **9**: 598–605.

Dozois RR, Goldberg SM, Rothenberger DA, Utsonomiya J, Nicholls RJ, Cohen Z, Hutten L, Moskowitz RL, Williams NS (1986) Restorative proctocolectomy with ilial reservoir. *Int J Colorectal Dis* **1**:2–19.

Duthie GS, Bartolo DCC (1990) Nocturnal leakage is related to high pressure pouch waves following restorative proctocolectomy. *Br J Surg* **77**:A699.

Duthie GS, Bartolo DCC (1992) Abdominal rectopexy for rectal prolapse: a comparison of techniques. *Br J Surg* **79**: 107–113.

Duthie HL, Bennett RC (1963) The relation of sensation in the anal canal to the functional anal sphincter: a possible factor in anal continence. *Gut* **4**:179–182.

Duthie HL, Gairns FW (1960) Sensory nerve endings and sensation in the anal region in man. *Br J Surg* **47**:585–595.

Everett WG (1989) Experience of restorative proctocolectomy with ileal reservoir. *Br J Surg* **76**:77–81.

Hatakeyama K, Yamai K, Muto T (1989) Evaluation of ileal W pouch anal anastomosis for restorative proctocolectomy. *Int J Colorectal Dis* **4**:150–155.

Heppell J, Belliveau P, Taillefer R, Dubé S, Derbekyan V (1987) Quantitive assessment of pelvic ileal reservoir emptying with a semisolid radionucleotide enema. *Dis Colon Rectum* **30**:81–85.

Holdsworth PJ, Johnston D (1988) Anal sensation after restorative proctocolectomy for ulcerative colitis. *Br J Surg* **75**:993–996.

Johnston D, Holdsworth PJ, Nasmyth DG *et al.* (1987) Preservation of the entire anal canal in conservative proctocolectomy for ulcerative colitis: a pilot study comparing end to end ileo-anal anastomosis without mucosal resection with proctectomy and endo-anal anastomosis. *Br J Surg* **74**:940–944.

Keighley MRB, Kmiot W (1990) Surgical options in ulcerative colitis: role of ileo-anal anastomosis. *Aust NZ J Surg* **60**: 835–848.

Keighley MRB, Winslet MC, Yoshioka K, Lightwood R (1987) Discrimination is not impaired by excision of the anal transition zone after restorative proctocolectomy. *Br J Surg* **74**:1118–1121.

Keighley MRB, Yoshioka K, Kmiot W, Heyen F (1988) Physiological parameters influencing function in restorative proctocolectomy and ileo-pouch-anal anastomosis. *Br J Surg* **75**:997–1002.

King DW, Lubowski DZ, Talley NA, Pryor DS (1987) Restorative proctocolectomy with ileal reservoir and ileoanal anastomosis: a clinico-physiological study. *Aust. NZ J Surg* **57**:555–558.

Kirwan WA, O'Riordan MG, Waldron R (1989) Declining indications for abdominoperineal resection. *Br J Surg* **76**: 1061–1063.

Kmiot WA, Pinho M, Yoshioka K, Keighley MRB (1989) Does anal function improve following restorative proctocolectomy? *Br J Surg* **76**:63–66.

Landi E, Fianchini A, Landa L *et al.* (1990) Proctocolectomy and stapled ileo-anal anastomosis without mucosal proctectomy. *Int J Colorectal Dis* **5**:151–154.

Laurberg S, Swash M (1989) Effects of aging on the anorectal sphincters and their innervation. *Dis Colon Rectum* **32**: 737–742.

Lavery IC, Tuckson WB, Easley KA (1989) Internal anal sphincter function after total abdominal colectomy and stapled ileal pouch-anal anastomosis without mucosal proctectomy. *Dis Colon Rectum* **32**:950–953

Levitt MD, Lewis AAM (1991) Determinants of ileoanal pouch function. *Gut* **32**:126–127.

Lewis W, Holdsworth PJ, Sagar P, Johnston D (1992) Results of restorative proctocolectomy in patients over the age of 50 years. *Gut* in press.

Lindquist K (1990) Anal manometry with microtransducer technique before and after restorative proctocolectomy. *Dis Colon Rectum* **33**:91–98.

Loening-Baucke V, Metcalf AM, Shirazi S (1989) Anorectal manometry in active and quiescent ulcerative colitis. *Am J Gastroenterol* **84**:892–897.

Luukkonen P (1988) Manometric followup of anal sphincter function after ileo-anal pouch procedure. *Int J Colorectal Dis* **3**:43–46.

McHugh SM, Diament NE (1987) Effect of age, gender, and parity on anal canal pressures: contribution of impaired anal sphincter function to fecal incontinence. *Dig Dis Sci* **32**:726–736.

Martin LW, Fischer JE (1982) Preservation of ano-rectal continence following total colectomy. *Ann Surg* **196**:700–704.

Miller R, Orrom WJ, Duthie G, Mortensen N (1990) Ambulatory anorectal physiology in patients following restorative proctocolectomy for ulcerative colitis: comparison with normal controls. *Br J Surg* **77**:895–897.

Miller R, Bartolo DCC, Cervero F, Mortensen NJ (1988a) Anorectal sampling: a comparison of normal and incontinent patients. *Br J Surg* **75**:44–47.

Miller R, Bartolo DCC, Roe AM, Mortensen NJMCC (1988b) Assessment of microtransducers in anorectal manometry. *Br J Surg* **75**:40–43.

Nasmyth DG, Johnston D, Godwin PGR, Dixon MF, Williams NS (1986a) Factors influencing bowel function after ileal pouch-anal anastomosis. *Br J Surg* **73**:469–473.

Nasmyth DG, Williams NS, Johnston D (1986b) Comparison of the function of triplicated and duplicated pelvic ileal reservoirs after mucosal proctectomy and ileo-anal ana-stomosis for ulcerative colitis and adenomatous polyposis. *Br J Surg* **73**:361–366.

Nicholls RJ (1984) Restorative proctocolectomy with ileal reservoir. *Ann R Coll Surg Engl* **66**:42–45.

Nicholls RJ, Lubowski DZ (1987) Restorative proctocolectomy: the four loop (W) reservoir. *Br J Surg* **74**:564–566.

Nicholls RJ, Pezim ME (1985) Restorative proctocolectomy with ileal reservoir for ulcerative colitis and familial adenomatous polyposis: a comparison of three designs. *Br J Surg* **72**:470–474.

O'Connell PR, Pemberton JH, Kelly KA (1987a) Motor function of the ileal J pouch and its relation to clinical outcome after ileal pouch-anal anastomosis. *World J Surg* **11**:735–741.

O'Connell PR, Stryker SJ, Metcalf AM, Pemberton JH, Kelly KA (1988) Anal canal pressure and motility after ileoanal anastomosis. *Surg Gynecol Obstet* **166**:47–54.

Öresland T, Fasth S, Akervall S, Nordgren S, Hultén L (1990) Manovolumetric and sensory characteristics of the ileoanal J pouch compared with healthy rectum. *Br J Surg* **77**:803–806.

Parks AG, Nicholls RJ, Belliveau P (1980) Proctocolectomy with ileal reservoir and anal anastomosis. *Br J Surg* **67**:533–538.

Pemberton JH (1991) Neorectum and assessment of anorectal function following surgery. In *Clinical Measurement in Coloproctology*. Kumar D, Waldron D, Williams NS (eds). London, Springer-Verlag, pp. 165–187.

Pemberton JH, Kelly KA, Beart RW, Dozois RR, Wolff BG, Ilstrup DM (1987) Ileal pouch-anal anastomosis for chronic ulcerative colitis: long term results. *Ann Surg* **206**:504–511.

Pemberton JH, Phillips SF, Ready RR, Zinsmeister AR, Beahrs OH (1989) Quality of life after Brooke ileostomy and ileal pouch anal anastomosis. *Ann Surg* **209**:620–628.

Pescatori M, Parks AG (1984) The sphincteric and sensory components of preserved continence after ileoanal reservoir. *Surg Gynecol Obstet* **158**:517–521.

Primrose JN, Holdsworth PJ, Nasmyth DG, Womack N, Neal DE, Johnston D (1987) Intact anal sphincter with end to

end ileoanal anastomosis for ulcerative colitis: comparison with mucosal proctectomy and pull-through anastomosis. *Br J Surg* **74**:539.

Read MG, Read NW (1982) Role of anal sensation in preserving continence. *Gut* **23**:345–347.

Roe AM, Bartolo DCC, Mortensen NJMcC (1986) New method for assessment of anal sensation in various anorectal disorders. *Br J Surg* **73**:310–312.

Rothenberger DA, Wong WD, Buls JG, Goldberg SM (1985) The S ileal pouch anal anastomosis. In *Alternatives to conventional ileostomy*. RR Dozois (ed) Chicago, Yearbook Medical Publishers.

Sagar PM, Holdsworth PJ, Johnston D (1991) Correlation between laboratory findings and clinical outcome after restorative proctocolectomy: serial studies in 20 patients with end to end pouch anal anastomosis. *Br J Surg* **78**:67–70.

Seow-Choen A, Tsunoda A, Nicholls RJ (1991) Prospective randomized trial comparing anal function after hand sewn ileoanal anastomosis with mucosectomy versus stapled ileoanal anastomosis without mucosectomy in restorative proctocolectomy. *Br J Surg* **78**:430–434.

Scott NA, Pemberton JH, Barkel DC, Wolff BG (1989) Anal and ileal pouch manometric measurements before ileostomy closure are related to functional outcome after ileal pouch-anal anastomosis. *Br J Surg* **76**:613–616.

Stryker SJ, Phillips SF, Dozois RR, Kelly KA, Beart RW (1986) Anal and neorectal function after ileal pouch anal anastomosis. *Ann Surg* **203**:55–61.

Williams NS, Johnston D (1985) The current status of mucosal proctectomy and ileo-anal anastomosis in the surgical treatment of ulcerative colitis and adenomatous polyposis. *Br J Surg* **72**:159–168.

Williams NS, Marzouk DEMM, Hallen RI, Waldron DJ (1989) Function after ileal pouch and stapled pouch anal anastomosis for ulcerative colitis. *Br J Surg* **76**:1168–1171.

Winckler G (1958) Remarques sur la morphologie et l'innervation du muscle releveur de l'anus. *Arch Anat Histol Embryol (Strasb)* **41**:77–95.

Chapter 7
Pelvic Pouch – Physiology vs. Function

LEIF HULTÉN, STIG FASTH AND TOM ÖRESLAND

Introduction

Most pelvic pouch patients establish a fairly good function with time. It is far from perfect, however. Although varying over a wide range, patients with a well established pelvic pouch have an average day-time stool frequency of about five, and almost half of the patients need to empty at night. Urgency is generally a rare problem encountered mainly during episodes of pouchitis. None of the patients have to evacuate using a catheter. Frank faecal incontinence rarely exists but about 20% of patients have occasional problems with soiling of underwear and perianal soreness and prefer therefore to use a protective pad, particularly at night (Table 7.1). A majority of patients also prefer to use anti-diarrhoeal agents. While stool frequency is higher and continence problems are more common during the immediate postoperative phase, function improves during the first year and it also seems that there is a continuous slow improvement even beyond that time (Öresland *et al.*, 1989; Wexner *et al.*, 1989).

Anal continence may be defined as the ability: to control defaecation voluntarily, to discriminate between solid and liquid faeces and wind, to defer evacuation to a time which is socially acceptable and to maintain control even during sleep. By strictly applying this definition it seems that only about half of the patients with a pelvic pouch are fully continent over a longer time period. The surgical approach has therefore been varied and several techniques are still evolving in an attempt to improve results, with different modifications employed both for the proctectomy and for construction of the reservoir. Whether such changes in technique have been beneficial is difficult to know, since comparisons are often made on historical controls or the results presented in such a way that they do not allow for comparison. Particularly the differences in criteria of assessment and mode of expression of the functional results contribute to the difficulties. Defaecation frequency, urgency, the ability to release gas safely, soiling of underwear, need for a protective pad and the need for constipating drugs, etc., are commonly used variables to define the results. Apart from a functional evaluation based on these individual markers each variable can also be alotted points where the total number is considered to reflect the overall functional result in each patient. While such an arbitrary score system may be appropriate particularly for comparative purposes (Table 7.2), the evaluation is still subjected to a considerable 'observer' variation.

Anal continence is maintained by a complex interaction between local reflex mechanisms and voluntary interventions, involving factors such as: sphincter function, anorectal sensation, the rectoanal inhibitory reflex, the anorectal angle, rectal capacity and the propulsive forces of the intestine. Anal manometry alone allows for an objective assessment of resting anal sphincter tone and the capacity of voluntary squeeze, while simultaneous recording of rectal volume and anal pressure in response to graded rectal distension is advantageous in that it allows also for assessment of rectal–pouch volume and compliance, reflex sphincter inhibition and the threshold for appreciation of rectal sensation. Such laboratory studies may be helpful in the interpretation and objective evaluation of the functional results after restorative proctocolectomy, allowing a more accurate comparison to be made between different surgical modifications.

Methodological considerations

The results presented here comparing normal rectoanal and pouch–anal physiology are based on a specially designed laboratory set up which allows for simultaneous recording of rectal/pouch volume and anal pressure on graded isobaric rectal/pouch distension (Åkervall *et al.*, 1988). The system consists of two units, one reflecting pouch volume at preset distension pressures and the other anal pressure (Fig. 7.1). The unit for distension and volume registration consists of

Table 7.1 Pelvic J pouch. Functional results at 1 year (n = 100).

	Evacuation frequency	Patients with symptom (%)
24-hour evacuation	4.5 (2–11)	
Daytime evacuation	≤4	50
	≥7	10
Night-time evacuation	≥1 week	40
Mucous soiling		20
Perineal soreness		16
Need for constipating drugs		79

Table 7.2 Functional score system.

	Score points		
	0	1	2
Number of bowel movements			
Daytime	≤4	5	≥6
Night-time	0	>1/week	≥2/night
Urgency (inability to defer evacuation >30 min)	No	Yes	
Evacuation difficulties (>15 min spent in toilet on any occasion during the week)	No	Yes	
Soiling, seepage			
Daytime	No	>1/week	
Night-time	No	>1/week	
Inability to safely release flatus	No	Yes	
Perianal soreness	No	Occasional	Permanent
Protective pad			
Daytime	No	>1/week	
Night-time	No	>1/week	
Dietary restrictions	No	Yes	
Medication (continuous or occasional)	No	Yes	
Social handicap (not able to resume full-time occupation or participate in social life)	No	Yes	

Score range 0–15. Patients with overall good function will score 0 points and those with poor function will score a maximum of 15 points.

a wide-diameter water-filled cylindrical vessel open to air and suspended on a force displacement transducer (Grass FT 10D) for continuous weight recording. This vessel is connected via a non-distensible tube to a closed air reservoir with a volume of 600 ml. The air reservoir is connected to the pouch volume balloon, a flaccid thin-walled polyethylene bag, 12 cm long, which is hermetically attached to an air tube. When the water reservoir is raised above the air reservoir, a pressure is generated in the air compartment of the air reservoir. When air is allowed to expand the rectal balloon by opening an air vent, water will flow into the air reservoir and the weight change of the water reservoir will reflect the volume of air in the pouch balloon (1 g of water is set equal to 1 ml). The pressure exerted on the pouch wall via the balloon is equal to the difference in the levels of the water in the reservoirs and is expressed in cmH_2O. The distension pressures used are 20, 40, 60 and 80 cmH_2O; additional distensions are performed at 5-cmH_2O intervals in the

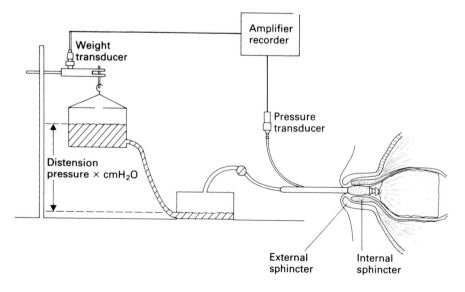

Fig. 7.1 Schematic illustration of the manovolumetry set up.

lower pressure range for a more precise estimation of sensory thresholds. Anal pressures are obtained from the water-filled balloon of an endotracheal tube (Mallincrodt N. 7 outer diameter 10 mm) threaded onto the air tube and connected to a pressure transducer (Statham P 23D). The recording system is disposable. Anal pressure and pouch volume are recorded on a Grass Polygraph.

This laboratory technique allows the following parameters to be studied:

1 *Resting anal pressure* (*RAP*). The mean level of the anal pressure recorded after a minimum of 5 minutes of adaptation is taken to reflect the function of internal anal sphincter at rest.

2 *Maximum squeeze pressure* (*MSP*). The highest of three consecutive squeezing efforts, representing external sphincter function.

3 *Pouch volume*. This refers to the maximal volume recorded during each 60-second distension.

4 *Pouch motility*. Refers to volume fluctuations dduring pppouch distensions.

5 *Maximal pouch volume*. The volume at a distension pressure of 80 cmH$_2$O.

6 *Pouch compliance* is defined as volume increase (ml)/pressure increase (cmH$_2$O) calculated in the four pressure intervals 0–20, 20–40, 40–60 and 60–80 cmH$_2$O.

7 *Rectoanal inhibition reflex* (*RAIR*) is defined as 20% reduction of RAP with concomitant disappearance of spontaneous anal motility on rectal distension.

8 *First sensation*. The threshold distension pressure and corresponding volume required to elicit a sensation of pouch filling.

9 *Urge to defaecate*. The threshold distension pressure and corresponding volume required to elicit urge to defaecate or any sensation signalling the need for pouch emptying.

Differences in methodology contribute greatly to the varying results reported on anal sphincter function. A multiplicity of methods such as station pull-through or continuous withdrawal of perfused catheters (Taylor *et al.*, 1983; Becker, 1984; Stryker *et al.*, 1986; Harms *et al.*, 1987; Sharp *et al.*, 1987; Keighley *et al.*, 1988b; Chaussade *et al.*, 1989) or microtransducers (Emblem et al., 1989a; Lindquist, 1990) or stationary or station pull-through air filled balloons or microballoons (Nicholls *et al.*, 1981; Neal *et al.*, 1982; Pescatori & Parks, 1984; Nasmyth *et al.*, 1986a; Keighley *et al.*, 1987) are currently used for anal pressure recordings.

While pressure sensitive catheters may have the advantage of minimal distortion of the anal canal they may still give unreliable results, particularly in serial measurements if differences in axial orientation are not corrected for. Although balloons may give a less accurate localization of the source of the pressure they are not sensitive to axial orientation and are also simple to use in repetitive studies. Differences in probe diameters influence the result of the pressure recording. It has been demonstrated convincingly (Gibbons *et al.*, 1986; McHugh *et al.*, 1987; Åkervall *et al.*, 1988) that the recorded pressures increase with increasing probe diameter. In a recent study by Lestar *et al.* (1989) it was also suggested that with increasing probe diameter the relative contribution of the internal sphincter neurogenic activity to the overall resting anal pressure diminishes as the relative contribution of internal sphincter myogenic activity and stretching of passive elements increases.

Comparisons of reports on pouch volumes and compliance are also made difficult because of substantial differences in methodology. The latex balloons of varying length, which are mostly used, may expand in a longitudinal direction to a varying degree giving unreliable volume estimations. For this reason, compliance calculations may also be more inaccurate, the more so as the inherent compliance of the balloon has to be subtracted. Non-compliant flaccid balloons of a fixed length as used in our laboratory should therefore be more accurate. Radiographic studies performed in our unit with contrast coated balloons, confirm that the technique used is a good estimate of pouch volume. Volume comparisons may also be unreliable due to variations of the definitions of the end-point at which the volume is recorded. In most studies this involves a subjective sensory component in terms of 'urge' or 'maximal tolerated volume', whereas we measure volume at fixed end-points in terms of predetermined pressure levels. From a functional point of view it can be argued which is the most relevant, but in longitudinal studies it seems that a fixed pressure end-point should be more reliable.

The system used in our laboratory also allows for a more accurate calculation of compliance in defined pressure intervals whereas others usually base the compliance calculations on a single estimation of pressure when patients perceive 'urge' or 'maximal tolerable volume'. The initial compliance, i.e. when calculating from zero level, is directly proportional to the registered volume and merely reflects the initial unfolding of the balloon. It is only when calculating

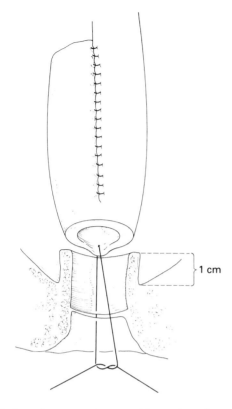

Fig. 7.2 Endoanal mucosectomy and J pouch anal anastomosis.

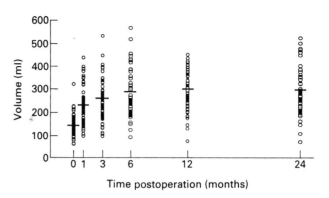

Fig. 7.3 Individual maximal pouch volumes (at 80 cmH$_2$O distension pressure) at intervals after loop ileostomy closure. Bars indicate median values.

compliance in intervals above the zero level that any additional information can be obtained (Madoff *et al.*, 1990).

Restorative proctocolectomy after endoanal mucosectomy

The importance of pouch design

The J configured pouch

The J pouch originally described by Utsunomiya *et al.* (1980) still appears to be the most popular model probably due to its simplicity in construction and lack of a potentially obstructing outlet segment.

The following results are based on regular clinical and functional assessment combined with mano-volumetric studies performed in 67 consecutively operated patients (Öresland *et al.*, 1990b). All these patients had a J pouch and proctectomy including mesorectum and a complete mucosectomy had been performed by endoanal approach transecting the muscle cuff just above the pelvic floor (Fig. 7.2).

Pouch volume and compliance

Maximal pouch volume increased from 132 ± 46 ml immediately before, to 282 ± 85 ml at 1 year after, ileostomy closure and the most marked expansion occurred within the first 6 months (Fig. 7.3). After 1 year there was no further volume increase. Pouch compliance also increased with time and at 1 year postoperatively, was 8.6 ml/cmH$_2$O in the pressure interval 0–20 cmH$_2$O, and 3.0, 1.3 and 1.1 ml/cmH$_2$O in the pressure intervals 20–40, 40–60 and 60–80 cmH$_2$O, respectively. The pouch volume recorded before ileostomy closure was predictive for the ultimate volume at 1 year, i.e. a low initial pouch volume was indicative of a subsequent low volume. A similar correlation appeared to exist between the length of ileum used for construction of the pouch and the subsequent maximal pouch volume (Fig. 7.4). Pouch volume and compliance also proved to be functional determinants. Thus, a high evacuation frequency correlated with a small pouch volume, and daytime soiling and the need for retarding drugs were also related to a low pouch volume. A high functional score reflecting a less satisfactory overall function, also correlated to a low pouch volume and a low pouch compliance. However, while a low initial pouch volume was predictive for a subsequent bad overall functional result, it was not predictive for a subsequent high stool frequency.

The expansion properties of the pelvic J pouch observed in this study are in concert with the reports from several other studies (Neal *et al.*, 1982; Harms *et al.*, 1987; Luukkonen, 1988), although differences in methodology do not always allow for reliable comparison of reported data on pouch capacity (Taylor *et*

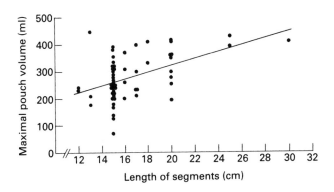

Fig. 7.4 Length of ileum segment used for construction versus ultimate pouch volume at 1 year. $r = 0.48$; $p < 0.001$ ($y = 12.3x + 77.7$).

al., 1983; Nicholls & Pezim, 1985; Becker & Raymond, 1986; Nasmyth et al., 1986a; Stryker et al., 1986). When compared with a study on J pouches from the Mayo Clinic, where a similar volume recording balloon was used, it appears that the final average maximal pouch volume (about 300 ml) in our series of patients is lower (O'Connell et al., 1987). It is very likely, however, that this discrepancy may be due to different definitions. In the Mayo study maximal volume was defined as maximal tolerable volume, whereas in our study maximal volume was recorded at a fixed distension pressure of 80 cmH₂O.

Although it was demonstrated that the capacity of the pouch increased with increasing length of intestine used for its construction, there was considerable variation in the final pouch volume, even in pouches constructed from equal lengths of ileum (Fig. 7.4). Patient and operative factors failed to explain this variance in pouch expansion. The fact that a continent ileostomy, constructed from equal lengths of ileum (30 cm) attains a final volume which is at least double that of a pelvic pouch (Berglund et al., 1984; Hallgren et al., 1989), suggests that the pelvic space itself or the actual pressure conditions within the pelvis may be important variables in determining pouch expansion. Variations in the formation of postoperative adhesions and/or fibrosis in the pelvis, and differences in viscoelasticity and/or neural tone of the intestine may be factors that affect pouch volume expansion. The observation that a low early pouch volume is predictive of a future low capacity might support this view.

Pouchitis, a common problem among the 67 J pouch patients, appeared to influence pouch function adversely by reducing its volume capacity. Patients

who had symptoms of pouchitis when investigated at the 1-year follow-up, proved to have significantly lower maximal pouch volume than those without pouchitis (215 ± 78 vs. 292 ± 82 ml; $p < 0.05$) and patients who had previously suffered episodes of pouchitis but were free of symptoms when investigated at the 2-year follow-up also had a lower reservoir volume than those who had never suffered from the condition. While Moskowitz et al. (1986) were unable to demonstrate any differences in compliance comparing pouches with and without inflammation, the results of the present study indicate that pouchitis is associated with a low reservoir capacity.

The functional outcome appears to be related to the volume and compliance of the pouch. The compliance of the pouch was highest in the lowest pressure interval (0–20 cmH₂O) amounting to about 8 ml/cmH₂O, implying that the J pouch can utilize at least 50% of its maximal volume at a distension pressure that is not appreciated by the patient (see below; sensory function). This finding is in agreement with recently published results (O'Connell et al., 1987). While most previous reports demonstrate that pouch volume is a determinant of evacuation frequency (Nicholls & Pezim, 1985; Becker & Raymond, 1986; Nasmyth et al., 1986a; O'Connell et al., 1987), a finding confirmed in the present study also, the correlation between volume and the continence function is commented upon more rarely. According to our results pouch volume appears also to be determinant for this function.

Pouch motility

The inherent smooth muscle tone and motility pattern of the ileum at rest and on distension might have an important impact on pouch function. The motility pattern on rapid graded pouch distension differs markedly from the normal rectum (Fig. 7.5). Distension of the ileal pouch generates a more pronounced and longlasting reflex contraction displacing about 35% of the pouch volume at 40 cmH₂O distension as compared to 10% in controls. Moreover, the initial contraction is followed by repetitive contractions in the vast majority of pouches. While such contractions disappear in the rectum on pressures exceeding 50 cmH₂O most ileal pouches still exhibit reflex contractions at a distension pressure of 80 cmH₂O. While the presence of such 'high pressure motility' correlates with a low maximal pouch volume, patients in whom pouch

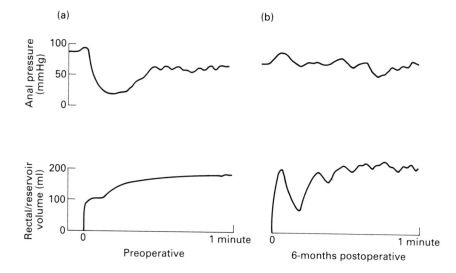

Fig. 7.5 Resting anal pressure (upper panel) and volume expansion profile (lower panel) on (a) rectal and (b) pelvic J pouch-distension. Note the pronounced motility pattern and lack of reflex sphincter inhibition on pouch distension.

motility does not exhibit this pattern have the best functional result.

This observation which is consonant with previous reports implies that the distension volume at which high pressure waves are generated, i.e. threshold volume, may be an important functional determinant (Stryker *et al.*, 1986; O'Connell *et al.*, 1987). This finding also reflects a fundamental physiological difference between the normal rectum and the ileal substitute. While the healthy rectum can accommodate increasing volumes with either none or only minor motor contractions, the ileal pouch lacks this physiological property of adaptive relaxation.

Other pouch designs

There is clinical evidence to show that the S shaped reservoir attains a larger capacity than the J shaped pouch, and that this is associated with a lower defaecation frequency and possibly also with a better continence function (Nicholls & Pezim, 1985). Moreover the W configurated pouch is reported to be superior both to the J and S pouch (Nicholls & Lubowski, 1987; Everett, 1989). The favourable expanding properties of the S shaped pouch have been ascribed to a greater relative degree of outflow resistance while the spherical form of the W pouch is considered to be of great

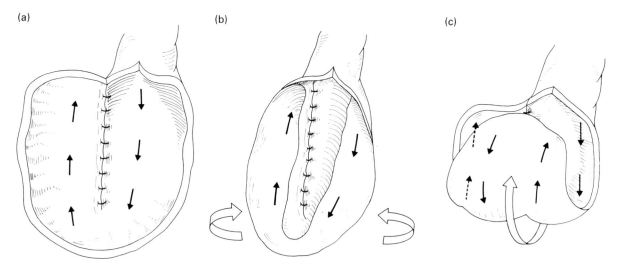

Fig. 7.6 Different folding principles for pouch construction.
(a) The J configurated ileum segment split longitudinally.
(b) Pouch closed along vertical axis (traditional J pouch).
(c) Pouch folded and closed according to Kock's original principle (K pouch).

advantage in providing the greatest volume for any given length of ileum (Nicholls & Lubowski, 1987; Thomson *et al.*, 1987). Experimenting with substitutes for the urinary bladder Kock became impressed by a pouch design (Fig. 7.6a,b) proposed by Tasker (1953). The motor activity in the two parts of ileum split and folded according to that technique was considered to counteract itself to some extent resulting in large volume capacity and relatively low pressure at filling. However, high pressures still developed at larger volumes and although patients generally remained continent during the day they usually leaked during sleep. Kock therefore developed his double-folded reservoir (Fig. 7.6c). After splitting of the intestinal segment at its anti-mesenteric border, it is folded into an upside down U, but instead of the pouch being closed from side-to-side, the bottom of the U is folded down and united to the ends of the segment and the reservoir is closed in this way. Kock (1969) proposed that this pouch configuration should have little or no inherent motility as the peristalsis of the reservoir segments were oriented in four different directions. The big initial circumference would also create advantageous compliance and volume characteristics as a relatively low pressure within the reservoir should create a wall tension that would favour rapid pouch expansion (Berglund *et al.*, 1987). This pouch folding technique has subsequently proven its merits in the continent urostomy and ileostomy (Kock, 1987).

However, whether differences in the ultimate pouch volume and function described above are in fact attributed to specific properties of the pouch types or simply due to different lengths of ileum used for their construction is controversial. The latter theory is supported by the fact that longer segments of ileum are required for construction of the functionally favourable W pouch, that increasing length of ileum for construction of a J pouch improves ultimate result and that the functional results of W pouches are less impressive when compared with J pouches constructed from equal length of ileum (Keighley *et al.*, 1988a). Comparative studies between different pouch models are scarce and their value limited as the series of patients are often heterogeneous and small and the comparisons mostly based on historical controls.

A comparative study on the manovolumetric characteristics and function in patients with an S pouch, a J pouch or a pouch double-folded according to Kock (Hallgren *et al.*, 1989), all pouches constructed from equal lengths of ileum, showed evidence that despite a

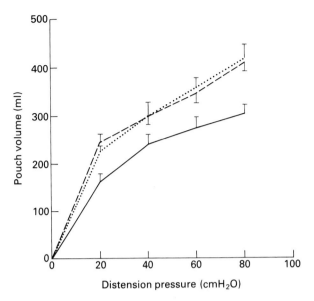

Fig. 7.7 The expansion properties of three different pouch types, mean ± SE. ———, J pouch; – – – –, K pouch; ·······, S pouch.

similar initial pouch volume (about 120–130 ml) the S and K pouches expanded more favourably and at 1 year the maximal volume in these two designs (420 and 410 ml respectively) was about 100 ml larger than in J pouches (305 ml) (Fig. 7.7). Moreover, the pouch volume in S and K pouches was bigger at all distension pressures. However the overall functional result at 1 year differed but little.

A recent controlled randomized and more detailed study comparing the J and K pouches confirmed these results demonstrating the superior expanding properties of the K pouch (Öresland *et al.*, 1990c). Moreover, while pouch compliance of the two designs was by and large similar in the pressure intervals above 20 cmH$_2$O it was significantly higher in the K pouch in the low pressure interval (7.3 vs. 10.8 ml/cmH$_2$O, $p < 0.001$) (Fig. 7.8). In contrast to the observations made by Kock *et al.* the motility pattern of the two pouch designs was similar and when studied at distension pressures up to 40 cmH$_2$O, both types exhibited volume reductions reflecting pouch wall tension that was in excess of the distension pressure used. The majority of the J and K pouches still exhibited these high pressure waves even when maximally distended at 80 cmH$_2$O, although these contractions appeared to be somewhat less frequent in the K pouches. Even in this study functional imperfections were on the whole equally distributed in the two groups of patients however (Fig. 7.9). Since pouch characteristics are perhaps of less importance

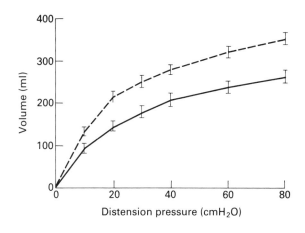

Compliance in pressure interval (ml/cmH₂O, mean ± S.E.)	J	7.3 ± 0.7	3.1 ± 0.3	1.5 ± 0.1	1.3 ± 0.1
	K	10.8 ± 0.6	3.3 ± 0.2	2.0 ± 0.2	1.5 ± 0.1
		$p < 0.001$	n.s.	$p < 0.05$	n.s.

Fig. 7.8 The volume expansion properties mean ± SE (upper panel) and calculated compliance in the pressure intervals 0–20, 20–40, 40–60 and 60–80 cmH₂O (lower panel) in J and K pouches. ——, J pouch; ----, K pouch; n.s., not significant.

compared to other as yet unexplored factors and known factors such as volume and quality of the ileal effluent (O'Connell *et al.*, 1986), it is not surprising that this study failed to show any difference in functional outcome between the two pouch models.

The fact that the volume of the K pouch is larger, and shows less variability than the J pouch, is in good keeping with Kock's hypothesis, and the observation that the compliance of the pouch is also significantly higher than that of the J pouch might also support such a view. However, this latter difference appears to be dependent mainly on the better 'unfolding' ability of the K pouch at lower pressures, while at higher pressures the compliance of the K and J pouch was mostly similar. Although the hypothesis proposed by Kock is very attractive, it is not quite convincing. The spherical form of the K pouch *per se* may well explain its superior expansion. According to geometrical formulae it can be calculated that the cylindrically shaped J pouch constructed from a 30-cm length of ileum would yield a volume that is approximately 30% lower than the spherical K pouch constructed from an equal length of ileum.

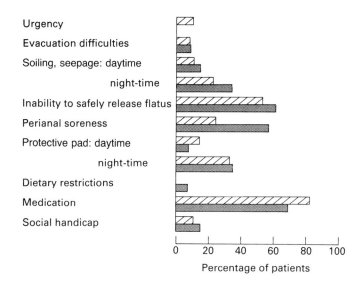

		J (n = 27)	K (n = 26)
Number of bowel movements daytime	≤4	52	39
	5	33	38
	≥6	15	23
Number of bowel movements night-time	0	56	38
	>1/week	33	50
	≥2/night	11	12

Fig. 7.9 Defaecation pattern and proportion of functional defects at one year after surgery. ▨, J pouch patients; ▩, K pouch patients.

The importance of anal sphincter function

Sphincter function is another determinant considered to be important for continence in pouch patients. Patients with a low resting anal pressure (RAP) are said to leak more often than those with a less pronounced reduction of sphincter tone and it is assumed that the endocavitary traumatizing technique for coring out of the anal mucosa may be the main cause for this. The impact of distal mucosectomy on anal sphincter function has been studied extensively. A permanent reduction in RAP is reported in most studies but its magnitude varies greatly (Stryker *et al.*, 1986; Keighley *et al.*, 1988b). Such wide variations may be due to the taking of measurements at different stages postoperatively, to differing methodology (see p. 103) or operative techniques.

In the series of 67 J pouches referred to above, the technique of endoanal mucosectomy starting from the pectinate line and using an anal retractor was employed in all patients (Fig. 7.10). It was demonstrated that RAP decreased markedly after surgery,

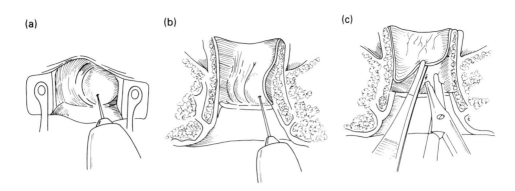

Fig. 7.10 Endoanal mucosectomy technique. (a) Submucous injection of adrenaline solution. (b) Dissection starts at pectinate line, and (c) proceeds just above the pelvic floor.

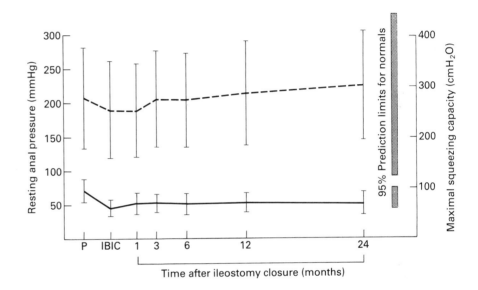

Fig. 7.11 Resting anal pressure —— and maximal squeezing capacity ———— at intervals. Shaded bars represent the 95% prediction limits for normals. IBIC, immediately before ileostomy closure; P, preoperative.

and remained lowered corresponding to a permanent reduction of about 25% after 1 year. However, preoperative RAP (70 ± 17 mmHg) in these patients proved to be significantly higher than in normal subjects (61 ± 8 mmHg), and at 1 year RAP was within the prediction limits for normals in two-thirds of patients (Fig. 7.11). These patients leaked to the same extent as those with lower RAP. Maximal squeeze pressure (MSP) decreased slightly after operation, recovering to preoperative levels 3 months after closure of the loop ileostomy. There was no correlation between overall functional results and the postoperative sphincter status.

Conflicting with many previous reports suggesting that a lowered RAP is associated with both poor continence (Nicholls *et al.*, 1981; Pescatori & Parks, 1984; Nasmyth *et al.*, 1986a; Keighley *et al.*, 1988b; O'Connell

et al., 1988) and a higher defaecation frequency (Lindquist, 1990) these observations would imply that the postoperative reduction in RAP *per se* may not be the principal cause of functional defects after restorative proctocolectomy. In fact, there is evidence to show that continence in ileoanal pouch patients in whom the internal sphincter has been partly or entirely removed is still reasonably well preserved (Pearl *et al.*, 1985; Ryan & Fink, 1988).

Whether the external sphincter may also contribute to poor functional results is controversial (Neal *et al.*, 1982; Stryker *et al.*, 1985). Abnormal EMG registrations and morphological abnormalities of the external sphincter have been demonstrated after restorative proctocolectomy (Emblem *et al.*, 1989a). The fact that the squeeze capacity appears to be fairly well preserved and that stress incontinence is an uncommon defect in these patients speaks against any major damage however.

There is evidence that the cause of sphincter pressure reduction after endoanal proctectomy is due to the operative trauma with over-distension of the sphincter. Even if this may well be so, the moderate reduction of resting anal tone does not fully explain the functional imperfection. Concomitant removal of the transitional zone of mucosa, loss of anal cushions, the presence of full-thickness ileum and postoperative deformation of the anal canal may, however, each or in combination contribute to the deterioration of anal continence.

Pouch–anal sensory function

Sphincter inhibition

Reflex sphincter inhibition on rectal distension is elicited by stimulation of mechanoreceptors in the rectal wall, but may also be elicited by electrical or thermal stimulation (Nagasaki et al., 1989). The pathway of the reflex is considered dependent on an intact myenteric nerve plexus and the reflex is absent in Hirschsprung's disease. Controversy exists as regards the fate of reflex sphincter inhibition after mucosal proctectomy. While some authors report that it is abolished in all patients (Heppel et al., 1982; Grant et al., 1986; Harms et al., 1987; Keighley et al., 1988b), others have demonstrated its presence or reappearance in a varying proportion of patients (Nicholls et al., 1981; Neal et al., 1982; Taylor et al., 1983; Pescatori & Parks, 1984; Becker et al., 1985; Stryker et al., 1985; Sharp et al., 1987; Holdsworth & Johnston, 1988; O'Connell et al., 1988; Slors et al., 1989; Chaussade et al., 1989; Emblem et al., 1989b). Variations in follow-up time and methodology for studying reflex inhibition may to some extent explain the divergent results.

The rectoanal inhibition reflex (RAIR) demonstrated before operation in all of our 67 patients was completely abolished after surgery, but with the passage of time a similar reflex inhibitory response on pouch distension reappeared in 15 patients. However, the distension pressure required to elicit the response in these patients was significantly higher than in controls (34 ± 22 vs. 12 ± 3 cmH$_2$O; $p < 0.05$), and higher also when compared with preoperative figures (17 ± 9; $p < 0.05$). The patients' ability to release flatus safely, which should be a specific and closely related functional variable, was not dependent on the presence of reflex inhibition and the overall functional results were

not convincingly better in patients in whom sphincter inhibition had reappeared.

It is difficult to understand the mechanism by which the reflex inhibition is elicited in these patients. Lane and Parks (1977) who demonstrated reappearance of reflex inhibition in patients subjected to rectal excision and coloanal anastomosis suggested that the intramural nerve plexus of the colon might regenerate across the anastomosis. The observation in our study that the reflex was abolished after surgery and reappeared subsequently often several months or a year later would support such a view. However, it may well be so that the reduction of sphincter tone observed on pouch distension in these patients does not reflect a true reflex inhibition at all. It seems unlikely that the myenteric plexus of the small intestine could establish connections with the internal anal sphincter at the level of the pectinate line where it is in fact also devoid of ganglia cells. The observation that the pressure threshold needed to elicit sphincter inhibition is considerably higher than in controls would imply that the response is an artifact rather than a true reflex (Grant et al., 1986).

Perception

An important facet of anorectal function is the ability to perceive rectal filling and urge to defaecate. Mano-volumetric and sensory characteristics of the ileoanal pouch as compared to the healthy rectum are in these respects markedly different. When studied by the technique used in our unit, the volume and pressure threshold for first sensation of pouch filling was significantly higher than in the normal rectum (30 cmH$_2$O

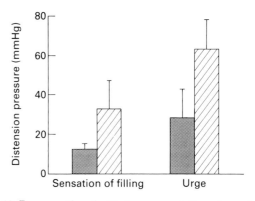

Fig. 7.12 Pressure thresholds for appreciation of rectal or pouch-filling sensation and appreciation of defaecation urge. ▨ normal rectum; ▨, ileal pouch.

vs. 15 cmH$_2$O). Defaecation urge was also experienced at a significantly higher distension volume and the pressure threshold was about 60 cmH$_2$O compared to 30 cmH$_2$O in the rectum (Fig. 7.12). It should be emphasized in this context that the problem in assessing any sensation, which is essentially a personal experience on the part of the patient, is notoriously difficult. When interrogating patients more specifically as regards these sensory modalities the majority of patients stated that they were unable to specify the sensation calling them to stool. Sixty percent of the patients referred to a diffuse abdominal discomfort, bloating or a feeling of suprapubic distension combined with borborygmi, sometimes with a poorly defined pressure sensation deep in the pelvis. Ten percent of the patients did not experience the urge sensation at all. Only one-third of the patients stated that the sensation was 'normal' or similar to that they thought they had experienced before they had their disease. Still more confusing however was the statement that the subjective sensation experienced on pouch distension in the laboratory was not always equal to the sensation that called to stool in their daily life (Öresland et al., 1990a).

While a high volume at perception of pouch filling proved to be directly related to a large maximal pouch volume, and also correlated positively to the functional results there was neither correlation to the pressure threshold for this sensation nor to the sensory thresholds for urge to defaecate. In fact, patients with suprapubic or undetermined vague localization of the 'urge' signal had a lower daytime evacuation frequency, suffered less from soiling and had a significantly better overall function.

The findings indicate that there are fundamental differences between the sensory function of the ileal pouch and the healthy rectum, significantly higher pressures and volumes being required to elicit sensations in the pouch. Keighley et al. (1988b) found no differences when comparing the volumes required to elicit sensations, whereas our findings are in agreement with those reported by O'Connell et al. (1987) who also demonstrated a blunted sensation in pouch patients as compared to controls. Considering the extensive operation with full-thickness proctectomy, mucosal stripping of the anal canal and replacement of the rectum with an ileal substitute, it is hard to believe that the nervous pathways conveying true 'rectal' sensations would remain preserved. Nor could the ileal pouch supplied by vagal and sympathetic nerve fibres, possibly mediate such qualities. The results there-

fore cast doubt on the hypothesis that the receptors necessary for the appreciation of rectal filling and urge of defaecation are located in the levator ani muscle as postulated by Scarli and Kiesewetter (1970) and Lane and Parks (1977). The markedly different volume and pressure thresholds would imply a nerve fibre set with other neurophysiological properties, such as sympathetic visceral afferents or pain fibres. The fact that a substantial proportion of the patients are unable to specify the sensation calling them to stool or stating that they experience a vague intra-abdominal discomfort or pain would also support such a view.

Taken together these observations clearly indicate that storage, evacuation, and sensory function of the pelvic pouch are controlled by mechanisms other than those regulating normal rectal function. The rectum is replaced by an ileal substitute without connections, neither to the motor nor to sensory pathways in the pelvic nerves. The motor component of the autonomous defaecation reflex is certainly absent and most patients have to evacuate by straining. The reflex sphincter inhibition which is supposed to play an important role for continence disappears in all patients after surgery. Although reappearing in some patients its absence appears not to influence results adversely.

Proctectomy with preservation of the entire anal canal and a stapled ileoanal anastomosis

Heald and Allen (1986) described how the rectum could be excised and an ileoanal anastomosis con-

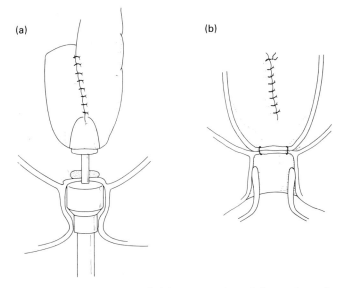

Fig. 7.13 Proctectomy with (a) preservation of the anal canal and (b) stapled ileoanal anastomosis.

structed entirely from the abdominal approach, stapling the pouch to the top of the anal canal. The principle difference compared to the traditional technique is that the anal canal with the transitional zone of mucosa is well preserved in this operation and that sphincter over-distension is also avoided (Fig. 7.13).

The procedure has later been popularized by Johnston *et al.* (1987) who showed evidence that resting anal pressure was only moderately reduced and that the functional outcome was significantly better than in those patients who had undergone endoanal proctectomy and mucosectomy. In a subsequent more detailed study (Holdsworth & Johnston, 1988) from the Leeds unit, the threshold of anal mucosal electro-sensitivity proved to be significantly greater in those who had undergone the mucosectomy with endoanal anastomosis, compared with those undergoing a stapled end-to-end anastomosis. Furthermore, patients in the latter group were better able to release flatus without fear of faecal soiling, and 75% of them regained a rectoanal inhibitory reflex. Less than one-third of those in whom endoanal mucosectomy had been done were able to release flatus safely and reflex sphincter inhibition was present in less than 25%. Prolonged and vigorous retraction on the anal sphincter required to permit the removal of the anorectal mucosa and the time consuming manual construction of the ileoanal anastomosis was considered to provide a plausible explanation for the decrease in sphincter tone and the resulting functional imperfections. Other studies have failed to confirm the favourable results after the stapled end-to-end anastomosis, however, Williams *et al.* (1989) demonstrated that the operation was still associated with a pronounced reduction of resting anal pressure and while night evacuation was significantly reduced this was the only functional variable to show a difference when compared to patients with a manual transanal anastomosis.

In our unit 30 patients with the pouch stapled to the top of the anal canal were compared with 30 age- and sex-matched patients operated by endoanal mucosectomy. All patients were followed for at least a year. The postoperative RAP reduction in patients with stapled pouches proved to be similar at each interval postoperatively (Fig. 7.14). The immediate RAP reduction 4–6 weeks after surgery amounted to about 35% in both groups of patients and at 1 year RAP remained still significantly lower than the preoperative level – 22% in the stapled and 25% in the mucosectomy group. However, at this stage the sphincter pressure

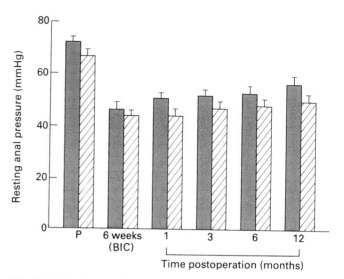

Fig. 7.14 Resting anal pressure, preoperatively (P), before ileostomy closure (BIC), and at monthly intervals postoperatively, in ▨, stapled pouch–anal anastomosis and ▨, handsewn.

Table 7.3 Reflex sphincter inhibition vs. ability to release gas safely in stapled and handsewn pouch-anal anastomosis (1-year follow-up).

	Mucosectomy	Stapled
Reflex inhibition	1/30 (3%)	7/30 (23%)
Ability to release gas safely	12/30 (40%)	14/30 (47%)

still remained within the 95% prediction limit of healthy controls in the majority of patients (Hallgren *et al.*, 1990).

Sphincter inhibition was completely abolished after surgery in all patients irrespective of technique used. At 1 year a sphincter tone reduction on rectal distension similar to the preoperative inhibitory reflex was present only in one out of 30 (3%) of the mucosectomy patients and in seven out of 30 stapled patients (23%). Twelve out of 30 patients (40%) in the former group and 14 out of 30 (47%) in the stapled group considered they were able to release gas safely (Table 7.3). The distension pressure required to elicit the response was 30–35 cmH_2O compared to 15 cmH_2O in normals (Fig. 7.15).

The functional results as reflected in individual functional variables proved to be largely the same in patients with stapled pouches as for patients operated with endoanal mucosectomy (Table 7.4).

To date, it is therefore unclear whether the stapled anastomosis is functionally much better than the original

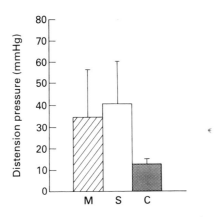

Fig. 7.15 The distension pressure thresholds for sphincter inhibition in stapled and handsewn ileoanal anastomosis compared to controls. ▨, mucosectomy (M); ▢, stapled (S); ▓, controls (C). $p < 0.05$.

Table 7.4 Functional results at 1 year.

	Mucosectomy ($n = 30$)	Stapled ($n = 30$)
Evacuation frequency 24 hours	4, 8 (1–8)	4, 8 (1–7)
Need for night-time evacuation (>1/week) (%)	10	10
Soiling		
Daytime	7	7
Night-time	21	10
Ability to release gas safely (%)	40	47
Use of pad (%)		
Daytime	10	10
Night-time	30	10
Medication (%)	75	45

technique with endoanal complete mucosectomy and sutured anastomosis. Johnston's favourable results should be interpreted with caution since in many of his patients part of the lower rectum appears to have been preserved implying that the operation was not always a pouch–anal but rather a pouch–rectal anastomosis (Sagar et al., 1990). The observation in the present study and in others (Williams et al., 1989; Seow-Choen et al., 1991) that there is still a significant and permanent reduction of RAP when stapling the anastomosis on top of the anal canal despite a minimal anal dilatation, would imply that other factors than sphincter over-distension may be involved. One explanation might be that the pelvic dissection and/or the transection of the rectum at the level of the levator ani muscle

may interfere with the extrinsic innervation to the sphincter muscles. There is experimental evidence supporting such a view (Carlstedt et al., 1988; Hallgren et al., 1992).

Other measures of improving function

Apart from modifications in operative technique pharmacological treatment for modulating intestinal motility and/or anal sphincter tone play an important role by modifying the quantity and the quality of the ileal effluent and improving sphincter tone. Loperamide has been extensively used, and a substantial number of pelvic pouch patients consider the drug beneficial and use it constantly. It has been convincingly demonstrated in ileostomy patients and patients with an ileorectal anastomosis that loperamide significantly decreases daily faecal volume, wet weight, water content and excretion rate, and that bulk density and viscosity of faeces is increased (Tytgat et al., 1977; King et al., 1982). A recent randomized double-blind study in our laboratory showed evidence that the drug reduced defaecation frequency in pelvic pouch patients by 50% and decreased significantly problems with soiling. The study also showed evidence that sphincter pressure increased significantly confirming previous suggestions that loperamide may also have a specific action on sphincter smooth muscles (Read et al., 1982). Clinical experience also speaks in favour of anti-cholinergic drugs used to improve continence especially in patients with night soiling and night evacuations. In a recent study atropine sulphate and benzilonium bromide were demonstrated to exert their effects by damping pouch motility, increasing pouch volume and raising luminal pressure thresholds for sense of filling and urge (Hallgren et al., 1991), while the anal sphincter was unaffected. Unfortunately effective treatment cannot be obtained without anti-cholinergic side effects but these problems may be reduced by administrating drugs at bedtime. Telander et al. (1981) used balloon dilatations in the early postoperative phase in young patients with a straight ileoanal anastomosis in an attempt to increase ileal volume capacity, and was able to demonstrate improved functional outcome. We accordingly in a randomized study employed both reservoir dilatations combined with sphincter exercises with the aim of improving the early functional results after loop ileostomy closure, but were unable to demonstrate any such effect (Öresland et al., 1988).

Which factors determine the functional outcome?

The presumptive functional determinants analysed in the presented studies could only explain a fraction of the total variability in functional outcome, and pouch volume was shown to be the only predictive factor for subsequent function which can be influenced by the surgeon. Stepwise regression analysis revealed that pouch volume and compliance (in the interval above 20 cmH$_2$O) accounted for only about 20% of the total variability of the functional score, however. Similar observations have been made by Becker & Raymond (1986) who found that diagnosis, ulcerative colitis or polyposis, and pouch capacity taken together accounted for only 10% of the total variance of stool frequency. Another clearly distinguishable determinant is patient's age; at all follow-up occasions elderly patients had a statistically significant higher, i.e. worse functional score than younger patients. However, several other factors related to the functional results were established, thereby elucidating the mechanisms controlling continence in these patients. As yet, the relative importance of each of these factors remains unclear and no obvious avenue can be pointed out for further development in attempting to improve the functional results. However, for the individual patient with a malfunctioning pouch, the acquired knowledge may be of immediate importance revealing probable and perhaps amendable defects.

A number of other functional determinants, not specifically dealt with in the present study should also be considered. Stool volume (O'Connell et al., 1987) and impairment of pouch emptying (Nasmyth et al., 1986a; Stryker et al., 1986) have been demonstrated to influence stool pattern and continence. Pouch emptying is not considered to be dependent on pouch design (Nasmyth et al., 1986b; O'Connell et al., 1986; Nicholls, 1987) nor is the occurrence of pouchitis, although Fonkalsrud using the lateral isoperistaltic design (Stelzner et al., 1988) reports an increased incidence in larger pouches. However, outlet obstruction may well contribute to the complication in that series. While no specific bacteriological changes have been demonstrated in patients with pouchitis, it has been shown that patients with bacterial overgrowth in the upper small intestine have an increased stool volume (O'Connell et al., 1986).

Rectoanal versus pouch–anal function, integrative aspects

Normal continence is dependent on a complex interaction between local reflex mechanisms and voluntary intervention. Important factors are the sensation of rectal filling and urge to defaecate, and the ability to discriminate between gas, and fluid and firm faeces. The internal anal sphincter is normally in a state of near maximal contraction. The muscle is responsible for about 85% of resting anal pressure (Frenckner & v.Euler, 1975) and is considered of importance for continence during sleep. The external anal sphincter and the puborectalis contract briskly on voluntary demands or reflexly in response to postural changes, for example, when lifting heavy objects, or in other situations which are associated with rapid increases in intra-abdominal pressure such as coughing. It is apparent from daily life and from several clinical situations that the demand on the sphincter muscles will also be dependent on the quality and quantity of the faeces.

Moderate balloon distension of the rectum will evoke a vague sensation of filling sometimes appreciated as a sensation of passing wind, whereas a more pronounced distension will evoke defaecation urge or pain. These sensations are supposed to be evoked by stimulation of free nerve endings in the rectal wall and mediated through afferent pelvic nerve fibres (Goligher & Hughes, 1951). Stretch receptors of the levator ani muscle, external sphincter and/or perirectal tissue have also been suggested to contribute to rectal sensory function (Scarli & Kiesewetter, 1970; Lane & Parks, 1977). The immediate response to rectal distension is a relaxation of the internal anal sphincter (the RAIR). The relaxation allows rectal contents to come into contact with the sensory epithelium of the transitional zone in the upper anal canal. The distension also gives rise to a shortlasting external sphincter contraction (the guarding reflex) which allows firm faeces to be kept in the rectum. The combined response is considered important for sampling (Duthie & Bennett, 1963), e.g. to discriminate between flatus and faeces but still defer passage of rectal content. The RAIR is closely dependent on the intact intrinsic innervation. The reflex is absent in patients with Hirschsprung's disease which is characterized by the absence of enteric ganglion cells. The reflex may also be absent if the rectum has been severed and an anastomosis constructed between the site of the distension and the sphincter (Gaston, 1948; Schuster et al., 1963; Fasth & Hultén, 1987).

Specific for the rectal musculature is the property of receptive relaxation. Given a slow filling rate the intra-luminal pressure does not increase until the maximal tolerated volume is approached. This accommodative capacity of the rectum is considered an important factor in maintaining faecal continence. On rapid distension of the rectum, however, a rectal contraction can be demonstrated in the majority of normal subjects even before the maximal volume is reached. The contribution of such contractions to the act of defaecation has been debated. According to traditional physiology a mass peristalsis moving the content of the left colon into the rectum is considered to be the phenomenon which initiates the sequence of events in defaecation. The filling sensation and the urge to defaecate occur when residues accumulate and distend the rectum. The autonomous part of the defaecation reflex, considered to be mediated by the pelvic nerves, is reinforced voluntarily by an increase in intra-abdominal pressure, i.e. straining and a relaxation of the pelvic floor. Opinions differ regarding the importance of rectal contraction and it has been suggested that there are two main patterns of defaecation, one group of normal subjects exhibiting a reflex type of defaecation with little straining, whereas in the other group the bowel can only be emptied with considerable straining (Rutter & Riddell, 1975). It seems reasonable to assume that defaecation in the latter group has become habitual in the sense that urge of defaecation is not necessarily the sign of evacuation but rather a social act. Such factors might also explain why defaecation frequency in healthy subjects varies between three per day to once every third day despite the fact that the daily faecal volumes vary little (for review see Goligher, 1984; Henry & Swash, 1991).

The physiological and clinical data observed in our study imply that despite ostensible similarities fundamental differences also exist between the healthy rectum and the pelvic J pouch. This is hardly surprising considering that the ileal substitute lacks not only the properties inherent in the rectal musculature but also its specific nervous supply (Fig. 7.16). Neither receptive relaxation on distension nor active reflex emptying exist in this artificial setting. Nevertheless, the terminal ileum when folded and converted to a pouch still behaves as a reservoir organ, and in the presence of a compliant reservoir and an adequate outlet resistance most patients can adopt a specific defaecation pattern with maintenance of an acceptable continence function.

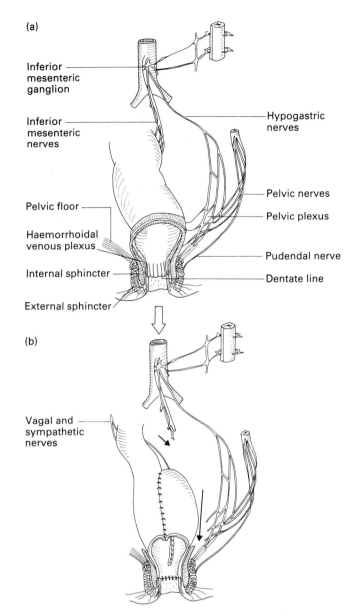

Fig. 7.16 (a) Schematic representation of anorectal anatomy and nerve supply. (b) After restorative proctocolectomy the ileal pouch replacing the rectum lacks many of the efferent and afferent nervous pathways controlling normal anorectal function, as indicated by the arrows.

Loss of, or defects in one or more of the factors involved in normal anorectal continence may possibly be compensated for by others; for example, a large pouch volume may compensate for a sphincter with a low resistance to leakage, or a small pouch may be compensated for by a low faecal volume, etc. Such factors might also to some extent explain the difficulties in identifying any single defect with an overall poor continence. These overlapping mechanisms controlling continence are perhaps not as effective with increasing age which might explain the observation that age correlated with functional outcome. There was also a gradual improvement in function beyond the time where no further changes were seen in the measured physiological variables, implying that there probably are several other patient-related factors, not as easily recognized as age, that are of immense importance for functional outcome. For example, it appears very likely that patients will learn by trial and error to adopt dietary restrictions to make firmer stools and change the timing of meals to gain control over defaecation habits. Many patients find that they can avoid night evacuations by bringing forward the timing of the final evening meal. Such measures, as well as the use of motility retarding drugs and bulk agents, may have an important impact on continence.

It is obvious that an ileal pouch cannot replace the normal rectum with its unique reservoir properties, it is merely an alternative to the conventional and continent ileostomy (Hultén 1985, 1986, 1988a,b,c, 1989, 1990). As such restorative proctocolectomy has definitely proven its merits and is now considered the main alternative for curative treatment for ulcerative colitis and familial polyposis. Although there is the possibility of further refinements, the major achievement was probably that made by the early pioneers who put this operation into clinical practice. However, the last word has not been said as regards the definite place of restorative proctocolectomy since the long-term results are unknown. Age has been demonstrated to be a functional determinant after restorative proctocolectomy. Incontinence is known to be a problem of the aged, and an important question is whether these patients will still have an acceptable continence when they become elderly. It also remains to be seen what will happen in the long run considering the substantial number of patients that are prone to develop pouchitis. Only further careful follow-up over decades will answer these and similar questions.

References

Åkervall S, Fasth S, Nordgren S, Öresland T, Hultén L (1988) Manovolumetry: a new method for investigation of anorectal function. *Gut* **529**:614–623.

Becker JM (1984) Anal sphincter function after colectomy, mucosal proctectomy and endorectal ileoanal pull-through. *Arch Surg* **119**:526–531.

Becker JM, Raymond JL (1986) Ileal pouch-anal anastomosis. A single surgeon's experience with 100 consecutive cases. *World J Surg* **10**:375–383.

Becker JM, Hillard AE, Mann FA, Kestenberg A, Nelson JA (1985) Functional assessment after colectomy, mucosal proctectomy, and endorectal pull-through. *World J Surg* **9**:598–605.

Berglund B, Brevinge H, Kock NG, Lindholm E (1987) Expansion of various types of ileal reservoirs in situ. An experimental study in rats. *Eur Surg Res* **19**:298–304.

Berglund B, Kock NG, Myrvold HE (1984) Volume capacity and pressure characteristics of the continent ileostomy reservoir. *Scand J Gastroenterol* **19**:683–690.

Carlstedt A, Nordgren S, Fasth S, Appelgren L, Hultén L (1988) Sympathetic nervous influence on the internal anal sphincter and rectum in man. *Int J Colorect Dis* **3**:90–95.

Chaussade S, Verduron A, Hautefeuille M *et al.* (1989) Proctocolectomy and ileoanal anastomosis without conservation of a rectal muscular cuff. *Br J Surg* **76**:273–275.

Duthie HL, Bennett RC (1963) The relation of sensation in the anal canal to the functional anal sphincter: a possible factor in anal continence. *Gut* **4**:179–182.

Emblem R, Erichsen AA, Mörkrid L, Ganes T, Stien R, Bergan A (1989a) Failed ileoanal anastomoses: correlation between clinical findings and anal canal neurophysiologic and histologic examinations. *Scand J Gastroenterol* **24**:623–631.

Emblem R, Stien R, Mørkrid L (1989b) Anal sphincter function after colectomy, mucosal proctectomy, and ileoanal anastomosis. *Scand J Gastroenterol* **24**:171–178.

Everett WG (1989) Experience of restorative proctocolectomy with ileal reservoir. *Br J Surg* **176**:77–81.

Fasth S, Hultén L (1987) Functional results after sphincter saving operations for low rectal tumors. In *Disordered Defaecation*, HG Gooszen, HO ten Cate Hoedemaker, IT Weterman, MRB Keighley (eds). Dordrecht, Matinus Nijhof Publishers, pp 195–206.

Frenckner B, v.Euler CHR (1975) Influence of pudendal block on the function of the anal sphincters. *Gut* **16**:482–489.

Gaston EA (1948) Fecal continence following resections of the rectum with preservation of the anal sphincters. *Surg Gynecol Obstet* **87**:669–678.

Gibbons CP, Bannister JJ, Trowbridge EA, Read NW (1986) An analysis of anal sphincter pressure and anal compliance in normal subjects. *Int J Colorect Dis* **1**:231–237.

Goligher JC (1984) *Surgery of the Anus, Rectum and Colon*, 5th edition. London, Bailliére Tindall Press.

Goligher JC, Hughes ESR (1951) Sensibility of the rectum and colon, its role in the mechanism of anal continence. *Lancet* **1260**:513–517.

Grant D, Cohen Z, McHugh S, McLeod R, Stern H (1986) Restorative proctocolectomy. Clinical results and manometric findings with long and short rectal cuffs. *Dis Colon Rectum* **29**:27–32.

Hallgren T, Fasth S, Nordgren S, Öresland T, Hallsberg L, Hultén L (1989) Manovolumetric characteristics and functional results in three different pelvic pouch designs. *Int J Colorect Dis* **4**:156–160.

Hallgren T, Fasth S, Nordgren S, Öresland T, Hultén L (1990) The stapled ileal pouch-anal anastomosis. A randomized study comparing two different pouch designs. *Scand J*

Gastroenterol **25**:1161–1168.

Hallgren T, Fasth S, Nordgren S, Öresland T, Hultén L (1991) The effect of atropine and bensilonium bromide on pelvic pouch and anal sphincter function. *Scand J Gastroenterol* **216**:563–571.

Hallgren T, Fasth S, Öresland T, Hultén L (1992) Damage of the autonomous nervous pathways – The principle cause of postoperative sphincter impairment after restorative proctocolectomy. *Brit J Surg* (in press).

Harms BA, Hamilton JW, Yamamoto DT, Starling JR (1987) Quadruple-loop (W) ileal pouch reconstruction after proctocolectomy: Analysis and functional results. *Surgery* **102**:561–567.

Heald RJ, Allen DR (1986) Stapled ileo-anal anastomosis: a technique to avoid mucosal proctectomy in the ileal pouch operation. *Br J Surg* **73**:571–572.

Henry MM, Swash M (1991) *Coloproctology and the Pelvic Floor. Pathophysiology and Management.* London, Butterworths.

Heppel J, Kelly KA, Phillips SF, Beart RW, Telander RL, Perrault J (1982) Physiologic aspects of continence after colectomy, mucosal proctectomy, and ileo-anal anastomosis. *Ann Surg* **195**:435–443.

Holdsworth PJ, Johnston D (1988) Anal sensation after restorative proctocolectomy for ulcerative colitis. *Br J Surg* **75**:993–996.

Hultén L (1985) The continent ileostomy (Kock's pouch) versus the restorative proctocolectomy (Pelvic pouch). *World J Surg* **69**:952–959.

Hultén L (1986) Restorative proctocolectomy with ileal reservoir. (Symposium.) *Int J Colorect Dis* **1**:2–19.

Hultén L (1988a) Surgical options in the treatment of ulcerative colitis and Crohn's colitis. *Schweitz Med Wochenschr* **118**:743–749.

Hultén L (1988b) Die kontinente Ileostomie – Kock'scher Pouch. *Chirurg* **59**:143–149.

Hultén L (1990) Some facts about restorative proctocolectomy with ileo-pouch anal anastomosis. Proktokolektomie und ein pelvines Ileum-Reservoir. In *Das kolorektake karzinom und seine Präkanzerosen*, Izbicki JR, Wilker DK, Schweiberer L (eds). Berlin, de Gruyter, pp. 173–188.

Hultén L, Fasth S, Nordgren S, Öresland T (1988c) Kock's pouch converted to a pelvic pouch – a case report. *Dis Colon Rectum* **31**:467–469.

Johnston D, Holdsworth PJ, Nasmyth DG et al. (1987) Preservation of the entire anal canal in conservative proctocolectomy for ulcerative colitis: a pilot study comparing end-to-end ileo-anal anastomosis without mucosal resection with mucosal proctectomy and endo-anal anastomosis. *Br J Surg* **74**:940–944.

Keighley MRB, Winslet MC, Yoshioka K, Lightwood R (1987) Discrimination is not impaired by excision of the transitional zone after restorative proctocolectomy. *Br J Surg* **74**:1118–1121.

Keighley MRB, Yoshioka K, Kmiot W (1988a) Prospective randomised trial to compare the stapled double lumen pouch and the sutured quadruple pouch for restorative proctocolectomy. *Br J Surg* **75**:1008–1011.

Keighley MRB, Yoshioka K, Kmiot W, Heyen F (1988b) Physiological parameters influencing function in restorative

proctocolectomy and ileo-pouch-anal anastomosis. *Br J Surg* **75**:997–1002.

King RFGJ, Norton T, Hill G (1982) A double blind crossover study of the effect of loperamide hydrochloride and codeine phosphate on ileostomy output. *Aust NZ J Surg* **52**:121–124.

Kock NG (1969) Intra-abdominal 'reservoir' in patients with permanent ileostomy. *Arch Surg* **99**:223–231.

Kock NG (1987) The development of the continent ileal reservoir (Kock pouch) and application in patients requiring urinary diversion. In *Bladder Reconstruction and Continent Urinary Diversion*, R Lowell, LT King (eds). Chicago, London, Year Book, Publ. Inc.

Lane RHS, Parks AG (1977) Function of the anal sphincters following colo-anal anastomosis. *Br J Surg* **64**:596–599.

Lestar B, Penninckx F, Kerremans R (1989) The composition of anal basal pressure. An in vivo and in vitro study in man. *Int J Colorect Dis* **4**:118–122.

Lindquist K (1990) Anal manometry with microtransducer technique before and after restorative proctocolectomy. Sphincter function and clinical correlations. *Dis Colon Rectum* **33**:91–98.

Luukkonen P (1988) Manovolumetric follow-up of anal sphincter function after an ileo-anal pouch procedure. *Int J Colorect Dis* **3**:43–46.

McHugh SM, Diamant NE (1987) Effect of age, gender, and parity on anal canal pressures Contribution of impaired anal sphincter function to fecal incontinence. *Dig Dis Sci* **732**:726–736.

Madoff RD, Orrom WJ, Rothenberger DA, Goldberg SM (1990) Rectal compliance: a critical reappraisal. *Int J Colorect Dis* **5**:37–40.

Moskowitz LR, Shepherd NA, Nicholls RJ (1986) An assessment of inflammation in the reservoir after restorative proctocolectomy with ileoanal ileal reservoir. *Int J Colorect Dis* **1**:167–174.

Nagasaki A, Ikeda K, Sumitomo K (1989) Rectoanal reflex induced by H_2O thermal stimulation. *Dis Col Rect* **32**:765–768.

Nasmyth DG, Johnston D, Godwin PGR, Dixon MF, Smith A, Williams NS (1986a) Factors influencing bowel function after ileal pouch-anal anastomosis. *Br J Surg* **73**:469–473.

Nasmyth DG, Williams NS, Johnston D (1986b) Comparison of the function of triplicated and duplicated pelvic ileal reservoirs after mucosal proctectomy and ileo-anal anastomosis for ulcerative colitis and adenomatous polyposis. *Br J Surg* **73**:361–366.

Neal DE, Williams NS, Johnston D (1982) Rectal, bladder and sexual function after mucosal proctectomy with and without a pelvic reservoir for colitis and polyposis. *Br J Surg* **69**:599–604.

Nicholls RJ (1987) Restorative proctocolectomy with various types of reservoirs. *World J Surg* **11**:751–762.

Nicholls RJ, Lubowski DZ (1987) Restorative proctocolectomy: the four loop (W) reservoir. *Br J Surg* **74**:567–568.

Nicholls RJ, Pezim ME (1985) Restorative proctocolectomy with ileal resevoir for ucerative colitis and familial adenomatous polyposis: a comparison of three reservoir designs. *Br J Surg* **72**:470–474.

Nicholls RJ, Belliveau P, Neil M, Wilks M, Tabaqchali S (1981) Restorative proctocolectomy with ileal reservoir: a pathophysiological assessment. *Gut* **22**:462–468.

O'Connell PR, Pemberton JH, Brown ML, Kelly KA (1987) Determinants of stool frequency after ileal pouch-anal anastomosis. *Am J Surg* **153**:157–164.

O'Connell PR, Rankin DR, Weiland LH, Kelly KA (1986) Enteric bacteriology, absorption, morphology and emptying after ileal pouch-anal anastomosis. *Br J Surg* **73**:909–914.

O'Connell PR, Stryker SJ, Metcalf AM, Pemberton JH, Kelly KA (1988) Anal canal pressure and motility after ileoanal anastomosis. *Surg Gynecol Obstet* **166**:47–54.

Öresland T, Fasth S, Åkervall S, Nordgren S, Hultén L (1990a) Manovolumetric and sensory characteristics of the ileoanal J pouch compared with healthy rectum. *Br J Surg* **77**:803–806.

Öresland T, Fasth S, Nordgren S, Åkervall S, Hultén L (1990b) Pouch size: the important functional determinant after restorative proctocolectomy. *Br J Surg* **77**:265–269.

Öresland T, Fasth S, Hultén L, Nordgren S, Swensson L, Åkervall S (1988) Does balloon dilatation and anal sphincter training improve ileoanal-pouch function? *Int J Colorectal Dis* **3**:153–157.

Öresland T, Fasth S, Nordgren S, Hallgren T, Hultén L (1990c) A prospective randomized comparison of two different pelvic pouch designs. *Scand J Gastroenterol* **25**:986–996.

Öresland T, Fasth S, Nordgren S, Hultén L (1989) The clinical and functional outcome after restorative proctocolectomy. A prospective study in 100 patients. *Int J Colorectal Dis* **4**:50–56.

Pearl RK, Nelson RL, Prasad ML, Abcarian H, Schuller N (1985) Ileoanal anastomosis 24 years after total proctocolectomy for ulcerative colitis. *Dis Colon Rectum* **328**:180–182.

Pescatori M, Parks AG (1984) The sphincteric and sensory components of preserved continence after ileoanal reservoir. *Surg Gynecol Obstet* **158**:517–521.

Read M, Read NW, Barber DC, Duthie HL (1982) Effects of loperamide on anal sphincter function in patients complaining of chronic diarrhea with fecal incontinence and urgency. *dig Dis Sci* **27**:807–814.

Rutter KRP, Riddell RH (1975) The solitary ulcer syndrome. *Bailliere's Clin Gastroenterol* **4**:505–530.

Ryan P, Fink R (1988) New rectum and new anal canal: two cases of ileal reservoir-cutaneous anastomosis. *Aust NZ J Surg* **58**:161–165.

Sagar PM, Holdsworth PJ, Johnston D (1993) Quality of life after restorative proctocolectomy. A comparison of two methods. *Dis Colon Rectum* (in press).

Scarli AF, Kiesewetter WB (1970) Defecation and continence: some new concepts. *Dis Colon Rectom* **213**:81–107.

Schuster MM, Hendrix TR, Mendeloff AI (1963) The internal anal sphincter response: Manometric studies on its normal physiology, neural pathways, and alteration in bowel disorders. *J Clin Invest* **42**:196–207.

Seow-Choen A, Tsunoda A, Nicholls RJ (1991) Prospective randomized trial comparing anal function after hand sewn ileoanal anastomosis with mucosectomy versus stapled ileoanal anastomosis without mucosectomy in restorative proctocolectomy. *Br J Surg* **78**:430–434.

Sharp FR, Bell GA, Seal AM, Atkinson KG (1987) Investigations of the anal sphincter before and after restorative proctocolectomy. *Am J Surg* **5153**:469–472.

Slors JFM, Taat CW, Brummelkamp WH (1989) Ileal pouch-anal anastomosis without rectal muscular cuff. *Int J Colorectal Dis* **4**:178–181.

Stelzner M, Fonkalsrud EW, Lichtenstein G (1988) Significance of reservoir length in the ileal pullthrough with ileal reservoir. *Arch Surg* **10123**:1265–1268.

Stryker SJ, Daube JR, Kelly KA *et al.* (1985) Anal sphincter electromyography after colectomy, mucosal rectectomy, and ileoanal anastomosis. *Arch Surg* **120**:713–716.

Stryker SJ, Phillips SF, Dozois RR, Kelly KA, Beart RW (1986) Anal and neorectal function after ileal pouch-anal anastomosis. *Ann Surg* **1203**:55–61.

Tasker JH (1953) A new technique: an experimental study with report of a case. *Br J Urol* **25**:349–352.

Taylor BM, Cranley B, Kelly KA, Phillips SF, Beart RW, Dozois RR (1983) A clinico-physiological comparison of ileal pouch-anal and straight ileoanal anastomosis. *Ann Surg* **4198**:462–468.

Telander RL, Perrault J, Hoffman AD (1981) Early development of the neorectum by balloon dilations after ileoanal anastomosis. *J pediatr Surg* **16**:911–916.

Thomson WHF, Simpson AHRW, Wheeler JL (1987) Mathematical prediction of ileal pouch capacity. *Br J Surg* **74**:567–568.

Tytgat GN, Huibregtse K, Dagevos J, Van den Ende A (1977) Effect of loperamide on fecal output and composition in well-established ileostomy and ileorectal anastomosis. *Dig Dis Sci* **22**:669–675.

Utsunomiya J, Iwama T, Imagio M *et al.* (1980) Total colectomy, mucosal proctectomy, and ileoanal anastomosis. *Dis Colon Rectum* **23**:459–466.

Wexner SD, Jensen L, Rothenberger DA, Wong WD, Goldberg SM (1989) Long-term functional analysis of the ileoanal reservoir. *Dis Colon Rectum* **32**:275–281.

Williams NS, Marzouk DEMM, Hallan RI, Waldron DJ (1989) Function after ileal pouch and stapled pouch-anal anastomosis for ulcerative colitis. *Br J Surg* **76**:1168–1171.

Chapter 8
Pouchitis – Acute Inflammation in Ileal Pouches

NEIL J. McC. MORTENSEN AND MICHAEL V. MADDEN

Introduction

Pouchitis is the commonest late complication of restorative proctocolectomy (Pemberton *et al.*, 1987). It is characterized by macroscopic inflammation of the ileal pouch mucosa (Tytgat & Van Deventer, 1988; Scott & Phillips, 1989; Madden *et al.*, 1990). The term pouchitis was first used by Kock *et al.*, (1977) to describe the syndrome of acute ileal reservoir inflammation which occurred in some of their patients with ulcerative colitis who had undergone proctocolectomy with a continent ileostomy (Kock pouch). Pouchitis was subsequently described in patients with ileal pouches (Handelsman *et al.*, 1983; Kelly *et al.*, 1983; Hultén & Svaninger, 1984; Moskowitz *et al.*, 1986; O'Connell *et al.*, 1986; Fonkalsrud, 1987; Pemberton *et al.*, 1987; Fleshman *et al.*, 1988; Everett, 1989; Curran & Hill, 1990; de Silva *et al.*, 1991). In the early 1950s the procedure of choice for patients with ulcerative colitis was a proctocolectomy and end ileostomy. Ileitis developing in the terminal ileum immediately proximal to the end ileostomy was recognized at that time (Warren & McKittrick, 1951; Lyons & Garlock, 1954; Thayer & Spiro, 1962). It was usually relieved by stomal dilatation and lavage with a catheter and it was thought that the ileitis occurred secondarily to chronic ileostomy obstruction (Warren & McKittrick, 1951; Counsell, 1956). With the introduction of the Brooke ileostomy involving everting the ileum to make a spout, ileostomy obstruction is now rare, as is ileostomy ileitis (Scott & Phillips, 1989). Some of the reported cases of ileostomy ileitis may also originally have been patients with Crohn's disease rather than ileitis.

Diagnosis

There is no agreed definition of pouchitis and uniform criteria have not been used. There is therefore, a wide variation in the reported incidence of pouchitis ranging from 13 to 30% in studies of Kock pouches (Kock *et al.*, 1985; Jarvinen *et al.*, 1986), and 7 to 14% in pelvic pouches (Dozois *et al.*, 1986). Some regard pouchitis as a purely clinical diagnosis based on change in symptoms with or without histological or endoscopic evidence of inflammation (O'Connell *et al.*, 1986). Most agree however that for an unequivocal diagnosis, suggestive symptoms should be accompanied by acute mucosal inflammation seen on endoscopy, together with evidence of a polymorphonuclear leukocyte infiltration (Moskowitz *et al.*, 1986; Tytgat & Van Deventer, 1988; Meuwissen *et al.*, 1989; Madden *et al.*, 1990; Shepherd, 1990). Using these more strict criteria, the incidence of pouchitis varies between 10 and 20% (Moskowitz *et al.*, 1986; Kock, 1987; Zuccaro *et al.*, 1989).

Symptoms and signs

The main symptom is usually diarrhoea, often stained pink or bright red by blood. This can be associated with abdominal pain, bloating and generalized symptoms such as malaise and fever. In a minority of cases there may also be extra-intestinal manifestations such as arthralgia, arthritis, iritis and pyoderma gangrenosum (Klein *et al.*, 1983; Knobler *et al.*, 1986; O'Connell *et al.*, 1986; Hultén, 1989; Zuccaro *et al.*, 1989; Lohmuller *et al.*, 1990). Since diarrhoea, with the frequent passage of loose stools, can occur after restorative proctocolectomy in the absence of pouch inflammation, for example where there is a stricture or a long distal ileal segment, such as in the early S reservoirs, the symptom alone is not sufficient to make a diagnosis. Routine physical examination is important to rule out anastomotic stricture. Most anastomoses admit an index finger, but even if a little finger passes comfortably, then the patient probably does not have a functionally significant stenosis. Pouchitis may be misdiagnosed by both clinician and pathologist in a patient with an anastomosis above the dentate line and persistent proctitis in the remaining rectal mucosa. In this situation careful endoscopic examination of the pouch outlet is necessary to establish that the abnormal mucosa lies distal to the anastomosis as the pathologist will find a biopsy from this area hard to distinguish from pouchitis. In the early postoperative period when pouchitis is most unusual, a rare but important cause of bloody diarrhoea is an ischaemic reservoir (see below).

In view of these conditions which can mimic pouchitis, the reservoir must be examined endoscopically. It is normal for the mucosal vascular pattern to disappear within a few weeks of construction although this does not always happen. At endoscopy there must be changes of inflammation including mucosal oedema, erythema, friability and sometimes mucosal erosions or frank ulceration (Tytgat & Van Deventer, 1988; Meuwissen *et al.*, 1989; Tytgat 1989; Zuccaro 1989; Madden *et al.*, 1990). The changes can be patchy but more commonly involve the whole pouch mucosa (Meuwissen *et al.*, 1989; Madden *et al.*, 1990). Two studies have shown that only about half the patients with symptoms suggesting pouchitis actually have pouch inflammation on endoscopy (Church *et al.*, 1987; Meuwissen *et al.*, 1989).

The terminal ileum just proximal to the pouch is usually but not always spared. It was affected in three out of 14 episodes studied by Di Febo *et al.* (1990). Severe terminal ileum involvement can sometimes be seen in patients with chronic pouchitis.

Natural history

It is generally accepted that exposure of the pouch mucosa to the faecal stream is necessary for the development of pouchitis. It can develop from as early as 3 months after ileostomy closure, the incidence falling after 2–3 years. It may behave in a similar manner to colitis with episodes of exacerbation and remission. There may be recurrent acute episodes or even a persisting chronic illness. Öresland *et al.* (1989) studied the cumulative incidence of pouchitis in 99 patients with an ileoanal reservoir, followed over a mean period of 2 years from ileostomy closure. There were 23 patients who developed an episode of pouchitis, out of whom 11 (48%) had only a single attack. The remainder had intermittent recurrent episodes, only two of them (9%) experiencing prolonged chronic pouchitis (Fig. 8.1). By 3 years over 30% of the patients had experienced at least one attack. This incidence is similar to that estimated to occur in patients with a continent ileostomy, where about 35% of patients

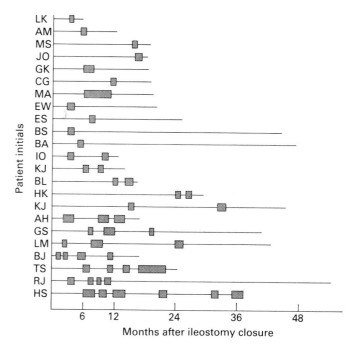

Fig. 8.1 Number and length of pouchitis episodes (–▦–) in 23 out of 99 patients with ileoanal reservoir. From Öresland *et al.* (1989) with permission.

had had pouchitis within 10 years from construction (Hultén, 1989).

Incidence

A few systematic attempts have been made to define the true incidence of pouchitis; in the study of Moskowitz *et al.* (1986) there were 6 (11%) patients out of 55 cases studied. This was a retrospective analysis and did not examine the incidence of the condition. In a retrospective review of 734 cases seen over a mean follow-up period of 41 months, 210 (29%) patients had symptomatic pouchitis whilst 128 (17%) had recurrent symptoms (Lohmuller *et al.*, 1990). Different criteria for the diagnosis of pouchitis were used here, there being no endoscopic or histological confirmation. Nonetheless, this incidence is similar to that reported by Öresland *et al.*, 1989. The mean interval between ileostomy closure however and the development of pouchitis was different, ranging from 6 months (Hultén, 1989 and Öresland *et al.*, 1989) to 17 months (Pemberton *et al.*, 1987).

When a more stringent definition of pouchitis is used including endoscopic and histological criteria, true cases of pouchitis in patients with polyposis are rare. In previous series with Kock pouches, pouchitis was rarely seen in the polyposis group (Hultén, 1989). Only a few poorly documented cases have been reported in patients with familial adenomatous polyposis (FAP) (Kmiot & Keighley, 1990; Gustavsson et al., 1987; Dozois et al., 1989; Dube & Heyen, 1990; Lohmuller et al., 1990). In a retrospective study of 37 patients having restorative proctocolectomy for FAP, none had developed pouchitis after a mean follow-up period of 5 years (Madden et al., 1991). All these patients had been examined regularly by endoscopy and biopsy. In two studies, the diagnosis of pouchitis was mainly clinical, and even though routine endoscopy and biopsy were not always employed, pouchitis was significantly more frequent in colitis patients compared with those with polyposis. Becker and Raymond (1986) reported incidences of 23 and 0% and Lohmuller et al. (1990) 31 and 6%, respectively.

Pouchitis is much more common in those patients who had had extensive colitis compared with left sided or distal disease (Farrands et al., 1988). There is no predisposition however to develop pouchitis in patients who had backwash ileitis at the time of their colectomy (Gustavsson et al., 1987).

A rare syndrome of pouch inflammation occurs prior to ileostomy closure (Meuwissen et al., 1989; Warren et al., 1990). It is likely that the aetiology of the inflammation in these cases is different from that of pouchitis in functioning pouches. Possible mechanisms include mucosal ischaemia (Shepherd, 1990) or a mechanism similar to that occurring in diversion colitis. Since faecal diversion is advocated in the management of severe pouchitis not responding to medical therapy, this probably does represent a different problem.

The reservoir mucosa

Histological studies have shown that both acute and chronic inflammatory changes are common following the construction of an ileal reservoir (Kelly et al., 1983; Philipson et al., 1985; Moskowitz et al., 1986; Nasmyth et al., 1986; Nilsson et al., 1980; Shepherd et al., 1987; Luukkonen et al., 1988a).

Chronic inflammation

Changes of chronic inflammation are so common that they are almost a normal feature of an established pouch. The changes take the form of a chronic inflammatory cell infiltrate and villous atrophy (Moskowitz et al., 1986; Nasmyth et al., 1986; O'Connell et al., 1986;

Kock et al., 1977; Shepherd et al., 1987; de Silva et al., 1990). The chronic inflammatory changes do not however correlate with function (Moskowitz et al., 1986). These changes are also accompanied by several features suggesting colonic metaplasia, including elongation of the crypts (Lersch et al., 1989, de Silva et al., 1990), a change in mucus production from mainly sialomucin (typical of small bowel) to predominately sulphomucin (characteristic of colonic mucosa) (Shepherd et al., 1987; Ojerskog et al., 1990; de Silva et al., 1990) and an increase in goblet cells (Lersch et al., 1989; Ojerskog et al., 1990). These features of colonic metaplasia have persisted without dysplasia in 15 continent ileostomies biopsied some 15–20 years after their construction (Ojerskog et al., 1990). In pouchitis the villi are flatter and the crypts deeper than in normal reservoirs. Despite these features of colonic metaplasia, half of the eight inflamed reservoirs studied by de Silva et al. (1990) retained a small bowel pattern of mucin. It is interesting that this tendency to produce small bowel mucin should have persisted despite other evidence of colonic metaplasia. There is therefore a partial, rather than a complete 'colon'-ization of the pouch mucosa. The same pattern of mucin production was reported in rectal biopsies from a high proportion (over 50%) of patients with active ulcerative colitis and was seldom evident in those in remission (Ehsanullah et al., 1982). Another important histological feature is the low intra-epithelial lymphocyte density (IEL) (Philipson et al., 1975; Shepherd et al., 1987; Shepherd, 1989). Whereas IEL densities are greatly increased in untreated coeliac disease (Fergusson, 1977), densities have been found to be strikingly low in pouches, but do not increase even when pouchitis develops (Shepherd et al., 1987; 1989).

Acute inflammation

Mild acute inflammatory changes are also common in normal reservoirs. Unlike chronic inflammation, acute inflammation does correlate with function. In a survey of 53 patients having biopsies from the reservoir taken between 5 and 62 months after ileostomy closure, severe acute inflammatory changes were restricted to patients with both a high stool frequency and endoscopically inflamed reservoir mucosa. The severity of acute inflammation was estimated blind by the pathologist and graded using the features shown in Table 8.1. Frequency of evacuation correlated significantly with the histological acute inflammation score. This was largely accounted for by the six patients

Table 8.1 Scoring system for histopathological changes in reservoir muscosa.

Histological feature	Score
Acute	
Polymorph infiltration	
None	0
Mild and patchy infiltrate in the surface epithelium	1
Moderate with crypt abscesses	2
Severe with crypt abscesses	3
Ulceration	
None	0
Mild superficial	1
Moderate	2
Extensive	3
Chronic	
Chronic inflammatory cell infiltration	
None	0
Mild and patchy	1
Moderate	2
Severe	3
Villous atrophy	
None	0
Minor abnormality of villous architecture	1
Partial villous atrophy	2
Subtotal villous atrophy	3

From Shepherd *et al.* (1987).

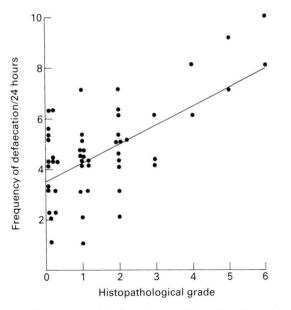

Fig. 8.2 Frequency of defaecation and histological grade of inflammation in 55 patients examined by one clinician. Correlation coefficients of linear regression: *r*, 0.65; *p*, 0.001. From Moskowitz *et al.* (1986) with permission.

of the 53 with a score of 4 to 6, all of whom passed six or more stools per 24 hours (Fig. 8.2). Among the 40 patients who passed less than six stools per 24 hours, 25 (63%) showed mild or moderate inflammatory changes (Moskowitz *et al.*, 1986). In a further study an acute infiltrate in the lamina propria was found in five (38%) out of 13 reservoirs in the absence of endoscopic abnormality and without any correlation with function, whilst out of 10 conventional ileostomies none showed any histological inflammation (Nasmyth *et al.*, 1986). Thus there is some variation in the reported prevalence of acute inflammatory changes related to function and endoscopic appearances. These again must represent differences in diagnostic criteria.

The presence of acute inflammation in the reservoir is more common in patients with ulcerative colitis than in those with familial adenomatous polyposis. This was observed in Kock continent ileostomies (Ojerskog *et al.*, 1990) and has been confirmed for ileoanal reservoirs. Thus in a comparison between 72 patients with ulcerative colitis and 12 with polyposis the mean histological acute inflammation score in the colitis group was 1.87, (Fig. 8.3) significantly higher than that of 0.15 in the polyposis group (Moskowitz *et al.*, 1986). In the same study however, the difference between chronic inflammatory scores (2.46 vs. 1.54) was not significant. No significant differences have been found between the degree of mucosal inflammation and the different pouch designs (Moskowitz *et al.*, 1986; Nasmyth *et al.*, 1989a). Although there are rare reports of the isolation of pathogens, such as *Campylobacter jejuni* (Meuwissen *et al.*, 1989; O'Connell *et al.*, 1986) and *Clostridium difficile* (Nicholls *et al.*, 1989; O'Connell *et al.*, 1986) from the pouch stool, no known intestinal pathogen has been incriminated consistently in pouchitis (Nasmyth *et al.*, 1989b). Diagnostic criteria should therefore require the exclusion of known intestinal pathogens.

Aetiology

The cause of pouchitis remains unknown and there may be more than one cause (Zuccaro *et al.*, 1989; Shepherd, 1990).

Crohn's disease

Crohn's disease is a contraindication to restorative proctocolectomy (Dozois *et al.*, 1986; Beart, 1988; Mortensen, 1989; Pezim *et al.*, 1989). Patients with equivocal clinical

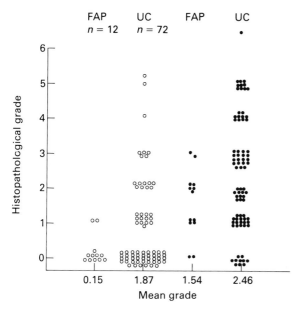

Fig. 8.3 Histological grade of inflammation in patients with an original diagnosis of familial adenomatous polyposis (FAP) and ulcerative colitis (UC). o, acute inflammation, *p*, 0.05; •, chronic inflammation, n.s. From Moskowitz *et al.* (1986) with permission.

and pathological features, that is those with indeterminate colitis seem to do as well functionally following pouch formation and have a similar incidence of pouchitis to patients with unequivocal ulcerative colitis (Pezim *et al.*, 1989). Most large series have a small number of cases of pouches which have been excised for Crohn's disease which was not suspected at the time of the reservoir formation (Nicholls & Pezim, 1985; Pemberton *et al.*, 1987; Everett, 1989; Wexner *et al.*, 1989; Zuccaro *et al.*, 1989). Although this has led to suggestions that pouchitis may be a manifestation of Crohn's disease, the majority of patients have no histological features to support this diagnosis (Tytgat, 1989). Subramani *et al.* (1990) reviewed the histology of colectomy specimens originally diagnosed as ulcerative colitis in 33 patients with ileal pouches. Fifteen of these had pouchitis and 18 did not. The original diagnosis of ulcerative colitis changed to Crohn's disease in equal numbers of colectomy specimens (three each) in the two groups with and without pouchitis, suggesting that pouchitis does not reflect underlying Crohn's disease. Even the presence of mucosal granulomata and fissure ulceration, features which have sometimes been reported in pouchitis, are not considered to be definitive evidence of Crohn's disease. These fissures may arise from surgical manipulation or high intra-

luminal pressure within the pouch (Lohmuller *et al.*, 1990; Shepherd, 1990). Granulomas probably occur as a reaction of the ileal mucosa to an altered luminal environment or foreign material (Shepherd, 1989, 1990).

Stasis and bacterial overgrowth

Since stasis is the main functional difference between pouches and conventional ileostomies it has long been implicated in the pathogenesis of pouchitis. A number of pouch emptying studies using both radioisotope and non-isotope methods have been used to investigate pouch emptying. None has shown any association between incomplete emptying and pouchitis (Moskowitz *et al.*, 1986; Nasmyth *et al.*, 1986; O'Connell *et al.*, 1986; Heppell *et al.*, 1987; Nasmyth *et al.*, 1989a; de Silva, 1991). Bacterial overgrowth follows stasis, and certainly total bacterial counts are higher in pouch stool compared to the effluent of a conventional ileostomy. Ileostomy effluent itself is higher in bacterial counts than normal faecal material (Philipson *et al.*, 1975; Brandberg *et al.*, 1972; Hill & Fernandez, 1989; Nasmyth *et al.*, 1985; Go *et al.*, 1988). Bacteriological studies have not shown any quantitative or qualitative difference in the stools of pouches with and without pouchitis (Luukkonen *et al.*, 1988a; Hill & Fernandez, 1989). A syndrome of *jejunal* bacterial overgrowth has also been described in patients with pouches (O'Connell *et al.*, 1986), but although this was associated with a poor functional result it was not associated with pouchitis. Furthermore, apart from a few case reports none of the known intestinal pathogens have been consistently implicated in pouchitis. The speed with which some cases of pouchitis respond to antibiotics, chiefly metronidazole, would suggest a bacteriological aetiology for pouchitis (Hultén & Svaninger, 1984; Fleshman *et al.*, 1988; Jarvinen *et al.*, 1986; Kock, 1987; Everett 1989; Öresland *et al.*, 1989; Zuccaro *et al.*, 1989). It is unlikely that bacteria are directly responsible for the occurrence of pouchitis, but it has been suggested that changes in the bacterial profile may play a part in the pathogenesis of pouchitis either by provoking an immune response in susceptible individuals (O'Connell *et al.*, 1986; Hill & Fernandez, 1989; Hultén, 1989; Scott & Phillips, 1989) or by an effect on faecal bile acids (Madden *et al.*, 1990).

High levels of deconjugated and secondary bile acids both of which are potentially mucosally toxic are to be found in pouches (Hill & Owen, 1989; Nasmyth *et al.*,

1989b). One study (Hill & Owen, 1989) has shown that although the concentration of secondary bile acids following dehydroxylation of primary bile acids is similar in pouches constructed for ulcerative colitis and FAP, there was a significant reduction in the concentration of conjugated bile acids in patients with pouchitis, all of whom had had previous ulcerative colitis. This would suggest an increased deconjugation of bile acids in pouchitis, although the authors recognized that their study was poorly controlled for standardization of patients' diets. Further evidence against this hypothesis is that the local instillation of cholestyramine is ineffective in the treatment of pouchitis (Hultén, 1989). Deconjugated bile salts are detergents and deoxycholic acid has been shown to pass into the colonic mucosa of rats, dissolving the lipids in cell membranes (Breuer et al., 1983). Reduced concentrations of tauro conjugated bile salts in the faeces in patients with pouchitis have been reported (Hill & Owen, 1989), but there could be a bacterial factor causing increased conjugation (Go et al., 1988; Nasmyth et al., 1989b). An association between pouchitis and low intragastric pH has been reported (Dube & Heyen, 1990) and this would suggest that an alteration of intraluminal microflora is the possible factor in pouchitis.

Recent studies in Oxford using in vivo dialysis of pouch fluid have demonstrated that a factor is present in pouches with a molecular weight of less than 1000 which is highly toxic to cultured colonic cell lines. Since this toxicity is partly inhibited by cholestyramine it may well be a bile acid and it could be this which causes the initial colonic metaplasia which is then subsequently involved in an immunologically mediated acute inflammation (Merrett et al., 1991).

Faecal short chain fatty acids

In the human colon carbohydrate from dietary fibre is broken down by anaerobes to volatile short chain fatty acids (SCFAs) (Roediger, 1980). An overgrowth of anaerobic bacteria could therefore alter the SCFA composition of ileal pouch contents. Since short chain fatty acids may suppress the growth of bacteria which produce toxic metabolites, and low luminal SCFA concentrations seem to play a part in the development of diversion colitis (Harig et al., 1989; Nasmyth et al., 1989b) it is worth noting both studies which have looked at SCFA concentrations in pouches. Nasmyth et al. (1989b) found SCFA concentrations in pouch stool

to be significantly higher than in conventional ileostomy effluent and similar to those in normal faeces. They also found an inverse correlation between butyrate concentrations and the degree of villous atrophy. Ambroze et al. (1989, 1990) however found that there was a 40% reduction in total SCFA concentrations in pouch stool compared to normal faeces. There was also a significant reduction in all the individual SCFAs measured (butyrate, isobutyrate, valerates, isovalerates and propionates) with the exception of acetate. In a further study from the same group total SCFA concentrations were now found to be similar to those found in normal faeces. No studies have yet been reported measuring SCFAs in the presence of pouchitis, but pouchitis does not respond to treatment with SCFA enemas (de Silva et al., 1989). This could indicate that reduced concentrations of SCFAs do not play a role in the pathogenesis of pouchitis. It does not however, exclude the possibility that the failure of pouch epithelial cells to metabolize SCFAs rather than a reduction in the concentration of SCFAs may be responsible. SCFAs do seem to have a trophic effect on terminal ileum epithelium as well as colonic mucosa (Goodlad et al., 1987, 1989; Sakata, 1987) and a failure of colonocytes to metabolize SCFAs, especially butyrate has been suggested as a possible pathogenic mechanism for the development of ulcerative colitis (Roediger, 1980).

Ischaemia

Ischaemic changes can be seen after pouch formation before closure of the loop ileostomy. Occasionally it may be so severe that the pouch needs to be excised or revised. Certainly milder forms of ischaemia have endoscopic appearances similar to those of pouchitis (Wong & Goldberg, 1987; Keighley et al., 1988; Pescatori et al., 1988; Tytgat, 1989; Shepherd, 1990). Hosie et al. (1989) measured pouch mucosal blood flow using a laser doppler probe, and found it to be lower in pouchitis when compared with healthy pouches or with conventional ileostomies. They also claimed patients with pouchitis had had more vascular division during the formation of their pouch than patients with healthy pouches, and they suggested that ischaemia may therefore be an aetiological factor in the pathogenesis of pouchitis. This work has not been substantiated and it is unlikely that ischaemia is important as it does not explain either the chronic relapsing nature of the condition or its predilection for patients with ulcerative colitis. The histological changes of pouchitis are also not the characteristic features of chronic ischaemia (Brandt *et al.*, 1981; Dixon, 1989; Lott & Wright, 1989).

Immunologically mediated acute inflammation

The development of pouchitis in an ileal reservoir may be a two-step process. In response to the new luminal environment the pouch may undergo adaptive colonic metaplasia (Wolfstein *et al.*, 1982; Go *et al.*, 1987; Shepherd *et al.*, 1987; Lerch *et al.*, 1989; Shepherd, 1990). This would then make the pouch mucosa vulnerable to immune damage in susceptible individuals, implying that pouchitis has an immunological basis, and its aetiology and pathogenesis are related to those of ulcerative colitis. Such a hypothesis would explain the apparent specificity of pouchitis for patients who had previously had ulcerative colitis.

Colonic metaplasia in ileal reservoirs

The histological changes in ileal pouches are dealt with in detail in Chapter 10. Villous atrophy, crypt hyperplasia and goblet cell hyperplasia which occur in functioning pouches produce a morphological change from the villous architecture typical of small intestine to the glandular changes typical of colonic mucosa. Studies of the ileal pouch mucosa and experimental models have also shown similar changes (Luukkonen *et al.*, 1988a; O'Byrne *et al.*, 1989). Not only does the pouch mucosa resemble colonic mucosa histologically, but there are changes in pouch mucin from a small bowel type sialomucin to a colorectal type sulphomucin (Go *et al.*, 1987; Shepherd *et al.*, 1987; de Silva *et al.*, 1990). The pouch epithelium may also acquire immuno reactivity against a colon specific monoclonal antibody (Shepherd, 1990; de Silva *et al.*, 1990). These changes all occur irrespective of the original diagnosis and have been reported in both pelvic and Kock ileal pouches (de Silva *et al.*, 1990; Shepherd *et al.*, 1987). In the experimental model using rats O'Byrne *et al.* (1989) showed that similar changes could be induced in ileal pouches and segments of ileum transposed to the distal colon. This experiment supports the view that colonic metaplasia occurs in response to exposure of the ileal mucosa to faecal stasis.

Further indirect evidence for colonic metaplasia is the occurrence of adenomatous polyps occurring *de novo* in pouches of patients who have had FAP (Beart *et al.*, 1982; Wolfstein *et al.*, 1982; Shepherd *et al.*, 1987; Stryker *et al.*, 1987; Hultén, 1989). Small numbers of polyps have been reported in the ileum of patients with FAP (Hamilton *et al.*, 1979), but there are now reports of pouches being carpeted by hundreds of adenomatous polyps, though none have developed in the ileum proximal to the pouch (Wolfstein *et al.*, 1982; Stryker *et al.*, 1987). These changes to a colonic type of mucosa are not complete however. De Silva *et al.* (1990) have demonstrated that small bowel specific sucrase-isomaltase activity persists in pouch epithelium regardless of morphological change, mucin type, or immunoreactivity against a colon specific monoclonal antibody. This together with the evidence that ileal pouches retain the ability to absorb vitamin B_{12}, D-xylose, phenylalanine, and bile acids, suggest that the colonic metaplasia in ileal pouches is incomplete (Jagenburg *et al.*, 1975; Philipson *et al.*, 1975; Gadacz *et al.*, 1977; Go *et al.*, 1988; Nasmyth *et al.*, 1989b).

Immune mechanisms in pouchitis

Rather than pouchitis being due to faecal stasis, the observation that equivocal pouchitis has been diagnosed almost exclusively in patients with previous pouchitis suggests that pouchitis and ulcerative colitis may share mechanisms in common. Episodes of pouchitis can also be associated with a number of extra-intestinal manifestations characteristic of inflammatory bowel disease (Klein *et al.*, 1983; Knobler *et al.*, 1986; O'Connell *et al.*, 1986; Hultén, 1989; Zuccaro *et al.*, 1989; Lohmuller *et al.*, 1990). There also appears to be an association between the occurrence of extra-intestinal manifestations of ulcerative colitis before restorative proctocolectomy and the subsequent development of pouchitis (Lohmuller *et al.*, 1990; de Silva *et al.*, 1991). There are marked histological similarities between pouchitis and active ulcerative colitis including the prominent polymorphonuclear cell infiltrate in the lamina propria and epithelium, with crypt abscess formation occurring together with marked chronic inflammatory cell infiltrates in the lamina propria, a low intra epithelial lymphocytes (IEL) density, crypt distortion and mucus depletion (Hirata *et al.*, 1986; Riddell, 1988). Immunohistochemical studies in pouchitis have shown an increase in the immunoglobulin G (IgG) isotype of plasma cells (Meuwissen *et al.*,

1989) and an increase in Royal Free D9 (RFD9) positive macrophages (de Silva *et al.*, 1990) in the pouch mucosa. Both these are features of active ulcerative colitis and do not occur as a non-specific response to an acute infective process (Van Spreeuel *et al.*, 1985; Allison *et al.*, 1988; Brandtzaeg *et al.*, 1989; Mahida *et al.*, 1989). This raises the possibility that effector mechanisms similar to those triggering the original ulcerative colitis are also operating in pouchitis. There are many reports of pouchitis responding to treatments active in ulcerative colitis and this further strengthens the association between pouchitis and ulcerative colitis.

Inflammatory mediators

Gertner *et al.* (1989) demonstrated that leukotriene B4 (LTB4) release in biopsies obtained from non-inflamed functioning ileal pouches in patients with previous ulcerative colitis was significantly higher than for biopsies from pouches formed for FAP. Furthermore LTB4 release in tissue obtained from defunctioned pouches and conventional ileostomies in patients with previous ulcerative colitis was as high as levels found in functioning pouches. These results suggest that there is increased ileal 5-lipo-oxygenase activity in patients with ulcerative colitis. Platelet activating factor (PAF) concentrations in the stools from patients with pouchitis have also been found to be significantly higher than in the stools of those without pouchitis (Chaussade *et al.*, 1990). PAF concentrations in the stools from pouches without pouchitis however were also found to be significantly higher than those found in normal faeces. This might reflect the milder degree of microscopic inflammation which is seen even in pouches which do not have pouchitis. Thus LTB4 and PAF may have a role in the mediation of inflammation in ileal pouches.

Treatment

The treatment of pouchitis still remains empirical. As we have already emphasized, it is important to rule out other common causes of a high stool frequency, such as a small reservoir, an anastomotic stricture, habitual frequent defaecation and incidental enteric infection. In the absence of an identifiable cause, frequent evacuation usually responds to an anti-diarrhoeal drug such as loperamide or codeine. Bulk laxatives such as ispaghula may make loose stools more formed, but

may also on occasion increase frequency. Of those patients with proven pouchitis, a minority with inflamed pouches retain good function and do not need treatment. Most others can be treated satisfactorily as an out-patient, and intravenous rehydration is seldom needed.

Metronidazole

There are many reports of the efficacy of metronidazole which is the most commonly used treatment (Hultén & Svaninger, 1984; Becker & Raymond, 1986; Jarvinen *et al.*, 1986; Moskowitz *et al.*, 1986; Fleshman *et al.*, 1988; Fonkalsrud, 1987; Luukkonen *et al.*, 1988b; Tytgat & Van Deventer, 1988; Everett, 1989; Öresland *et al.*, 1989; Curran & Hill, 1990; Lohmuller *et al.*, 1990). Metronidazole has immunosuppressive properties (suppression of cell mediated immunity) (Grove *et al.*, 1977) and a recent study has found it to be at least as effective as sulphasalazine in maintaining remission in patients with ulcerative colitis (Gilat *et al.*, 1989).

In a recent study (Madden *et al.*, unpublished observations), 13 patients who had undergone procto-colectomy for ulcerative colitis were entered into a double blind placebo cross over study. The end-point of this study was diarrhoea, but endoscopic inflammation, histological acute inflammation and serum C-reactive protein were also studied. All the patients were passing more than six stools per 24 hours or had consistently bloody stools or all had at least four out of six possible endoscopic criteria of mucosal acute inflammation (Moskowitz *et al.*, 1986). One patient did not relapse after responding to the first course of treatment and another was withdrawn because of an episode of bowel obstruction. The remaining 11 patients were evaluated after completing the course of metronidazole and placebo. Out of these, 10 (91%) had chronic unremitting symptoms of pouchitis before the study and one had an acute illness. Patients were randomly allocated to either receive metronidazole 400 mg by mouth three times a day, or placebo for 2 weeks. They then stopped the drug and if after 1 week pouchitis was still present, or when it later recurred, a further 2 weeks' treatment was given with the alternative drug. Assessments were made at the beginning and end of each 2-week period. To assess whether metronidazole would reduce stool frequency independently of an effect on pouchitis, 12 patients without clinical endoscopic or histological features of pouchitis were also studied before and after a 2-week course of

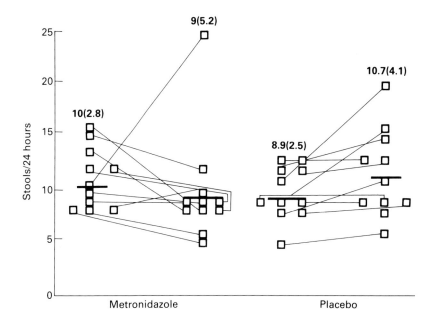

Fig. 8.4 Comparison of stool frequency for patients taking metronidazole compared with a placebo group, over 2 weeks. Numbers in bold, mean (SD) stools/24 h. Bars representative of median values.

metronidazole. They had all undergone restorative proctocolectomy, six for ulcerative colitis and six for familial polyposis.

On metronidazole the mean number of bowel actions decreased from 10 to 9 per 24 hours (Fig. 8.4) whilst on placebo frequency rose from 8.9 to 10.7 per 24 hours. When compared with the placebo, metronidazole improved diarrhoea significantly ($p < 0.05$, Student's paired one tail t test). Metronidazole therapy was associated with a slight improvement in endoscopic mucosal inflammation score (Fig. 8.5) the median score change being 0.5, but this did not differ significantly from placebo. Serum C-reactive protein levels improved on metronidazole but were not significantly different from a slight deterioration following placebo. The histological grade of acute inflammation fell slightly after metronidazole but again was not altered by placebo; this difference was not statistically significant. Metronidazole had no significant effect on stool frequency in the normal reservoirs of six out of the 12 patients with pouches but without pouchitis.

Other treatments

Other antibiotics such as Augmentin and vibramycin have also been used successfully (Hultén, 1989; Everett, 1989) although not all cases of pouchitis respond to antibiotics (Meuwissen *et al.*, 1989; Tytgat, 1989; Zuccaro *et al.*, 1989). Pouchitis can also be treated with enemas containing steroids or 5-aminosalicylic acid

derivatives, oral sulphasalazine, or short courses of prednisolone (Moskowitz *et al.*, 1986; Kock, 1987; Tytgat & Van Deventer, 1988; Hultén, 1989; Meuwissen *et al.*, 1989; Miglioli *et al.*, 1989; Tytgat, 1989; Zuccaro *et al.*, 1989). The repeated drainage of incompletely-emptying pouches may also contribute to rapid healing (Kock, 1987; Tytgat & Van Deventer, 1988; Meuwissen *et al.*, 1989). The xanthine oxidase inhibitor, allopurinol has been tested in an uncontrolled study which reported seven out of 12 patients with chronic pouchitis and four out of eight with acute pouchitis responding well (Levin *et al.*, 1990).

These various forms of treatment can be used either individually or in combination and are often effective. Rarely pouchitis is intractable and necessitates a diverting loop ileostomy. In a group of 28 patients with pouchitis, three had had a loop ileostomy. This was reversed in one after remission, but the patient later had brief further attacks, and one further patient was also converted to an ileostomy (Hultén, 1989). In intractable cases, the pouch may have to be excised (Halvorsen *et al.*, 1978; Fleshman *et al.*, 1988; Tytgat & Van Deventer, 1988; Hultén, 1989; Scott & Phillips, 1989; Wexner *et al.*, 1989).

Although the cause of pouchitis remains unknown (Tytgat & Van Deventer, 1988; Scott & Phillips, 1989; Madden *et al.*, 1990) there seem to be several clues. Firstly, the association with ulcerative colitis suggests that it may be a similar process or alternatively patients with familial adenomatous polyposis may produce

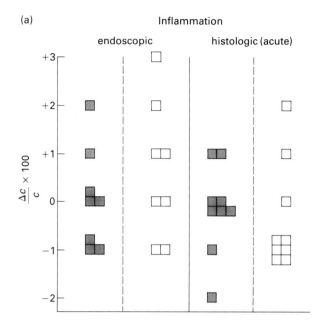

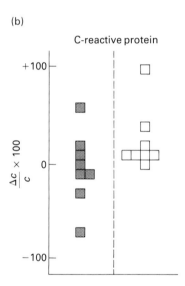

Fig. 8.5 (a) Endoscopic appearances and histological inflammation, and (b) C-reactive protein levels in metronidazole-treated patients and controls. Δc, difference between pre- and post-treatment values; c, pretreatment values; ▨, placebo patient; □, metronidazole patient.

a substance which suppresses pouchitis. Secondly, its absence from conventional ileostomies strongly suggests that a bacterial metabolite may play a causative role.

References

Allison MC, Cornwall S, Poulter LW, Dhillon AP, Pounder RE (1988) Macrophage heterogeneity in normal colonic mucosa and in inflammatory bowel disease. *Gut* **29**: 1531–1538.

Ambroze WL, Pemberton JH, Bell AM, Haddad AC, Philips SF (1989) Faecal short chain fatty acids after ileal pouch-anal anastomosis. (Abstract.) *Gastroenterology* **96**:A11.

Ambroze WL, Pemberton JH, Bell AM, Haddad AC, Phillips SF (1990) Faecal short chain fatty acid concentrations and effect on ileal pouch function. (Abstract.) *Gastroenterology* **29**:AS22.

Beart RW (1988) Proctocolectomy and ileoanal anastomosis. *World J Surg* **12**:160–163.

Beart RW, Fleming CR, Banks PM (1982) Tubulovillous adenomas in a continent ileostomy after proctocolectomy for familial polyposis. *Dig Dis Sci* **27**:553–556.

Becker JM, Raymond JL (1986) Ileal pouch-anal anastomosis. A single surgeon's experience with 100 consecutive cases. *Ann Surg* **204**:375–383.

Brandburg A, Kock NG, Phillipson B (1972) Bacterial flora in intra-abdominal ileostomy reservoir. *Gastroenterology* **64**: 413–416.

Brandt LJ, Boley SJ, Goldberg L, Mitsudo S, Berman A (1981) Colitis in the elderly: a reappraisal. *Am J Gastroenterol* **76**: 239–245.

Brandtzaeg P, Haltensen TS, Kett K *et al.* (1989) Immunobiology and immunopathology of human gut mucosa: humoral immunity and intraepithelial lymphocytes. *Gastroenterology* **97**:1562–1584.

Breuer NF, Rampton DS, Tammar A, Murphy GM, Dowling RH (1983) Effect of colonic perfusion with sulfated and non-sulfated bile acids on mucosal structure and function in the rat. *Gastroenterology* **84**:969–977.

Chaussade S, Denziot Y, Nicoli J *et al.* (1990) Stool PAF-acetor (PAF) is increased in patients with pouch ileo-anal anastomosis (IAA) and pouchitis. (Abstract.) *Gastroenterology* **98**:A164.

Church JM, Fazio VW, Lavery IC (1987) The role of fibreoptic endoscopy in the management of the continent ileostomy. *Gastrointest Endosc* **33**:203–209.

Counsell B (1956) Lesions of the ileum associated with ulcerative colitis. *Br J Surg* **44**:276–290.

Curran FT, Hill GL (1990) Results of 50 ileo-anal J pouch operations. *Aust NZ J Surg* **60**:579–683.

de Silva HJ, Ireland A, Kettewell M, Mortensen N, Jewell DP (1989) Short chain fatty acid irrigation in severe pouchitis. *N Engl J Med* **321**:1416–1417.

de Silva HJ, de Angelis CP, Soper N, Kettlewell MGW, Mortensen NJMcC (1991) Clinical and functional outcome following restorative proctocolectomy. *Br J Surg* **78**:1039–1044.

de Silva HJ, Millard PR, Kettlewell M, Mortensen NJ, Prince C, Jewell DP (1990) Mucosal characteristics of pelvic ileal pouches. *Gut* **32**:61–65.

Di Febo G, Miglioli M, Lauri A *et al.* (1990) Endoscopic assessment of acute inflammation of the ileal reservoir after restorative ileo-anal anastomosis. *Gastrointest Endosc* **36**: 6–96.

Dixon MF (1989) Vascular disorders, abnormalities, ischaemia, vasculitis: small intestine. In *Gastrointestinal and Oesophageal Pathology*. R Whitehead (ed). London, Churchill

Livingstone, pp. 561–580.

Dozois RR, Goldberg SM, Rothenberger DA *et al.* (1986) Restorative proctocolectomy with ileal reservoir. (Symposium.) *Int J Colorectal Dis* **1**:14–15.

Dozois RR, Kelly KA, Welling DR *et al.* (1989) Ileal pouch anal anastomosis: comparison of results in familial adenomatous polyposis and chronic ulcerative colitis. *Ann Surg* **210**: 268–273.

Dube S, Heyen F (1990) Pouchitis and gastric hyposecretion: cause or effect? *Int J Colorectal Dis* **5**:142–143.

Ehsanullah M, Filipe MI, Gazzard B (1982) Mucin secretion in inflammatory bowel disease: correlation with disease activity and dysplasia. *Gut* **23**:485–489.

Everett WG (1989) Experience of restorative proctocolectomy with ileal reservoir. *Br J Surg* **76**:77–81.

Farrands PA, Shepherd NA, Nicholls RJ (1988) Ileal reservoir inflammation (pouchitis) after restorative proctocolectomy ileal reservoir. (Abstract.) *Gut* **29**:A1486.

Fergusson A (1977) Intraepithelial lymphocytes of the small intestine. *Gut* **18**:921–937.

Fleshman JW, Cohen Z, McLeod RS, Stern H, Blair J (1988) The ileal reservoir and ileo-anal anastomosis procedure. Factors affecting technical and functional outcome. *Dis Colon Rectum* **31**:10–16.

Fonkalsrud EW (1987) Update on clinical experience with different surgical techniques of the endorectal pull-through operation for colitis and polyposis. *Surg Gynecol Obstet* **165**: 309–316.

Gadacz TR, Kelly KA, Phillips SF (1977) The continent ileal pouch: absorptive and motor features. Gastroenterology **72**:1287–1291.

Gertner DJ, Madden MV, De Nucci G, Rampton DS, Cynk E, Nicholls RJ, Lennard-Jones JE (1989) Increased leukotriene B4 release from ileal pouch mucosa in ulcerative colitis compared with familial adenomatous polyposis. (Abstract.) *Gut* **30**:A1481.

Gilat T, Leichtman G, Delpre G, Eschbar J, Bar Meir S, Fireman Z (1989) A comparison of metronidazole and sulphasalazine in the maintenance of remission in patients with ulcerative colitis. *J Clin Gastroenterol* **11**:392–395.

Go PMNYH, Lens J, Bosman FG (1987) Mucosal alterations in the reservoir of patients with rocks continent ileostomy. *Int J Colorect Dis* **4**:205–229.

Go PMNYH, Van Diejen-Visser MP, Davies BI, Lens J, Brombacher PJ (1988) Microbial flora and bile acid metabolism in patients with an ileal reservoir. *Scand J Gastroenterol* **23**:229–236.

Goodlad RA, Lenton W, Ghatei MA, Adrian TE, Bloom SR, Wright NA (1987) Effects of an elemental diet, inert bulk and different types of dietary fibre on the response of the intestinal epithelium to refeeding in the rat and relationship to plasma gastrin, enteroglucagon and PYY concentrations. *Gut* **28**:171–180.

Goodlad RA, Ratcliffe B, Fordham JP, Wright NA (1989) Does dietary fibre stimulate intestinal epithelial cell proliferation in germ free rats? *Gut* **30**:820–825.

Gorbach SL, Nahas L, Weinstein L (1967) Studies of intestinal microflora. IV. The microflora of ileostomy effluent: a unique microbiological ecology. *Gastroenterology* **53**: 874–880.

Grove I, Mahmoud AAF, Warren KS (1977) Suppression of cell-mediated immunity by metronidazole. *Int Arch Allergy Appl Immunol* **54**:422–427.

Gustavsson S, Weiland LH, Kelly KA (1987) Relationship of backwash ileitis to ileal pouchitis after ileal pouch-anal anastomosis. *Dis Colon Rectum* **30**:25–22.

Halvorsen JF, Hoch R, Nygaard K (1978) The continent reservoir ileostomy: review of a collective series of thirty-six patients from three surgical departments. *Surgery* (*St Louis*) **83**:252–259.

Hamilton SR, Bussey HJR, Mendlesohn GET *et al.* (1979) Ileal adenomas after colectomy in nine patients with adenomatous polyposis coli/Gardner's syndrome. *Gastroenterology* **77**:1252–1257.

Handelsman JC, Fishbein RH, Hoover HE, Smith GW, Haller JA (1983) Endorectal pull-through operation in adults after colectomy and excision of rectal mucosa. *Surgery* **93**: 247–253.

Harig JM, Soergel KH, Komorowski RA, Wood CM (1989) Treatment of diversion colitis with short-chain fatty acid irrigation. *New Engl J Med* **320**:23–28.

Heppell J, Belliveau P, Taillefer R, Dube S, Derbekyan V (1987) Quantitative assessment of pelvic ileal reservoir emptying with a semisolid radionuclide enema. A correlation with clinical outcome. *Dis Colon Rectum* **30**:81–85.

Hill MJ, Fernandez F (1989) Bacteriology (II). Pouchitis. (Workshop.) *Int J Colorectal Dis* **4**:204–229.

Hill MJ, Owen RW (1989) Faecal bile acids in pouch and pouchitis patients. Pouchitis. (Workshop.) *Int J Colorectal Dis* **4**:204–229.

Hirata I, Berrebi G, Austin LL, Keren DF, Dobbins WO (1986) Immunohistological characterization of intraepithelial and lamina propria lymphocytes in control ileum and colon and in inflammatory bowel disease. *Dig Dis Sci* **31**:593–603.

Hosie K, Sachaguchi M, Tudor R, Gourevitch D, Kimiot W, Keighley MRB (1989) Pouchitis after restorative proctocolectomy is associated with mucosal ischaemia. *Gut* **30**: A1471–1472.

Hultén L (1989) Workshop Pouchitis. *Int J Colorect Dis* **4**:205–229.

Hultén L, Svaninger G (1984) Facts about the continent ileostomy. *Dis Colon Rectum* **27**:553–557.

Jagenburg R, Kock NG, Philipson B (1975) Vitamin B$_{12}$ absorption in patients with continent ileostomy. *Scand J Gastroenterol* **10**:141–144.

Jarvinen HJ, Makitie A, Sivula A (1986) Long-term results of continent ileostomy. *Int J Colorectal Dis* **1**:40–43.

Keighley MRB, Yoshioka K, Kmiot W (1988) Prospective randomized trial to compare the stapled double lumen pouch and the sutured quadruple pouch for restorative proctocolectomy. *Br J Surg* **75**:1008–1111.

Kelly DG, Phillips SF, Kelly KA, Weinstein WM, Gilchrist MJ (1983) Dysfunction of the continent ileostomy: clinical features and bacteriology. *Gut* **24**:193–201.

Klein K, Stenzel P, Katon RM (1983) Pouch ileitis: report of a case with severe systemic manifestations. *J Clin Gastroenterol* **5**:149–153.

Kmiot WA, Keighley MRB (1990) Pouchitis following

colectomy and ileal reservoir construction for familial adenomatous polyposis. *Br J Surg* **77**:1283.

Knobler H, Ligumsky M, Okon E, Ayalon A, Nesher R, Rachmilewitz D (1986) Pouch ileitis – recurrence of inflammatory bowel disease in the ileal reservoir. *Am J Gastroenterol* **81**:199–201.

Kock NG (1987) Continent ileostomy. In *Surgery Inflammatory Bowel Disorders*. ECG Lee (ed). Edinburgh, Churchill Livingstone, pp. 65–80.

Kock NG, Darle N, Hultén L, Kewenter J, Myrvold H, Phillipson B (1977) Ileostomy. *Curr Probl Surg* **14**:36–38.

Kock NG, Myrvold HE, Nillson LO, Phillipson BM (1985) Continent ileostomy: the Swedish experience. In *Alternatives to Conventional Ileostomy*. RR Dozois (ed). Chicago, Year Book Medical Publishers, pp. 163–175.

Lerch MM, Braun J, Harder M, Hofstadter F, Schumpelick V, Matern S (1989) Postoperative adaption of the small intestine after total colectomy and J-pouch-anal anastomosis. *Dis Colon Rectum* **32**:600–608.

Levin KE, Pemberton JH, Phillips SF, Zinsmeister AR, Pezim ME (1990) Effect of a xanthine oxidase inhibitor (allopurinol) in patients with pouchitis after ileal pouch-anal anastomosis. *Gut* **31**:A1168.

Lohmuller JL, Pemberton JH, Dozois RR, Ilstrup D (1990) The relationship between pouchitis after ileal pouch-anal anastomosis and extra-intestinal manifestations of chronic ulcerative colitis. *Ann Surg* **211**:622–629.

Lott M, Wright NA (1989) Epithelial kinetics, control and consequences of alterations in disease. In *Gastrointestinal and Oesophageal Pathology*, R Whitehead (ed). London, Churchill Livingstone, pp. 91–105.

Luukonen P, Jarvinen H, Lehtola A, Sipponen P (1988a) Mucosal alterations in pelvic ileal reservoirs. A histological and ultrastructural evaluation in an experimental model. *Ann Chir et Gyn* **77**:91–96.

Luukonen P, Valtonen V, Sivonen A, Sipponen P, Jarvinen H (1988b) Faecal bacteriology and reservoir ileitis in patients operated on for ulcerative colitis. *Dis Colon Rectum* **31**: 864–867.

Lyons AS, Garlock JH (1954) Complications of ileostomy. *Surgery* **36**:784–788.

Madden MV, Farthing MJG, Nicholls RJ (1990) Inflammation in ileal reservoirs – 'pouchitis'. *Gut* **31**:247–249.

Madden MV, Neale KF, Nicholls RJ *et al.* (1991) Comparison of morbidity and function after colectomy with ileo-rectal anastomosis or restorative proctocolectomy for familial adenomatous polyposis. *Br J Surg* **78**:789–792.

Madden MV, McIntyre A, Nicholls RJ. Unpublished observations.

Mahida YR, Patel S, Gioncetti P, Vaux D, Jewell DP (1989) Macrophage subpopulations in the lamina propria of normal and inflamed colon and terminal ileum. *Gut* **30**: 826–834.

Merrett MN, Crotty BJ, Mortensen NJ, Jewell DP (1991) Ileal pouch dialysate is cytoxic to 1-407 and HT 29 cells: bile may be the active factor. *Gut* **32**:A1205.

Meuwissen SGM, Hoitsma H, Boot H, Seldenrijk CA (1989) Pouchitis (pouch ileitis). *Neth J Med* **35**:S54–S66.

Miglioli M, Barbara L, Di Febo G *et al.* (1989) Topical administration of 5-aminosalicylic acids: a therapeutic proposal for the treatment of pouchitis. *New Engl J Med* **320**:257.

Mortensen NJ (1989) Progress with the pouch – restorative proctocolectomy for ulcerative colitis. *Gut* **29**:561–565.

Moskowitz RL, Shepherd NA, Nicholls RJ (1986) An assessment of inflammation in the reservoir after restorative proctocolectomy with ileo-anal ileal reservoir. *Int J Colorectal Dis* **1**:167–174.

Nasmyth DG, Godwin PGR, Dixon MF, Williams NS, Johnston D (1985) The relationship between mucosal structure and intestinal flora in ileal reservoirs. *Brit J Surg* **72**: S129.

Nasmyth DG, Johnston D, Godwin PGR, Dixon MF, Smith A, Williams NS (1986) Factors influencing bowel function after ileal pouch-anal anastomosis. *Brit J Surg* **73**:469–473.

Nasmyth DG, Godwin PGR, Dixon MF, Williams NS, Johnston D (1989a) Ileal ecology after pouch-anal anastomosis or ileostomy. A study of mucosal morphology, faecal bacteriology, faecal volatile fatty acids, and their interrelationship. *Gastroenterology* **96**:817–824.

Nasmyth DG, Johnston D, Williams NS, King RFGJ, Burkinshaw L, Brooks K (1989b) Changes in the absorption of bile acids after total colectomy in patients with an ileostomy or pouch-anal anastomosis. *Dis Colon Rectum* **32**: 230–234.

Nicholls RJ, Pezim ME (1985) Restorative proctocolectomy with ileal reservoir for ulcerative colitis and familial adenomatous polyposis: a comparison of three reservoir designs. *Br J Surg* **72**:470–474.

Nicholls RJ, Holt SD, Lubowski DZ (1989) Restorative proctocolectomy with ileal reservoir. Comparison of 2-stage vs 3-stage procedures and analysis of factors that might affect outcome. *Dis Colon Rectum* **32** (4):323–326.

Nicholls RJ, Moskowitz RL, Shepherd NA (1985) Restorative proctocolectomy with ileal reservoir. *Br J Surg* **72**(suppl): S76–79.

O'Byrne JM, O'Connell PR, Nolan N, Marks P, Tanner WA, Keane FBV (1989) Colonic metaplasia of ileal mucosa: an experimental model [abstract]. *Gut* **30**:A1477.

O'Connell PR, Rankin DH, Weiland LH, Kelly KA (1986) Enteric bacteriology, absorption, morphology and emptying after ileal pouch-anal anastomosis. *Br J Surg* **73**: 909–914.

Ojerskog B, Kock NG, Nilsson LO, Philipson BM, Ahren C (1990) Long term follow-up of patients with continent ileostomies. *Dis Colon Rectum* **33**:184–189.

Öresland T, Fasth S, Nordgren S, Hultén L (1989) The clinical and functional outcome after restorative proctocolectomy. *Int J Colorectal Dis* **4**:50–56.

Pemberton JH, Kelly KA, Beart RW, Dozois RR, Wolff BG, Ilstrup DM (1987) Ileal pouch-anal anastomosis for chronic ulcerative colitis. Long term results. *Ann Surg* **206**:504–513.

Pescatori M, Mattana C, Castagneto M (1988) Clinical and functional results after restorative proctocolectomy. *Br J Surg* **75**:321–324.

Pezim ME, Pemberton JH, Beart RW (1989) Outcome of 'indeterminate' colitis following ileal pouch-anal anastomosis. *Dis Colon Rectum* **32**:653–658.

Philipson B, Brandberg A, Jagenburg R, Kock NG, Lager I,

Ahren C (1975) Mucosal morphology, bacteriology and absorption in intra-abdominal ileostomy reservoir. *Scan J Gastroenterol* **10**:145–153.

Riddell RH (1988) Pathology of idiopathic inflammatory bowel disease. In *Inflammatory Bowel Disease*. JB Kirsner, RG Shaler (eds) Philadelphia, Lea Ferbiger, pp. 329–350.

Roediger WEW (1980) The colonic epithelium in ulcerative colitis – an energy deficiency disease? *Lancet* **2**:712–5.

Sakata T (1987) Stimulatory effects of short chain fatty acids on epithelial cell proliferation in the rat small intestine: a possible explanation for tropic effects of fermentable fibre, gut microbes and luminal tropic factors. *Br J Nutr* **58**: 95–103.

Scott AD, Phillips RKS (1989) Ileitis and pouchitis after colectomy for ulcerative colitis. *Br J Surg* **76**:668–669.

Shepherd NA (1989) Workshop pouchitis. *Int J Colorect Dis* **4**:205–229.

Shepherd NA (1990) The pelvic ileal reservoir: pathology and pouchitis. *Neth J Med* **37**:S57–S64.

Shepherd NA, Jass JR, Duval I, Moskowitz RL, Nicholls RJ, Morson BC (1987) Restorative proctocolectomy with ileal reservoir: pathological and histochemical study of mucosal biopsy specimens. *J Clin Pathol* **40**:601–607.

Stryker SJ, Carney JA, Dozois RR (1987) Multiple adenomatous polyps arising in a continent reservoir ileostomy. *Int J Colorectal Dis* **2**:43–45.

Subramani K, Sachar DB, Harpaz, N, Bilotta J, Rubin PH, Janowitz HD (1990) Resistant pouchitis: does it reflect underlying Crohn's disease? (Abstract.) *Gastroenterology* **98**: A205.

Thayer WR, Spiro HM (1962) Ileitis after ileostomy: prestomal ileitis. *Gastroenterology* **42**:547–554.

Tytgat GNJ (1989) Pouchitis. (Workshop.) *Int J Colorectal Dis* **4**:205–229.

Tytgat GNJ, Van Deventer SJH (1988) Pouchitis. *Int J Colorectal Dis* **3**:226–228.

Van Spreeuel JP, Lindeman J, Meijer CLJM (1985) A quantitative study of immunoglobulin containing cells in the differential diagnosis of acute colitis. *J Clin Pathol* **38**:774–777.

Warren BF, Bartolo DCC, Collins CMP (1990) Preclosure pouchitis – a new entity. (Abstract.) *J Pathol* **160**:170A.

Warren R, McKittrick LS (1951) Ileostomy for ulcerative colitis: technique, complications and management. *Surg Gynecol Obstet* **93**:555–567.

Wexner SD, Jensen L, Rothenberger DA, Wong WD, Goldberg SM (1989) Longterm functional analysis of the ileoanal reservoir. *Dis Colon Rectum* **32**:275–281.

Wolfstein IH, Bat L, Neumann G (1982) Regeneration of rectal mucosa and recurrent polyposis coli after total colectomy and ileoanal anastomosis. *Arch Surg* **117**: 1241–1242.

Wong WD, Goldberg SM (1987) The 'S' pouch. In *Surgery of Inflammatory Bowel Disorders*. ECG Lee (ed). Edinburgh, Churchill Livingstone, pp. 81–95.

Zuccaro G, Fazio VW, Church JM, Lavery IC, Ruderman WB, Farmer RG (1989) Pouch ileitis. *Dig Dis Sci* **34**:1505–1510.

Chapter 9
Pouch Ecology

D. GEORGE NASMYTH AND NORMAN S. WILLIAMS

Introduction

From the point of view of avoiding the physical and psychosexual problems associated with a permanent ileostomy, the case for preserving anal continence might appear self-evident. On the other hand the physiological basis for constructing a faecal reservoir at the end of the small bowel is less clear. Knowledge of the normal ecology of the terminal ileum, that is the relationship between its bacterial flora, ileal motility and the structure and function of ileal mucosa, offers little support for its use as a reservoir organ. In practice, however, the consequences of a reservoir at the end of the small bowel have not been as deleterious as might have been anticipated from the expected, and the observed, changes in the bacterial flora.

The gastrointestinal tract has been described as an enormously complex and dynamic ecosystem (Abrams, 1983). The components of this ecosystem include not only the microbial flora, but the specialized tissues of the whole gastrointestinal tract and its principal derivatives: the liver and pancreas. Mucosal structure, absorption and secretion of luminal contents, intestinal motility and diet may all influence the bacterial flora and vice versa. In the normal state, mechanisms exist to ensure that the components within this system are fairly constant and the equilibrium thus established is a stable one. Following restorative proctocolectomy many of the components within the system change and hence a new equilibrium is established in the terminal ileum. These alterations in the ecology of the terminal ileum which occur after restorative proctocolectomy, their stability, their implications for gastrointestinal function, and their implications for the patient, will be discussed in this chapter.

Bacterial ecology of the ileum

Normal microflora

There are many inherent limitations in the methods available for the analysis of intestinal flora. Transport under anaerobic conditions, the avoidance of delay in establishing cultures, and homogenization of the specimen are important facets of such studies which may influence the results. Even when the greatest care has been taken with microbiological technique, it must be recognized that *in vitro* culture represents a very different environment to the lumen of the intestine. In the former situation, bacterial metabolites accumulate and the conditions for bacterial growth will rapidly be altered, whereas the situation within the lumen of the gut is one of continuous flux: there is influx of nutrient from the proximal bowel as well as efflux of the bacteria and their metabolic waste distally (Donaldson, 1964). Another consideration is that *in vivo* the growth of bacteria may be limited by competitive interaction between species, whereas *in vitro* a profuse growth of bacteria may be obtained which does not reflect the situation in the gut. Similarly failure to use the appropriate selective media may result in failure to identify important bacteria which are not numerically dominant (Finegold *et al.*, 1983). Surprisingly, in view of the limitations of the techniques available for analysis of the gut flora, the results of different investigators have been remarkably consistent.

Gastric acid destroys most bacteria entering the gut from the oropharynx, and gastric concentrations of bacteria are usually less than 10^3 colony forming units/ml (cfu/ml). The pH in the proximal jejunum is between 6.0 and 7.0 and the flora does not differ greatly from that in the stomach. The upper small bowel is sparsely populated by Gram-positive aerobes with very few anaerobes. The concentration of bacteria in the upper small bowel is low, 10^3-10^4 cfu/ml, and the predominant genera are *Streptococci*, *Staphylococci* and *Lactobacilli*. Progress distally along the small bowel is associated with a gradual change in the flora (Table 9.1) which is accompanied by an increase in luminal pH and a reduction in the oxidation–reduction potential (Simon & Gorbach, 1986). Distally, in the terminal ileum, the pH rises to 7.5 and the oxidation–reduction potential falls to $-150\,\text{mV}$. Both of these changes

Table 9.1 Human gastrointestinal flora.

	Stomach	Jejunum	Ileum	Faeces
Aerobic or facultative anaerobic bacteria				
Enterobacteria	$0-10^2$	$0-10^3$	10^2-10^6	10^4-10^{10}
Streptococci	$0-10^3$	$0-10^4$	10^2-10^6	10^5-10^{10}
Staphylococci	$0-10^2$	$0-10^3$	10^2-10^5	10^4-10^7
Lactobacilli	$0-10^3$	$0-10^4$	10^2-10^5	10^6-10^{10}
Fungi	$0-10^2$	$0-10^2$	10^2-10^3	10^2-10^6
Anaerobic bacteria				
Bacteroides	Rare	$0-10^2$	10^3-10^7	$10^{10}-10^{12}$
Bifidobacteria	Rare	$0-10^3$	10^3-10^5	10^8-10^{12}
Gram-positive cocci	Rare	$0-10^3$	10^2-10^5	10^8-10^{11}
Clostridia	Rare	Rare	10^2-10^4	10^6-10^{11}
Eubacteria	Rare	Rare	Rare	10^9-10^{12}
Total bacterial count	$0-10^3$	$0-10^5$	10^3-10^7	$10^{10}-10^{12}$

From Simon & Gorbach (1984).

favour the growth of anaerobic bacteria. Compared with the jejunum the terminal ileum contains increased numbers of organisms, with a total bacterial count of 10^5-10^8 cfu/ml. There is also a qualitative change with a slight anaerobe predominance and greater numbers of coliforms, *Clostridia*, *Bifidobacteria* and *Bacteroides* which are often absent from the proximal small intestine. In spite of these changes, the flora of the ileum is usually considered as transitional between the relatively sparse flora of the jejunum and the flora of the caecum in which the total bacterial counts rise to $10^{11}-10^{12}$ cfu/ml and the ratio of anaerobes to aerobes is more than $1000:1$. The predominant genera in the caecum are *Bacteroides*, *Bifidobacteria*, *Eubacteria* and anaerobic Gram-positive cocci such as *Clostridia* and *Enterococci* (Simon & Gorbach, 1984; 1986).

Microflora of ileostomy effluent

Colectomy and the formation of an end ileostomy results in a change in the flora of the terminal ileum: the number of organisms isolated from ileostomy effluent (8×10^7/g) is approximately 80 times greater than that detected in the normal distal ileum (10^6/g), but only one twenty-fifth of that in faeces (2×10^9/g) (Gorbach *et al.*, 1967c). The change in the flora after ileostomy is largely quantitative with the ratio of aerobes to anaerobes remaining close to unity, although some

observers have reported a slight predominance of anaerobes (Nasmyth, *et al.*, 1989b) and others a predominance of aerobes (Brandberg *et al.*, 1972).

The reasons for the altered microbial ecology of the terminal ileum following formation of an ileostomy are unclear, and open to speculation. Alterations in ileal motility and 'adaptation' to an ileostomy may be relevant factors.

Table 9.2 Faecal bacteriology after proctocolectomy.

Bacteria ($\log^{10}$ cfu/ml; median (range))	Pouch ($n = 11$)	Ileostomy ($n = 12$)
Total aerobes	8.3 (6.4–9.9)	9.0 (6.5–10.7)
Total anaerobes	10.6 (8.5–11.9)	9.6 (6.0–10.7)
Anaerobes/aerobes*	100 (18621–1)	4 (120–0.1)
Coliforms	7.9 (4.3–9.2)	7.4 (6.4–10.7)
Streptococcus	5.5 (0–8.7)	6.0 (0–8.9)
Enterococcus	5.8 (3.2–8.7)	5.5 (0–8.9)
*Bacteroides***	9.8 (0–11.9)	5.7 (0–10.1)
Fusobacteria	4.3 (0–7)	0 (0–5.6)
Clostridia	4.7 (0–8.5)	5.3 (0–7.3)
Eubacteria	0 (0–8.8)	0 (0–3.8)
Lactobacilli	4.1 (0–10.6)	5.6 (0–9)
*Bifidobacteria**	8.7 (0–11.9)	0 (0–9.6)
Veillonella	7.0 (0–9.6)	7.1 (0–9.6)
Staphylococcus coagulase positive	2.3 (0–4.6)	0 (0–5.2)
coagulase negative	0 (0–4)	0 (0–4.1)
Yeasts	3.2 (0–8.3)	3.4 (0–5.4)

From Nasmyth DG *et al.* (1989b).
$*p < 0.05$, $**p < 0.01$.

Microflora of ileal pouches

As ileal content provides an excellent substrate for bacterial growth, temporary storage of ileal effluent in a pouch might be predicted to cause greater changes in the bacterial ecology of the terminal ileum than those observed in patients who have undergone proctocolectomy and ileostomy. Initial experience with ileal pouches was with the continent ileostomy reservoir (Kock pouch), and the predicted alteration in the ileal flora was shown to occur. The total number of bacteria isolated from the Kock pouches exceeded that from conventional ileostomies, and there was a predominance of anaerobes in the majority of isolates (Brandberg *et al.*, 1972). Among the anaerobes, *Bacteroides* were predominant and the commonest aerobes were coliforms and *Lactobacilli*. Similar results have been reported in patients with pelvic pouches following restorative proctocolectomy (Nicholls *et al.*, 1981; Luukkonen *et al.*, 1988; Nasmyth *et al.*, 1989b).

A comparison of the faecal bacteriology in pelvic pouches and ileostomies is shown in Table 9.2. Fewer aerobes are found in the pouches than in the ileostomies, whereas the situation for anaerobes is reversed and greater numbers of anaerobes occur in the pouches. Although these differences are small in bacteriological terms it is important to consider the ratio of aerobes to anaerobes in each environment. The ratio of aerobes to anaerobes is significantly greater in the pouches (100:1) than in the ileostomies (4:1) (Fig. 9.1). *Bacteroides* and *Bifidobacteria* are the genera which show the greatest numerical increase between the pouches and the

ileostomies. From the cumulative results of several studies, it would now appear that the flora of the ileal pouch occupies an intermediate position between that of ileostomy effluent and normal faeces.

Examination of faecal effluent from the pouch for recognized intestinal pathogens has been remarkable only for their sparsity (Hill & Fernandez, 1989; Nasmyth *et al.*, 1989b). *Clostridium difficile* was found in five out of 15 patients with a pelvic pouch, but there were no adverse clinical features associated with it (Luukkonen *et al.*, 1988). In another study, two patients were found to have *Cl. difficile* in the pouch, both had diarrhoea but in neither instance was the cytotoxin found, and both improved with vancomycin therapy (Keighley *et al.*, 1989).

Regulation of bacterial flora

Several factors, specific to the host and to the bacterial populations themselves, regulate the environment and maintain a relatively constant bacterial population in each part of the gastrointestinal tract. Of the factors specific to the host, gastric acid, normal peristaltic activity and diet are probably the most important.

Gastric acid

Gastric acid kills most ingested bacteria and provides a major defence mechanism against potential pathogens. Patients with achlorhydria, or hypochlorhydria induced either pharmacologically or as a result of surgery, have increased numbers of bacteria in the upper small bowel, including anaerobes, and this may result in overgrowth with consequent malabsorption and diarrhoea (Simon & Gorbach, 1986). Neither hypochlorhydria nor achlorhydria, whether induced surgically or pharmacologically, have been documented as a cause of bacterial overgrowth in the upper small bowel of patients with restorative proctocolectomy. Nonetheless in patients with a pouch who develop increased stool volumes secondary to jejunal bacterial overgrowth, a reduction in gastric acid output if present, may be a significant aetiological factor.

Intestinal motility

Small bowel motility is usually conveniently divided into the digestive and interdigestive phases. The duration of the digestive phase is determined by the caloric load of the meal, but the recognition and interpretation

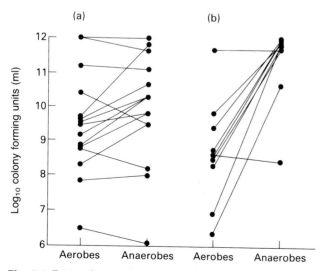

Fig. 9.1 Ratio of anaerobes/aerobes in ileal effluent. (a) After ileostomy, (b) after restorative proctocolectomy.

of patterns of motor activity during this phase remain poorly understood. By contrast the migrating motor complex (MMC) of the interdigestive phase is well recognized, and phase 3 of the MMC is a highly propulsive activity front which migrates along the jejunum into the ileum (Vantrappen et al., 1986). This activity front which is sometimes referred to as the interdigestive housekeeper is thought to be important in preventing stasis and bacterial overgrowth. Patients with disorders of interdigestive motor activity and an absence of phase 3 have been noted to have bacterial overgrowth (Vantrappen et al., 1977). The importance of phase 3 in relation to the clearance of luminal contents from the ileum is less clear as fewer than 10% of MMC's reach the ileocaecal sphincter. The terminal ileum, however, is characterized by intermittent propagated contractions of high amplitude, some of which cross the ileocaecal junction (Quigley et al., 1984).

Other mechanisms may operate in the terminal ileum to ensure propagation of luminal contents and the prevention of stasis. Short chain fatty acids (SCFA) which are the product of anaerobic bacterial fermentation of carbohydrate are not usually present in the ileum in significant quantities, although they are the predominant anions in the colon. In the absence of stasis and bacterial overgrowth the presence of SCFAs in the ileum is most likely to be associated with colo-ileal reflux. It has recently been shown that increased concentrations of SCFAs in the terminal ileum stimulate ileal motility and clearance of ileal contents (Kamath et al., 1988; Fich et al., 1989). It may well be, therefore, that this constitutes a method whereby the ileum can protect the small bowel against the effects of colo-ileal reflux by increasing the rate of forward transit of ileal contents. As the more recent observations on the terminal ileum have refuted the suggestion that the ileocaecal sphincter is tonically contracted (Quigley et al., 1984; Nasmyth & Williams 1985) it would seem reasonable to conclude that compartmentalization of ileal and caecal contents is dependent on locally propagated contractions in response to appropriate stimuli, and the concentration of SCFA in the ileum may be one such stimulus.

Jejuno-ileal motility shows relatively few changes after restorative proctocolectomy. Phase 3 of the MMC can be identified readily in the jejunum but it fades out in the ileum and never reaches the pouch. The principal difference in small bowel motility that has been observed after restorative proctocolectomy is the presence of prolonged propagated contractions which arise much more proximally than in normal subjects (Stryker et al., 1985). The significance of these contractions is unclear, they have been observed in the fasting state and it has been suggested that they may arise in reponse to distal ileal distension from prolonged storage of pouch contents (Stryker et al., 1985). However, it should not be construed from these observations on small bowel motility that gastrointestinal transit is increased after restorative proctocolectomy. In the majority of patients the reverse is the case, gastrointestinal transit is slowed (Soper et al., 1989), and the 'ileal brake' preserved after restorative proctocolectomy (Soper et al., 1990). If the normal patterns of small bowel motility after restorative proctocolectomy are largely unaltered, the question arises as to why jejunal bacterial overgrowth should develop in some patients giving rise to increased stool volumes (O'Connell et al., 1986). Similar findings of pouch dysfunction associated with proximal bacterial overgrowth have been reported in patients with a Kock pouch (Kelly et al., 1983). It is open to speculation whether those patients with jejunal bacterial overgrowth form a subgroup which is characterized by abnormal motility patterns. Vantrappen's studies in patients with small bowel overgrowth suggested that the overgrowth was secondary to a motility disorder rather than vice versa (Vantrappen et al., 1977; 1986). A unifying hypothesis might be that in some patients exaggerated reflex slowing of gastrointestinal transit permits bacterial overgrowth; it is noteworthy in this regard that small bowel transit may be slowed in patients with ulcerative colitis prior to any surgical procedure (Rao et al., 1987).

Another suggested explanation for jejunal overgrowth in patients with a pouch is reflux. Scintigraphic techniques have shown reflux from the pouch into the distal ileum as distension increases and large amplitude pressure waves are generated within the pouch (O'Connell et al., 1987). Onset of these high pressure waves is associated with filling of the pouch to the threshold volume at which an urge to defaecate is experienced. However, during evacuation of the pouch the scintigraphic studies showed that the pouch and the ileum immediately proximal to it were emptied as a single unit with no evidence of further reflux during evacuation (O'Connell et al., 1987). It would seem that the reflux that has been observed is limited in extent and there is no direct evidence to link it with jejunal bacterial overgrowth.

Diet

Diet is a factor which might be expected to have a significant effect on the composition of the intestinal flora, but using standard bacteriological techniques, surprisingly little effect has been demonstrated. On the other hand dietary variation has been shown to influence the activity of bacterial enzymes. This is primarily of interest in relation to the ecology of the colon, in particular colonic carcinogenesis (Simon & Gorbach, 1986). There are no published studies which show that diet has a significant effect on the composition or metabolic activity of the normal ileal flora. However, because the ecology of the ileal pouch more closely reflects that of the colon, the possibility that dietary factors may also influence the activity of bacterial enzymes in the pouch should be considered.

Microbial factors

Bacterial growth may be limited by direct competition for available substrates, production of an inimicable or stimulatory environment, and the production of bacteriocins (antibiotic like substances which inhibit the growth of other bacteria).

The role of competition for substrates, between bacteria of the same or different genera, as a mechanism controlling the growth of microbial populations is difficult to assess in relation to other environmental factors. This is particularly true of an environment as complex as the gastrointestinal tract. A few examples have been described such as the ability of coliforms to inhibit the growth of *Shigella flexneri*, which is due to competition for carbon sources in a reduced environment (Freter, 1962). It is unknown whether competition for substrates is an important regulator of the microbial flora of the ileal pouch.

Production of an environment which will inhibit or promote the growth of different organisms is another way in which bacteria can regulate their own environment. Two examples of this may well be relevant to the bacterial ecology of the ileal pouch. The growth of strict anaerobes may be facilitated by the presence of facultative bacteria which can grow aerobically or anaerobically. The latter bacteria will exhaust the environment of limited supplies of oxygen which would be inhibitory to the growth of strict anaerobes. Another way in which the resident microflora of the pouch may regulate their own environment is by production of SCFAs. Short chain fatty acids are by-products of anaerobic bacterial fermentation which may inhibit the growth of other bacteria when the pH of the luminal environment is <7.0. At this pH a significant proportion of the SCFA molecules will be in an undissociated state in which they can enter the bacterial cell where they act as inhibitors of bacterial metabolism (Simon & Gorbach, 1986).

Most, if not all bacteria produce substances, bacteriocins, which have antibiotic activity against other bacteria. A potential role for these substances can easily be demonstrated *in vitro*, but not *in vivo*. Bacteriocins in the gastrointestinal tract are probably rapidly inactivated and a role for these substances in the regulation of the intestinal flora has not been proven.

Stability of the microflora

Consideration of the various factors which regulate the gut microflora inevitably raises the question of the stability of the microflora with time. The faecal flora has been shown to be relatively constant over periods of several months (Gorbach *et al.*, 1967a), but studies on the flora of the normal ileum are much more difficult to perform and therefore data are limited. Duplicate samples on the same individual show no greater variations than may be accounted for by sampling and counting techniques (Gorbach *et al.*, 1967b). The stability of the pouch flora is implied by the relative consistency of bacteriological analysis from different centres. Analysis of further faecal samples from the same patients has been undertaken in a small number of patients, and the second sample showed a similar anaerobe predominance to the first sample. Some differences in the numbers of bacteria were observed, but there were no major qualitative differences (Nasmyth, 1987).

Interactions between the ileal microflora and the host

The mechanisms underlying the interactions between the gastrointestinal microflora and their host are poorly understood. Perhaps the most important reason for this is the difficulty that is presented to the investigator in attempting to study such an enormously complex ecosystem which cannot be satisfactorily reproduced *in vitro*, and is relatively inaccessible in the human. For this reason many of the observations on the relationship between the microflora of the gastrointestinal tract and its host have been made in animals. Obviously some caution must be used in drawing inferences from such studies about the interactions between the gut microflora and the human host, although in the majority of instances the basis for making such inferences is strong.

The interactions between the ileal microflora and the host can conveniently be considered under the following headings: intraluminal metabolism, mucosal morphology, and absorption.

Intraluminal metabolism: bile acids

Bacterial degradation of bile acids is one of the most well documented examples of intraluminal metabolism by the gut flora. In the normal host, conjugated bile acids are reabsorbed in the terminal ileum by an active transport mechanism. However, a small but significant proportion of conjugated bile acids reach the large intestine, where they undergo bacterial transformation. A wide range of intestinal bacteria, including *Bacteroides*, *Bifidobacteria*, *Fusobacteria*, *Lactobacillus* and *Clostridia* can hydrolyse conjugated bile acids. There is very little evidence of enzyme specificity for either taurine or glycine conjugates. Further transformations of the deconjugated bile acids then occur, the most important of which is 7α-dehydroxylation. 7α-Dehydroxylase is produced predominantly by *Clostridia* and *Eubacteria* and the 7α-dehydroxylating activity of these bacteria may be enhanced by *Bacteroides* (Hylemon & Glass, 1983). 7α-Dehydroxylation results in the transformation of cholic acid into deoxycholic acid and of chenodeoxycholic acid into lithocholic acid. A proportion of these secondary bile acids will be absorbed from the colon and re-enter the enterohepatic circulation, the remainder being excreted in the faeces.

The major significance of the bacterial degradation of bile acids for patients with an ileal pouch relates to the consequences of these bacterial transformations occurring in the ileum. Increased losses of bile acids from the enterohepatic circulation may be expected, as free bile acids and secondary bile acids are less well absorbed than the primary conjugated bile acids. The initial response to increased losses from the enterohepatic circulation is an increased synthesis of bile acids which may well be sufficient to compensate for relatively small losses. Greater losses will result in depletion of the bile acid pool and a reduced hepatic secretion of bile acids. This in turn may result in a degree of fat malabsorption and may also increase the lithogenicity of gallbladder bile (Heaton, 1972).

Impaired absorption of bile acids in patients with an ileal pouch may reflect increased intraluminal metabolism of primary conjugated bile acids by the microflora of the pouch, but it may also reflect a reduction in the activity of the mechanisms involved in the active transport of bile acids across the ileal mucosa. Faecal excretion of ^{14}C cholic acid has been shown to be greater in patients with a Kock pouch than in those with a conventional ileostomy. But as faecal excretion of ^{14}C cholic acid was greater in patients having a conventional ileostomy and a 50-cm ileal resection than in those with a Kock pouch it was assumed that significant ileal absorption was occurring from the Kock pouch in spite of a tendency to increased bacterial degradation of bile acids in the pouch (Andersson *et al.*, 1979). Analysis of bile acids in the effluent from ileostomies and pelvic ileal pouches has shown an increased proportion of secondary bile acids in the effluent from the pouches, which would support the contention that significant bacterial degradation of bile acids is occurring in the pouch (Nasmyth *et al.*, 1989a), although another study has reported no significant increase in secondary bile acids in the effluent from pelvic pouches but increased excretion of primary bile acids (Pedersen *et al.*, 1985). Increased excretion of primary bile acids in the effluent from pouches may be due to dysfunction of the ileal transport mechanisms, but it may also be due to bacterial deconjugation and the failure to demonstrate significant quantities of secondary bile acids in the pouch effluent does not preclude bacterial degradation of conjugated bile acids as a significant factor in their malabsorption.

The use of the ring-labelled bile acid ^{75}Se homotaurocholate (SeHCAT) might be expected to distinguish between ileal dysfunction and bacterial degradation of bile acids as the cause of bile acid malabsorption in patients with a pouch. In contrast to the naturally occurring bile acids and their radiolabelled analogues, bacterial deconjugation of SeHCAT is minimal (Ferraris *et al.*, 1984). Consequently active ileal transport is more closely reflected by the absorption of SeHCAT than ^{14}C cholic acid, as the latter is more susceptible to bacterial deconjugation.

Using SeHCAT there is evidence of bile acid malabsorption when pouch patients are compared with normal controls (Fiorentini *et al.*, 1987; Nasmyth *et al.*, 1989a). The SeHCAT test failed, however, to demonstrate a significant difference in bile acid absorption between patients with a conventional ileostomy and those with a pelvic pouch. In those patients with an

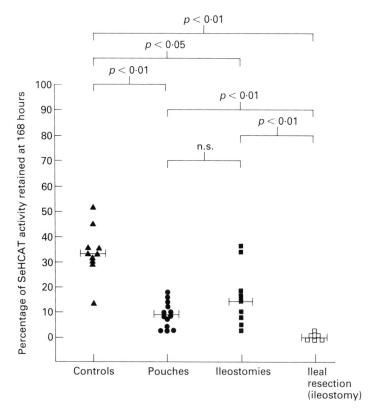

Fig. 9.2 The percentage of ^{75}Se homotaurocholate (SeHCAT) retained in the body 1 week after ingestion is an index of bile acid absorption by the ileal mucosa. Retention of SeHCAT was greater in patients with a pouch than in those with an ileostomy who had undergone resection of a length of terminal ileum equivalent to that used in construction of a pouch. From Nasmyth *et al.* (1989a).

ileostomy, who had undergone an ileal resection of more than 20 cm, retention of SeHCAT was less than that in the pouch patients (Fig. 9.2) (Nasmyth *et al.*, 1989a). This observation suggests that the ileal pouch mucosa retains a significant absorptive capacity for bile acids, as the rate at which bile acids were excreted was significantly increased by resection of a similar length of ileum to that used in the construction of the pouch. The observations of increased faecal excretion of secondary bile acids together with the absence of a significant difference in SeHCAT retention between patients with pouches and those with ileostomies tend to support the hypothesis that bacterial degradation of bile acids is the major cause of increased bile acid excretion in patients with an ileal pouch. Further evidence from *in vitro* studies showing normal taurocholate absorption by pouch mucosa supports this hypothesis (Hosie *et al.*, 1990).

Intraluminal metabolism: vitamin B$_{12}$

Tests of vitamin B$_{12}$ absorption also fail to distinguish between primary impairment of ileal transport mechanisms and secondary malabsorption due to intraluminal binding of B$_{12}$ by bacteria. It has been shown that *Bacteroides* will bind both cobalamin and the cobalamin–intrinsic factor complex (Welkos *et al.*, 1981), and since the numbers of *Bacteroides* are increased in ileal pouches, this together with jejunal bacterial overgrowth may explain the borderline values for B$_{12}$ absorption that have been reported in some pouch patients (Nicholls *et al.*, 1981; O'Connell *et al.*, 1986; Fiorentini *et al.*, 1987). Indirect evidence in support of bacterial binding of vitamin B$_{12}$ as the cause of abnormal Schilling Tests in some pouch patients, comes from the observation that treatment with metronidazole reverses this abnormality (Kelly *et al.*, 1983).

Intraluminal metabolism: short chain fatty acids

Anaerobic bacterial fermentation of both endogenous mucus and undigested carbohydrate (dietary fibre) occurs largely, if not exclusively, in the large intestine. The end products of this fermentation are SCFAs, of which the most important quantitatively are acetic, propionic and butyric acids. Short chain fatty acids are the principal anions in the colon and most of them are absorbed (Cummings, 1983). The alteration of the ileal flora after restorative proctocolectomy would be expected to result in increased production of SCFA in the pouch, and this has been confirmed (Nasmyth *et al.*, 1989b; Mortensen *et al.*, 1989). The significance of this change in the intraluminal milieu remains to be determined.

The role of SCFA production and absorption in the ecology of the colon is not yet fully understood, but a number of studies have indicated their importance. Butyrate and propionate have a stimulatory effect on the absorption of sodium from the human colon (Roediger & Rae, 1982), and isolated human colonocytes metabolize butyrate in preference to glucose (Roediger, 1980a). It has also been observed that the colonocytes from patients with ulcerative colitis show differences in their metabolism from those of normal subjects. In patients with ulcerative colitis, oxidation of butyrate by the colonocytes is impaired and there is increased oxidation of glucose and glutamine (Roediger, 1980b). In the rat, SCFAs stimulate colonic mucosal cell proliferation (Roediger, 1981), and the healing of colonic

Table 9.3 Faecal short chain fatty acids.

Short chain fatty acids	(mmol/kg), median (range)			
	Acetate	Propionate	Butyrate	Isobutyrate
Ileal pouch faeces ($n = 11$)	22 (2.5–83)	6 (0–10.4)	2.1 (0.4–29.2)	0.1 (0–0.7)
Ileostomy faeces ($n = 12$)	9.8 (1.2–74)	0.4 (0–10.7)	0.5 (0.1–15.6)	0 (0–0.5)
Normal faeces ($n = 17$)	6.3 (0.7–31.7)	2.1 (0.1–5.3)	2.4 (0.3–7.7)	0.3 (0–1.2)
Statistically significant differences				
Pouch:ileostomy	ns	$p < 0.05$	$p < 0.01$	ns
Pouch:normal	$p < 0.05$	ns	ns	ns
Normal:ileostomy	ns	$p < 0.05$	$p < 0.01$	$p < 0.01$

From Nasmyth DG *et al.* (1989b).
ns, not significant.

anastomoses (Rolandelli *et al.*, 1986). Production of SCFA in the normal ileum is low and instillation of SCFA into the terminal ileum results in increased ileal motor activity: a phenomenon which may represent a clearance mechanism occurring naturally in response to coloileal reflux (Kamath *et al.*, 1988).

As expected, the increased numbers of anaerobic bacteria in the pouch are associated with an increase in the concentration of SCFA in the pouch effluent (Mortensen *et al.*, 1989; Nasmyth *et al.*, 1989b). An analysis of faecal SCFA from normal subjects and patients with ileostomies and pelvic pouches is shown in Table 9.3. The ratios of individual short chain fatty acids in effluent from pouches and normal controls is very similar, although a difference in the concentration of acetate was noted in one study (Nasmyth *et al.*, 1989b). By contrast, the concentrations of faecal butyrate and propionate were significantly lower in patients with an ileostomy than in those with a pouch or normal subjects. The significance of differences in the concentration of SCFA in normal faeces and pouch effluent is unknown. In normal faeces the concentration of SCFA reflects not only production but also absorption, whereas the relative rates of production and absorption of SCFA in ileal pouches are unknown. Incubation of faecal suspensions from normal controls, pouches and ileostomies showed a lower rate of SCFA production by the faecal suspensions from the colectomized patients compared with controls, which would reflect known differences in the flora. However, the correlation coefficients between the rates of SCFA

production and the intestinal concentrations of SCFA were relatively weak and this inevitably raises questions about other mechanisms of SCFA regulation which cannot be reproduced *in vitro*, e.g. mucosal absorption (Mortensen *et al.*, 1989).

The consequences for the patient of increased concentrations of SCFA in the ileal pouch have not been fully investigated. The possibility that the motility patterns of the ileal pouch are influenced by the intraluminal concentrations of SCFA has been suggested (Phillips, 1987) but remains unproven. There is certainly no evidence that the frequency of defaecation in pouch patients can be related to the concentration of SCFA in pouch effluent. An association between mucosal structure and faecal SCFA has been observed but the mechanisms which may underlie this association have yet to be determined (Nasmyth *et al.*, 1989b).

Mucosal morphology

The effect of bacteria on intestinal mucosal structure is most apparent when the conventional digestive tract is compared with that of the germ-free host. The intestinal wall of the germ-free host is thinner with a reduced cellularity. The villi are narrower and elongated, the crypts are shallower and the total mucosal surface area is reduced (Gordon & Bruckner-Kardoss 1961). Labelling with ^{3}H thymidine shows a reduced turnover of epithelial cells with a prolonged crypt–villus transit time (Abrams *et al.*, 1963). The other principal difference between the conventional and

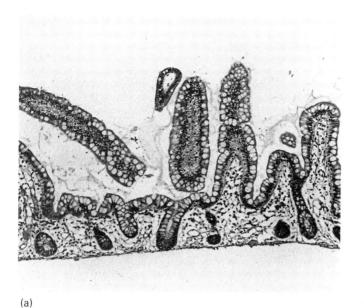

(a)

(b)

Fig. 9.3 Photomicrographs of ileal mucosa. (a) Illustrates ileal mucosal biopsy specimen obtained 10 cm proximal to an ileostomy, and shows preservation of normal villous architecture (magnification ×45). (b) Illustrates a biopsy specimen fron an ileal pouch with villous atrophy, crypt elongation and an increased infiltration of the lamina propria with chronic inflammatory cells (magnification ×73). From Nasmyth *et al.* (1989b).

germ-free host is the sparse lamina propria which contains very few lymphoid cells. When a normal bacterial flora is introduced to the germ-free animal, the gut mucosa rapidly takes on a conventional appearance and there is a marked increase in the cellularity of the lamina propria which is characterized by lymphocytes, polymorphonuclear leukocytes and plasma cells. In conditions of stasis in which there is bacterial overgrowth these mucosal changes become more pronounced.

Preliminary observations on the mucosal changes in the Kock pouch, within 12 months of the operation, showed similar changes to those observed in bacterial overgrowth of the proximal small bowel (Toskes *et al.*, 1975). There were varying degrees of villous atrophy in the pouch mucosa with reduced villous height, elongation of the crypts and increased infiltration of the lamina propria with acute and chronic inflammatory cells (Philipson, 1975). Similar changes were found in the pouches of patients who had undergone restorative proctocolectomy (Nicholls *et al.*, 1981) (Fig. 9.3).

Morphometry and histological grading

Assessment of the severity of histological change in the pouch and its relationship to other variables is clearly necessary if the significance of these changes is to be understood. Subjective assessment of serial mucosal biopsies for comparative purposes may vary considerably from one observer to the next (Corazza *et al.*, 1982). Attempts have therefore been made to introduce as much objectivity as possible into the assessment of ileal pouch biopsies. Eliminating subjectivity is much easier in relation to mucosal morphometry than mucosal cellularity. Two methods have been employed for morphometric assessment of pouch biopsies: stereological estimation of surface to volume ratio (Nilsson *et al.*, 1980) and computer aided microscopy (Nasmyth *et al.*, 1989b). Computer aided microscopy measures the ratio of mucosal surface length to area of lamina propria, and this has been shown to correlate well with measurements of volume to surface area using stereology (Corazza *et al.*, 1985). A further measure of mucosal cell turnover, which correlates well with morphometry, is the crypt cell production rate (CCPR). The CCPR is increased in the ileal pouch compared with normal ileal mucosa and correlates directly and inversely with crypt depth and villous height respectively. It is interesting to note that the CCPR is lower in the recently constructed and defunctioned

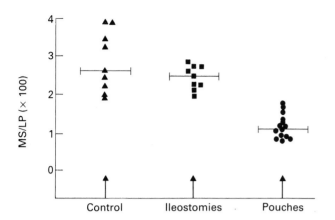

Fig. 9.4 Differences in the ratios of mucosal surface to area of lamina propria (MS/LP), an index of villous atrophy, in patients with an ileal pouch ($p < 0.01$), ileostomists and controls. From Nasmyth *et al.* (1986).

pouch than in the normal ileum, which emphasizes the profound effect that the bacterial flora have on mucosal kinetics (Kmiot *et al.*, 1989).

Morphometric assessment of biopsies from Kock pouches showed that villous height was diminished in the first few months after operation, but re-examination after 2 years and then again after 6–10 years showed that although these changes persisted, they were less marked. The hyperproliferative state of the mucosa appeared to subside and stabilize with time. In contrast the surface to volume ratio continued to increase with time, which appeared to be due to an increase in the volume of the lamina propria. This increase in volume of the lamina propria was not associated with any increase in its cellularity, in fact the converse was the case (Philipson *et al.*, 1975; Nilsson *et al.*, 1980). Morphometric assessment of biopsies from pelvic pouches has shown that all biopsies have some degree of villous atrophy compared with ileal mucosa from patients with an ileostomy or normal controls (Nasmyth *et al.*, 1986) (Fig. 9.4).

Eliminating subjectivity from the histological assessment of mucosal inflammation is much more difficult. Two quite similar systems of grading have been employed (Moskowitz *et al.*, 1986; Nasmyth *et al.*, 1986), in which the degrees of infiltration of the lamina propria with acute and chronic inflammatory cells, are graded according to whether they are absent, mild, moderate or severe. Other parameters such as epithelial ulceration, villous atrophy, crypt abscesses, crypt hyperplasia and fibrosis of the lamina propria have been graded similarly.

Despite the subjectivity of the techniques for histological grading the results reported by two groups are very similar. Moskowitz *et al.* (1986) showed that 30% of patients had some degree of acute inflammation in pouch biopsies. In many instances this inflammation was mild and in particular only 3.5% of patients showed severe acute inflammation. In a much smaller group Nasmyth *et al.* (1986) demonstrated that moderate or severe infiltration of the lamina propria with acute inflammatory cells was present in 38% of patients. In Moskowitz *et al.*'s (1986) study the histological grading was strongly correlated with the macroscopic grading on sigmoidoscopy, and the frequency of defaecation. It might have been expected that the morphometric measurements would correlate with the histological grading, in other words the more severe the inflammation, the greater the degree of villous atrophy. This was not the case (Nasmyth *et al.*, 1986), which is in fact consistent with the long-term observations on the Kock pouches in which the volume of the lamina propria increased but the infiltration with acute and chronic inflammatory cells subsided (Nilsson *et al.*, 1980).

Factors associated with mucosal change

Although there is clearly an association between the change in the flora of the pouch and the changes in the mucosa, the specific factors promoting structural mucosal change are unclear. The fact that the inflammatory cell infiltrate of the lamina propria appears to subside with time, whereas the changes in the mucosal surface to volume ratio do not, would suggest that the stimuli provoking these changes may be different. In respect of the inflammatory changes in the pouch mucosa it is important to consider the possibility that these are related to the underlying disease. The incidence of acute inflammatory change is significantly higher in patients with ulcerative colitis than in those with adenomatous polyposis, and pouchitis in which the most severe examples of acute inflammation are seen, occurs almost exclusively in patients with ulcerative colitis (Nicholls, 1989).

No correlation has been found between the histological grading of mucosal inflammation and the numbers of faecal bacteria, or the concentration of faecal SCFA. On the other hand an inverse correlation was found between the number of *Bacteroides* isolated from the pouch effluent and the degree of villous atrophy: the greater the numbers of *Bacteroides* isolated

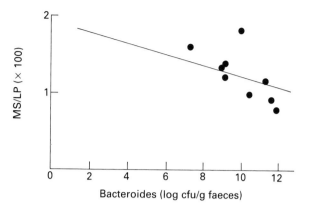

Fig. 9.5 Correlation between the ratio of mucosal surface length to area of lamina propria (MS/LP), an index of villous atrophy, and the numbers of *Bacteroides* in the pouch effluent. $p < 0.001$; Spearman rank correlation coefficient (r_s), -0.77.

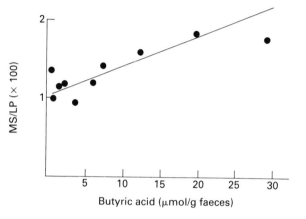

Fig. 9.6 Correlation between the ratio of mucosal surface length to area of lamina propria (MS/LP), an index of villous atrophy, and the concentration of butyric acid in the pouch effluent. $p < 0.05$; r_s, 0.73.

from the pouch effluent the lower was the morphometric index, indicating more severe villous atrophy (Fig. 9.5). The concentration of butyrate in the effluent from the reservoirs also correlated with the morphometric index. In this case the correlation was reversed, the higher the concentration of faecal SCFA the higher the morphometric index, indicating less severe villous atrophy (Nasmyth *et al.*, 1989b) (Fig. 9.6). Initially these findings may appear paradoxical. More severe villous atrophy was associated with increased numbers of *Bacteroides* in the pouch, yet higher concentrations of butyrate, a product of anaerobic fermentation, were associated with less severe villous atrophy. The apparent paradox can be explained: although *Bacteroides* are numerically important anaerobes, few species of

Bacteroides produce significant amounts of butyrate, although most species of *Bacteroides* do produce isobutyrate (Holdemann *et al.*, 1977). It would not, therefore, be expected that because there was a high count of *Bacteroides* there would concomitantly be a high concentration of butyrate.

It might be expected that the concentrations of faecal SCFA would reflect the relative numbers of anaerobic bacteria isolated from the faeces. In fact this was not the case, there was no correlation between faecal SCFA and the numbers of bacteria in the pouch. The concentration of SCFA in the pouch effluent depends not only upon the type and the number of bacteria present but also on the availability of appropriate substrates, the rates of fermentation and ileal absorption of SCFA.

There is no reason to suppose that increased production of SCFA will have a deleterious effect on ileal mucosa. Evidence from studies in animals suggests that SCFAs may suppress the growth of potentially enteropathic bacteria (Hentges, 1983), and are potent trophic factors for proliferation of small intestinal epithelium. Investigation of the latter effect in germ-free animals suggests that it is the SCFAs which are the appropriate stimulus and not bacteria (Sakata, 1987). The mechanism by which SCFAs mediate their effect on intestinal epithelial proliferation is unclear. A direct effect is unlikely as epithelial proliferation is observed remote from the site at which SCFAs are found within the lumen. Systemic mediators have been suggested, and more recent experiments would add credence to that suggestion (Sakata, 1989), although this mediator is unlikely to be either enteroglucagon, gastrin or peptide YY (Goodlad *et al.*, 1989). In the light of these observations the fact that higher concentrations of faecal butyrate were associated with less severe villous atrophy seems less surprising than it might at first.

More severe villous atrophy was associated with increased numbers of *Bacteroides*, but a mechanism whereby *Bacteroides* might influence mucosal structure is unknown. The potential of the altered flora to damage the ileal mucosa, both structurally and functionally requires further investigation. Most species of *Bacteroides* produce conjugated bile acid hydrolase and may also potentiate the production of 7β-dehydroxylase by *Eubacteria* (Hylemon & Glass, 1983). As deconjugated bile acids have been shown to cause extensive ultrastructural and functional damage to the small intestinal epithelium (Gracey *et al.*, 1973), this might be postulated as one mechanism whereby *Bacteroides* could induce deleterious structural change in the pouch mucosa.

Pouchitis – association with altered bacterial ecology

Pouchitis is a clinical syndrome characterized by a systemic illness, and severe acute inflammation of the pouch both macroscopically and microscopically. The question that inevitably arises, is what inferences can be drawn about the aetiology of this condition and, therefore, of its treatment from studies on the bacterial ecology of the pouch.

Pouchitis usually responds to medical treatment with metronidazole with or without steroids, depending on the severity of the attack. From this, it might be inferred that it is caused primarily by a change in the pouch flora. Attractive though this hypothesis might be, there is no bacteriological evidence to support it. No differences in the flora have been found between those patients with pouchitis and those without (Hill & Fernandez, 1989).

If pouchitis responds to antibiotic therapy, and no potential pathogen or consistent alteration in the flora can be identified, the possibility that pouchitis is related to the effects of altered bacterial metabolism should be considered. The two areas of bacterial metabolism worthy of consideration in this regard, are the production of SCFAs and the metabolism of bile acids.

As can be seen from the previous discussion, the role of SCFAs in the ecology of the colon is well established, and butyrate is the preferred substrate for the colonocyte (Roediger, 1980a). SCFAs augment healing of colonic anastomoses (Rolandelli et al., 1986) and colitis in the defunctioned rectum and left colon (which is histologically very similar to acute ulcerative colitis or pouchitis) has been shown to be an energy-deficiency disease which improves following infusion of SCFA (Harig et al., 1989). In view of the correlation between low concentrations of faecal butyrate and more severe villous atrophy it might be anticipated that pouchitis would respond as favourably as diversion colitis. Unfortunately this is not the case: infusions of SCFA did not ameliorate pouchitis, they made the situation worse (de Silva et al., 1989). This finding might appear to cast doubt on the significance of the relationship between villous atrophy and faecal butyrate and is worthy of further consideration. Diversion colitis is considered to be secondary to a nutritional deficiency in the colonic epithelium, but in patients with ulcerative colitis the problem is not one of substrate deficiency, but rather the inability of the colonic epithelium to utilize available substrate.

Isolated colonocytes from patients with active and quiescent ulcerative colitis are unable to oxidize butyrate to the same extent as normal colonocytes, and the magnitude of this metabolic defect is directly proportional to the activity of the disease (Roediger, 1980b).

As pouchitis is a disease which almost exclusively affects patients with ulcerative colitis, it may be that the same metabolic defect which is present in the large bowel is also present in the ileum, and hence it would seem unlikely that raising the luminal concentration of SCFA would be of value. Secondly, villous atrophy tends to be a feature of chronic inflammation rather than the severe acute inflammation which characterizes pouchitis. If raised intraluminal concentrations of SCFA were likely to be of therapeutic benefit in pouchitis, a correlation might be expected between the histological grading of acute inflammation and faecal SCFA, but none has been found (Nasmyth et al., 1989b). Finally the known effects of SCFA should be considered. In the rat they have a trophic effect on the mucosa of the small bowel (Sakata, 1987) and current evidence suggests that this effect is not a direct one but dependent on a humoral mediator (Sakata, 1987, 1989).

The involvement of a humoral mediator is suggested by the demonstration of increased epithelial proliferation in isolated, denervated jejunal loops when SCFAs are perfused into the hind gut (Sakata, 1989), and by the demonstration that butyrate inhibits the proliferation of cells in vitro (Kruh, 1982; Sakata, 1987). It would not, therefore, seem unreasonable to assume that if infusion of SCFA into the ileal pouch were to be associated with trophic effects on the pouch mucosa, that phenomenon would be dependent on either a mucosal receptor mechanism for SCFA, or absorption of SCFA. Both of these functions are likely to be markedly impaired in the presence of pouchitis.

A potential role for bacterial degradation of bile acids in the pathogenesis of pouchitis is based on rather circumstantial evidence, but would be worthy of further investigation. There is some evidence that deconjugation of bile acids is greater in faecal samples from patients with pouchitis (Madden et al., 1990), and it is known that there is a potential for deconjugated and secondary bile acids to damage intestinal epithelium (Gracey et al., 1973; Breuer et al., 1983). On this basis it would not seem unreasonable to investigate the hypothesis that pouchitis is a recurrence of ulcerative colitis in the pouch, which is precipitated by deconjugated and dehydroxylated bile acids.

Absorption from the pouch

Absorptive functions specific to the distal ileum are those of vitamin B_{12} and bile acids. In both instances there is some difficulty in distinguishing between dysfunction of active mucosal transport and intraluminal bacterial metabolism of the substrates, but the effects of the altered bacterial flora on mucosal structure must raise the possibility that mucosal transport is also impaired. Extensive absorption studies have been performed in patients with a continent reservoir ileostomy, and absorption of water and electrolytes appeared normal. Absorption of vitamin B_{12} was also normal provided intrinsic factor was present (Gadacz *et al.*, 1977). Malabsorption of bile acids and vitamin B_{12} may occur (Pedersen *et al.*, 1975; Fiorentini *et al.*, 1987; Nasmyth *et al.*, 1989a), but there is considerable indirect evidence that this is due to bacterial metabolism within the gut lumen rather than direct bacterial inhibition of active transport within the mucosa. Recent *in vitro* studies of taurocholate transport across pouch mucosa have failed to demonstrate a significant defect in active transport (Hosie *et al.*, 1990).

Summary

Following restorative proctocolectomy there are major changes in the microbial flora of the terminal ileum. The microflora of the pouch is characterized by a predominance of anaerobes, and is intermediate between that of ileostomy effluent and normal faeces. One of the consequences of the altered microbial ecology of the pouch is the bacterial metabolism of conjugated bile acids, undigested carbohydrate and other nutrients such as vitamin B_{12}. Intraluminal metabolism of bile acids and bacterial binding of vitamin B_{12} would appear to contribute significantly to impaired absorption of these substances from the pouch. Active transport across the ileal pouch mucosa may also be impaired, but it has proved very difficult to dissociate the effect of bacterial metabolism or binding of the substrates from defects in mucosal transport.

Short chain fatty acids, the end products of anaerobic bacterial fermentation, are essential to the normal ecology of the colon, but are not normally present in significant concentrations in the terminal ileum. The concentrations of SCFA in pouch effluent are much higher than in ileostomy effluent, but it is unknown to what extent SCFAs are absorbed from the pouch. The concentration of butyrate in the pouch has been related to structural change in the pouch mucosa, as have the number of *Bacteroides*, but it is unclear whether this reflects a direct effect of SCFA, or whether it is merely indicative of differences in the bacterial flora or other aspects of their metabolism.

The changes in ileal mucosal structure in the pouch appear to be an extension of those which occur when a bacterial flora is introduced into the germ-free digestive tract. The components of this change can be separated into the acute inflammation which in its most severe form is associated with pouchitis, and the changes of chronic inflammation: villous atrophy and increased infiltration of the lamina propria with chronic inflammatory cells. The latter changes appear to subside with time although widening of the lamina propria persists. Pouchitis is the commonest long-term complication of restorative proctocolectomy and in as much as the changes of pouchitis do not occur in patients with an ileostomy the altered microbial ecology of the pouch would appear to be implicated. However, specific bacterial pathogens have not been identified, neither is there any evidence of consistent quantitative or qualitative differences in the microbial flora of patients with pouchitis.

Current understanding of the ecology of the ileal pouch is poor and much is inferred from studies of intestinal flora and the products of their metabolism which have been conducted under different conditions. The need for further investigation of the ecology of the ileal pouch is paramount. If the factors influencing mucosal inflammation, structural change in the ileal mucosa and ileal absorption can be elucidated, the management of some of the postoperative problems that can arise in these patients, not least pouchitis, might be more effective than at present.

References

Abrams GD (1983) Impact of the intestinal microflora on intestinal structure and function. In *Human Intestinal Microflora in Health and Disease*, DJ Hentges (ed). New York, Academic Press pp. 291–310.

Abrams GD, Bauer H, Sprinz H (1963) Influences of the normal flora on mucosal morphology and cellular renewal in the ileum: a comparison of germ free and conventional mice. *Lab Invest* **12**:355–364.

Andersson H, Fasth S, Filipsson S *et al.* (1979) Faecal excretion of iv injected 14C-cholic acid in patients with continent ileostomy reservoir. *Scand J Gastroenterol* **14**:551–554.

Brandberg A, Kock NG, Philipson B (1972) Bacterial flora in intraabdominal ileostomy reservoir. A study of 23 patients provided with 'continent ileostomy'. *Gastroenterology* **63**: 413–416.

Breuer NF, Rampton DS, Tammar A, Murphy GM, Dowling RH (1983) Effect of colonic perfusion with sulfated and non-sulfated bile acids on mucosal structure and function in the rat. *Gastroenterology* **84**:969–977.

Corazza GR, Bonvicini F, Frazzoni M, Gatto M, Gasbarrini G (1982) Observer variation in assessment of jejunal biopsy specimens. A comparison between subjective criteria and morphometric measurement. *Gastroenterology* **83**: 1217–1222.

Corrazza GR, Frazzoni M, Dixon MF, Gasbarrini G (1985) Quantitative assessment of the mucosal architecture of jejunal biopsy specimens: a comparison between linear measurement, stereology and computer aided microscopy. *J Clin Pathol* **38**:765–770.

Cummings JH (1983) Fermentation in the human large intestine: evidence and implications for health. *Lancet* **i**:1206–1209.

de Silva HJ, Ireland A, Kettlewell M, Mortensen N, Jewell DP (1989) Short-chain fatty acid irrigation in severe pouchitis. *New Engl J Med* **321**:1416–1417.

Donaldson RM (1964) Normal bacterial populations of the intestine and their relationship to intestinal function. *New Engl J Med* **270**:938–945.

Ferraris R, Jazrawi R, Northfield TC (1984) Bile acid kinetics using a new gamma labelled bile acid. *Clin Sci* **66**:12pp.

Fich A, Phillips SF, Hakim NS, Brown ML, Zinsmeister AR (1989) Stimulation of ileal emptying by short chain fatty acids. *Dig Dis Sci* **34**:1516–20.

Finegold SM, Sutter VL, Mathisen GE (1983) Normal indigenous intestinal flora. In *Human Intestinal Microflora in Health and Disease*, DJ Hentges (ed). New York, Academic Press pp. 3–31.

Fiorentini MT, Locatelli L, Cecceopierri B *et al.* (1987) Physiology of ileoanal anastomosis with ileal reservoir for ulcerative colitis and adenomatosis coli. *Dis Colon Rectum* **30**:267–272.

Freter R (1962) *In-vivo* and *in-vitro* antagonism of intestinal bacteria against *Shigella flexnerii* II. The inhibitory mechanism. *J Inf Dis* **110**:38–46.

Gadacz TR, Kelly KA, Phillips SF (1977) The continent ileal pouch: absorptive and motor features. *Gastroenterology* **72**: 1287–1291.

Goodlad RA, Ratcliffe B, Fordham JP *et al.* (1989) Plasma enteroglucagon, gastrin and peptide YY in conventional and germ-free rats refed with a fibre-free or fibre-supplemented diet. *Q J Exp Physiol* **74**:437–442.

Gorbach SL, Nahas L, Lerner PI, Weinstein L (1967a) Studies of intestinal microflora I. Effects of diet, age and periodic sampling on numbers of fecal microorganisms in man. *Gastroenterology* **53**:845–855.

Gorbach SL, Plaut AG, Nahas L, Weinstein L, Spanknebel G, Levitan R (1967b) Studies of intestinal microflora II. Microorganisms of the small intestine and their relation to oral and faecal flora. *Gastroenterology* **53**:856–867.

Gorbach SL, Nahas L, Weinstein L, Levitan R, Patterson J (1967c) Studies of intestinal microflora IV. The microflora of ileostomy effluent: a unique microbial ecology. *Gastro-enterology* **53**:871–880.

Gordon HA, Bruckner-Kardoss E (1961) Effect of normal microbial flora on intestinal surface area. *Am J Physiol* **201**: 175–178.

Gracey M, Papadimitriou J, Burke V, Thomas J, Bower G (1973) Effects on small intestinal function and function induced by feeding a deconjugated bile salt. *Gut* **14**: 519–528.

Harig JM, Soergel KH, Komorowski RA, Wood CM (1989) Treatment of diversion colitis with short-chain-fatty acid irrigation. *New Engl J Med* **320**:23–28.

Heaton KW (1972) *Bile Salts in Health and Disease*. Edinburgh, Churchill Livingstone.

Hentges DJ (1983) Role of intestinal microflora in host defence against infection. In *Human Intestinal Microflora in Health and Disease*, DJ Hentges (ed). New York, Academic Press pp. 311–331.

Hill MJ, Fernandez F (1989) Bacteriology II. Pouchitis. (Workshop.) *Int J Colorectal Dis* **4**:205–209.

Holdeman LV, Cato EP, Moore WEC (1977) *Anaerobe Laboratory Manual*, 4th edn. Blacksburg, Anaerobe Laboratory, Virginia Polytechnic Institute and State University.

Hosie KB, Davie RJ, Panahamawa B, Birch NJ, Keighley MRB (1990) Bile acid absorption following restorative proctocolectomy. *Br J Surg* **77**:1420–21.

Hylemon PB, Glass TL (1983) Biotransformation of bile acids and cholesterol by the intestinal microflora. In *Human Intestinal Microflora in Health and Disease*, DJ Hentges (ed). New York, Academic Press pp. 189–213.

Kamath PS, Phillips SF, Zinsmeister AR (1988) Short chain fatty acids stimulate ileal motility in humans. *Gastroenterology* **95**:1496–1502.

Keighley MRB, Winslet MC, Flinn R, Kmiot W (1989) Multivariate analysis of factors influencing the results of restorative proctocolectomy. *Br J Surg* **76**:740–744.

Kelly DG, Phillips SF, Kelly KA, Weinstein WM, Gilchrist MJ (1983) Dysfunction of the continent ileostomy: clinical features and bacteriology. *Gut* **24**:193–201.

Kmiot WA, Youngs DJ, Winslet MC, Curran FT, Keighley MRB (1989) Ileal adaptation following restorative proctocolectomy. *Br J Surg* **76**:625.

Kruh J (1982) Effects of sodium butyrate, a new pharmacological agent, on cells in culture. *Mol Cell Biochem* **42**:65–82.

Luukkonen P, Vultonen V, Sivonen A, Sipponen P, Jarvinen H (1988) Faecal bacteriology and reservoir ileitis in patients operated on for ulcerative colitis. *Dis Colon Rectum* **31**: 864–67.

Madden MV, Farthing MJG, Nicholls RJ (1990) Inflammation in ileal reservoirs: 'pouchitis'. *Gut* **31**:247–249.

Mortensen PB, Hegnhoj J, Rannem T, Rasmussen HS, Holtug K (1989) Short-chain fatty acids in bowel contents after intestinal surgery. *Gastroenterology* **97**:1090–1096.

Moskowitz RL, Shepherd NA, Nicholls RJ (1986) An assessment of inflammation in the reservoir after restorative proctocolectomy with ileoanal ileal reservoir. *Int J Colorectal Dis* **1**:167–174.

Nasmyth DG (1987) *Mucosal proctectomy and ileal pouch-anal anastomosis: an investigation of factors influencing the functional result.* MS Thesis, University of London.

Nasmyth DG, Williams NS (1985) Pressure characteristics of the human ileocaecal region – a key to its function. *Gastroenterology* **89**:345–351.

Nasmyth DG, Johnston D, Godwin PGR, Dixon MF, Smith A, Williams NS (1986) Factors influencing bowel function after ileal pouch-anal anastomosis. *Br J Surg* **73**:469–473.

Nasmyth DG, Johnston D, Williams NS, King RFGJ, Burkinshaw L, Brooks K (1989a) Changes in the absorption of bile acids after total colectomy in patients with an ileostomy or pouch-anal anastomosis. *Dis Colon Rectum* **32**:230–234.

Nasmyth DG, Godwin PGR, Dixon MF, Williams NS, Johnston D (1989b) Ileal ecology after pouch-anal anastomosis or ileostomy. A study of mucosal morphology, fecal bacteriology, fecal volatile fatty acids, and their inter-relationship. *Gastroenterology* (1989) **96**:817–24.

Nicholls RJ (1989) Clinical diagnosis. Pouchitis. (Workshop.) *Int J Colorectal Dis* **4**:205–229.

Nicholls RJ, Belliveau P, Neill M, Wilks M, Tabaqchali S (1981) Restorative proctocolectomy with ileal reservoir a pathophysiological assessment. *Gut* **22**:462–468.

Nilsson LO, Kock NG, Lindgren I, Myrvold HE, Philipson BM, Ahren C (1980) Morphological and histochemical changes in the mucosa of the continent ileostomy reservoir 6–10 years after its construction. *Scand J Gastroenterol* **15**:737–747.

O'Connell PR, Pemberton JH, Kelly KA (1987) Motor function of the ileal J pouch and its relation to clinical outcome after ileal pouch-anal anastomosis. *World J Surg* **11**:735–741.

O'Connell PR, Rankin DR, Weiland LH, Kelly KA (1986) Enteric bacteriology, absorption, morphology and empty-ing after ileal pouch-anal anastomosis. *Br J Surg* **73**:909–914.

Pedersen BH, Simonsen L, Hansen LK *et al.* (1985) Bile acid malabsorption in patients with an ileal reservoir with a long efferent leg to an anal anastomosis. *Scand J Gastroenterol* **20**:995–1000.

Philipson B, Brandberg A, Jagenburg R, Kock NG, Lager I, Ahren C (1975) Mucosal morphology, bacteriology and absorption in intra-abdominal ileostomy reservoir. *Scand J Gastroenterol* **10**:145–153.

Phillips SF (1987) Biological effects of a reservoir at the end of the small bowel. *World J Surg* **11**:763–768.

Quigley EMM, Borody TJ, Phillips SF, Wienbeck M, Tucker RL, Haddad A (1984) Motility of the terminal ileum and ileocecal sphincter in healthy humans. *Gastroenterology* **87**:857–866.

Rao SSC, Read NW, Brown C, Bruce C, Holdsworth CD (1987) Studies on the mechanism of bowel disturbance in ulcerative colitis. *Gastroenterology* **93**:934–940.

Roediger WEW (1980a) The role of anaerobic bacteria in the metabolic welfare of the colonic mucosa in man. *Gut* **21**:793–798.

Roediger WEW (1980b) The colonic epithelium in ulcerative colitis: an energy deficiency disease. *Lancet* **ii**:712–715.

Roediger WEW (1981) Utilization of nutrients by isolated epithelial cells of the rat colon. *Gastroenterology* **83**:424–9.

Roediger WEW, Rae DA (1982) Trophic effect of short chain fatty acids on mucosal handling of ions by the defunctioned colon. *Br J Surg* **69**:23–25.

Rolandelli RH, Koruda MJ, Settle RG, Rombeau JL (1986) Effects of intraluminal infusion of short-chain fatty acids on the healing of colonic anastomosis. *Surgery* **100**:198–203.

Sakata T (1987) Stimulatory effect of short-chain fatty acids on epithelial cell proliferation in the rat intestine: a possible explanation for trophic effects of fermentable fibre, gut microbes and luminal trophic factors. *Br J Nutr* **58**:95–103.

Sakata T (1989) Stimulatory effect of short-chain fatty acids on epithelial cell proliferation of isolated and denervated jejunal segment of the rat. *Scand J Gastroenterol* **24**:886–890.

Simon GL, Gorbach SL (1984) Intestinal flora in health and disease. *Gastroenterology* **86**:174–93.

Simon GL, Gorbach SL (1986) The human intestinal microflora. *Dig Dis Sci* **31**(suppl):147S–162S.

Soper NJ, Chapman NJ, Kelly KA, Brown ML, Phillips SF, Go VLW (1990) The 'ileal brake' after ileal pouch-anal anastomosis. *Gastroenterology* **98**:111–116.

Soper NJ, Orkin BA, Kelly KA, Phillips SF, Brown ML (1989) Gastrointestinal transit after proctocolectomy with ileal pouch-anal anastomosis or ileostomy. *J Surg Res* **46**:300–305.

Stryker SJ, Borody TJ, Phillips SF, Kelly KA, Dozois RR, Beart RW (1985) Motility of the small intestine after proctocolectomy and ileal pouch-anal anastomosis. *Ann Surg* **201**:351–356.

Toskes PP, Gianella RA, Jervis HR, Nat DSc, Rout WR, Takeuchi A (1975) Small intestinal mucosal injury in the experimental blind loop syndrome. Light and electron microscopic and histochemical studies. *Gastroenterology* **68**:193–203.

Vantrappen G, Janssens J, Hellemans J, Ghoos Y (1977) The interdigestive motor complex of normal subjects and patients with bacterial overgrowth of the small intestine. *J Clin Invest* **59**:1158–66.

Vantrappen G, Janssens J, Coremans G, Jian R (1986) Gastrointestinal motility disorders. *Dig Dis Sci* **31**(suppl):5S–25S.

Welkos SL, Toskes PP, Baer H, Smith GW (1981) Importance of anaerobic bacteria in the cobalamin malabsorption of the experimental rat blind loop syndrome. *Gastroenterology* **80**:313–320.

Chapter 10
Pouch Pathology

BRYAN F. WARREN AND NEIL A. SHEPHERD

Introduction

The conception of the pelvic ileal reservoir and its popularity amongst surgeons and patients alike has effectively provided pathologists with an entirely new field of study. Although still very much in its infancy, pathological study of the reservoir has added important information for the management and prognosis of pouch patients. Pathological changes have been demonstrated which closely mirror those seen elsewhere in the gastrointestinal tract, particularly in the rectum. After all, the reservoir is sited in the position of the rectum and functions as a neorectum. For instance, mucosal prolapse changes are not infrequently seen on the anterior wall of the reservoir with almost identical clinical and pathological changes to those seen in the solitary ulcer (mucosal prolapse) syndrome of the rectum. The apposition of ileal mucosa adjacent to the anal canal with the inevitable changes of stasis and an altered intraluminal environment, particularly with regard to bacteriology, means that normal ileal-type mucosa is very rarely seen in the pouch. In fact, mucosal biopsies show an array of pathological changes that often belie the apparent lack of symptomatology and clinical abnormalities. In this chapter these pathological changes will be described, together with an account of specialized laboratory techniques that have been applied to reservoir mucosal biopsies. Finally the potential causes of these pathological changes and their possible long-term sequelae are discussed.

Histological features of reservoir mucosa

Inflammation and architectural changes

Histopathological analysis of mucosal biopsies has shown that chronic inflammatory changes and architectural abnormalities are almost universal in the pelvic ileal reservoir (Shepherd et al., 1987). Assessment of successive biopsies taken over a long period of time shows that less than 10% of patients will consistently show an entirely normal small intestinal-type mucosa (Shepherd et al., 1987). The chronic inflammatory cell infiltration of the lamina propria is often variable in individual biopsies, between biopsies taken from different parts of the reservoir and with time. The infiltrate is characterized by a predominance of lymphocytes and plasma cells although eosinophils may be a prominent feature, particularly soon after pouch construction (Shepherd et al., 1987). The inflammatory changes are usually associated with architectural abnormalities (Fig. 10.1) although there is not a constant relationship between these changes. The villous architecture of normal ileal mucosa becomes stunted: these changes show great variation in individual biopsies and in biopsies taken at different times and from different parts of the pouch. The architectural anomalies vary from mild villous atrophy through partial villous atrophy to subtotal atrophy (O'Connell et al., 1986; Shepherd et al., 1987; de Silva et al., 1991). When more severe villous atrophy is present, this is associated with crypt hyperplasia. The mucosa simulates that seen in coeliac disease, although it lacks the intra-epithelial lymphocyte infiltrate of that disease (Shepherd et al., 1987).

The morphological changes, both in terms of chronic inflammation and architectural abnormalities, are a feature of the reservoir mucosa in patients with ulcerative colitis, familial adenomatous polyposis and functional disorders of the colorectum. It is likely that these represent a response of the ileal mucosa to the altered environment and probably to stasis and changes in the bacterial flora of the ileum. These changes are probably the prerequisite for subsequent acute inflammatory changes that occur in pouchitis (Shepherd 1990a; de Silva et al., 1991). Acute inflammation is certainly much less common than the chronic changes and may be seen in several different circumstances, including mucosal prolapse, mucosal ischaemia and Crohn's disease. However, active inflammation is much more likely to be seen in association with the more chronic pathological changes as a non-specific phenomenon or

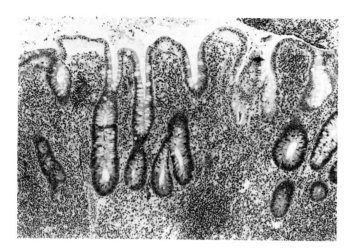

Fig. 10.1 Ileal reservoir mucosa from a patient with ulcerative colitis. There is diffuse chronic inflammation of the lamina propria in association with severe partial villous atrophy. H & E ×75.

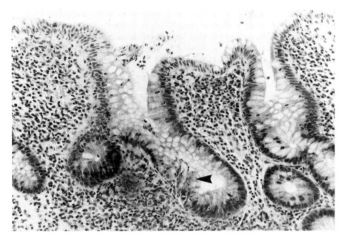

Fig. 10.2 Active inflammation in the pouch mucosa. The mucosa shows typical chronic inflammatory and architectural features but in addition there is a mild to moderate polymorph infiltrate in the crypt epithelium of the central crypt (arrowhead) and in the adjacent lamina propria. A small crypt abscess is beginning to form and polymorphs are being extruded into the pouch lumen (at top). H & E ×150.

Table 10.1 Scoring system for pathological changes in the ileal reservoir mucosa.

	Score
Acute changes	
Acute inflammatory cell infiltrate	
None	0
Mild and patchy infiltrate in the surface epithelium	1
Moderate with crypt abscesses	2
Severe with crypt abscesses	3
Ulceration	
None	0
Mild superficial	1
Moderate	2
Extensive	3
Maximum total	6
Chronic changes	
Chronic inflammatory cell infiltrate	
None	0
Mild and patchy	1
Moderate	2
Severe	3
Villous atrophy	
None	0
Minor abnormality of villous architecture	1
Partial villous atrophy	2
Subtotal villous atrophy	3
Maximum total	6

From Shepherd *et al.* (1987).

in association with pouchitis. Active inflammation is characterized by a polymorph infiltrate in the crypt and surface epithelium and sometimes in congeries in the lamina propria (Fig. 10.2). Ulceration may be present, particularly in pouchitis. The ulceration is usually superficial: deep ulceration with mucosal erosion is unusual and should raise suspicions of a more specific pathology such as Crohn's disease or ischaemic enteritis. A grading system has been introduced to score the acute and chronic features seen in the pouch

mucosa and this is given in Table 10.1. Scores for acute inflammation have been shown to correlate with the degree of macroscopic inflammation seen on sigmoidoscopy, the frequency of defaecation and with the presence of pouchitis (Moskowitz *et al.*, 1986). Acute inflammatory scores are also much higher in the ulcerative colitis patient group than those with familial adenomatous polyposis (Moskowitz *et al.*, 1986). Acute inflammation, in any form, is unusual in polyposis patients and when present is very rarely more than a very mild intra-epithelial polymorph infiltrate.

Although there is evidence of variation of the inflammatory and architectural changes within individual biopsies and in different parts of the pouch (see below), recent studies of serial mucosal biopsies indicate that the changes in the ileal pouch mucosa occur soon after faecal stream exposure, and once the changes have occurred, the mucosa appears to reach a steady state in terms of inflammation, architectural

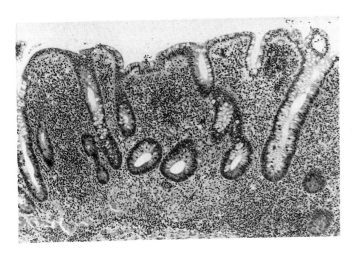

Fig. 10.3 Pouch mucosa with subtotal villous atrophy and diffuse chronic inflammation of the lamina propria. The histological appearances are reminiscent of those of large bowel mucosa. H & E ×75.

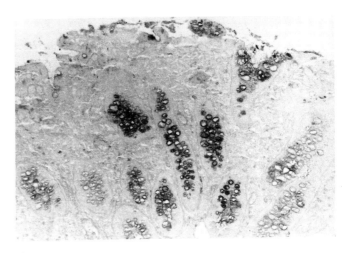

(a)

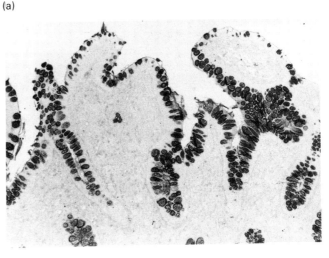

(b)

Fig. 10.4 Mucin histochemistry from two pouch mucosal biopsies of a patient with ulcerative colitis: (a) 6 months after ileostomy reversal. The mucosa which is grossly atrophic shows a mixed pattern of grey (blue) staining sialylated mucin and black (brown-black) staining sulphomucin. The mucin depletion relates to the presence of active inflammation; (b) 2 years after ileostomy reversal. The mucosa shows partial villous atrophy and a predominance of black (brown-black) staining indicating colonic-type sulphomucin. Both HIDAB ×150.

abnormality, histochemistry, and proliferation (de Silva *et al.*, 1990c). These findings would appear to confirm previous studies (Moskowitz *et al.*, 1986). Nevertheless marked fluctuation in these parameters with time is seen in pouchitis, a condition characterized by relapses and remissions particularly after drug therapy, and other inflammatory conditions of the pouch. Long-term studies of the pouch mucosa are required to confirm that the morphological changes in the pouch predate the onset of pouchitis and whether any of these changes will predict subsequent pouchitis. The long-term morphological changes in the pouch mucosa are completely unknown, but there is evidence from the Kock continent ileostomy reservoir at least that a return to relatively normal villous architecture can be expected in many cases (Helander *et al.*, 1990).

Metaplasia

The common occurrence of villous atrophy together with crypt hyperplasia creates a morphological appearance reminiscent of large bowel mucosa (Fig. 10.3): this phenomenon has been called colonic metaplasia (O'Connell *et al.*, 1986; Shepherd *et al.*, 1987; Nasmyth *et al.*, 1989). In addition when chronic inflammation is present, as it usually is, the appearances closely resemble those of chronic ulcerative colitis and, in association with active inflammation as seen in pouchitis, the pouch mucosa mimics active ulcerative colitis. These changes result from an adaptive response of the ileal mucosa to the altered intraluminal environment, especially stasis and alterations in faecal flora (Shepherd, 1990b). Similar alterations are seen in the ileal pouches of experimental animals (Luukkonen *et al.*, 1988a; O'Byrne *et al.*, 1989).

The evidence for colonic metaplasia is strongly supported by mucin histochemical studies, which have demonstrated a change from small intestinal type sialylated mucin to highly sulphated colorectal-type mucin, in a high proportion of cases (Fig. 10.4) (Shepherd *et al.*, 1987; de Silva *et al.*, 1991). The mucin

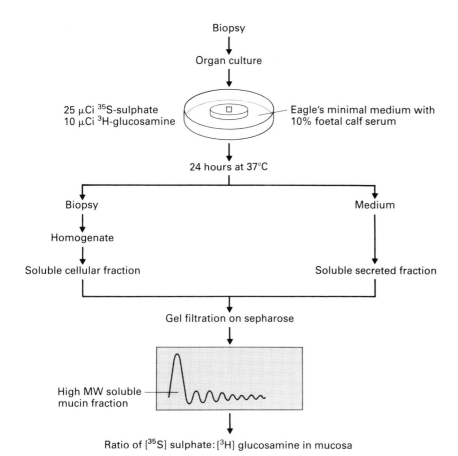

Biopsy

↓

Organ culture

25 μCi ^{35}S-sulphate
10 μCi ^{3}H-glucosamine

Eagle's minimal medium with
10% foetal calf serum

24 hours at 37°C

Biopsy   Medium

↓   ↓

Homogenate

↓

Soluble cellular fraction   Soluble secreted fraction

↓

Gel filtration on sepharose

↓

High MW soluble
mucin fraction

↓

Ratio of [^{35}S] sulphate: [^{3}H] glucosamine in mucosa

Fig. 10.5 The methodology of the ^{35}S–^{3}H glucosamine dual labelling technique for mucin in pouch mucosal biopsies.

change is independent of the original diagnosis, occurring in both ulcerative colitis and polyposis patients. The alterations in mucopolysaccharides have also been shown by the use of sophisticated biochemical techniques, in particular the ^{35}S sulphate:^{3}H glucosamine dual-labelling method which demonstrates the increased sulphation of both intracellular and secreted large intestinal-type mucus in the pouch (Fig. 10.5) (Corfield *et al.*, 1990). The technique is far more sensitive than standard histochemical methods and therefore may prove to be a useful way to monitor the amount and extent of colonic metaplasia.

The evidence for colonic metaplasia in the reservoir mucosa is further substantiated by the acquisition of immunoreactivity for putative colon-specific monoclonal antibodies (Fig. 10.6) (Shepherd *et al.*, 1990b; de Silva *et al.*, 1991) and it has been intimated that changes occur in the proliferative compartment such that it more closely resembles that of large bowel mucosa rather than small bowel mucosa (Paganelli *et al.*, 1989). Nevertheless, when there is colonic metaplasia, this is by no means complete: it appears

that all pouches retain evidence of small intestinal mucosal differentiation, specifically disaccharidase activity (de Silva *et al.*, 1991). The precise relationship between the metaplastic changes and inflammation is still unclear, and this is particularly so with active inflammation and pouchitis. Most of the evidence indicates that the chronic inflammatory changes with metaplasia predate acute inflammation and are the prerequisite for pouchitis in susceptible individuals (Shepherd 1990a; de Silva *et al.*, 1991).

Colonic metaplasia is a common and widespread feature of the reservoir mucosa. Less common is an epithelial change from small intestinal-type mucosa to that resembling antral-type gastric mucosa (Fig. 10.7). Recent studies of this pyloric metaplasia indicate that it is a non-specific response of intestinal epithelium to ulceration with highly characteristic morphological and immunohistochemical features (Wright *et al.*, 1990). It is a characteristic feature of small intestinal Crohn's disease but may also be seen in various inflammatory conditions of the small and large intestine. Pyloric metaplasia is seen in a small proportion of reservoirs

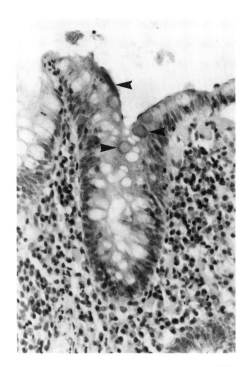

Fig. 10.6 Pouch mucosa showing expression of the monoclonal antibody PR 3A5 in goblet cells of the crypts and surface epithelium (arrowheads). Current evidence indicates that this antibody is specific to colorectal-type mucin (Richman & Bodmer, 1987). PR 3A5 immunohistochemistry ×300.

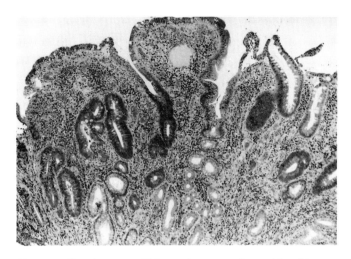

Fig. 10.7 Pouch mucosal biopsy from a patient with a history of chronic relapsing pouchitis now in remission. There is subtotal villous atrophy, chronic inflammation and widespread pyloric metaplasia, indicated by the pale staining glands present centrally and inferiorly. H & E ×75.

and in this situation is a useful marker of previous severe active inflammation and ulceration (Shepherd *et al.*, 1987).

Pathology of pouchitis

There is much confusion and controversy surrounding pouchitis, the chronic relapsing inflammatory condition of the pouch mucosa. This is predominantly because the term has, in the past, been too loosely applied: many different inflammatory diseases have been called pouchitis (Shepherd, 1990b). There is no doubt that many conditions can cause active inflammation in the reservoir. There is now considerable agreement that the definition of pouchitis should include: clinical (increase in stool frequency, urgency, discharge, fever and other systemic symptoms), endoscopic (increased vascularity, bleeding and ulceration) and histopathological criteria (Moskowitz *et al.*, 1986; Tytgat & van Deventer, 1988; Nicholls, 1989; Madden *et al.*, 1990; Warren & Shepherd, 1992). The pathological features of pouchitis are therefore of prime importance in assessing the patient with symptomatology from an ileal reservoir.

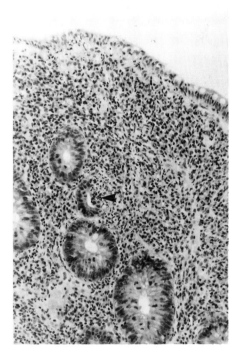

Fig. 10.8 Reservoir mucosal biopsy from a patient with pouchitis. There is subtotal villous atrophy with diffuse chronic inflammation. Active inflammation is present in the form of intraepithelial polymorphs and a crypt abscess is forming (arrowhead). Polymorphs are also present in the lamina propria. H & E ×150.

The histopathological features of pouchitis are highly characteristic but are not necessarily specific to the condition. The pouch mucosa shows chronic changes, such as chronic inflammation of the lamina propria and a variable, focal but often marked degree of villous atrophy (Shepherd *et al.*, 1987; de Silva *et al.*, 1991). It is the acute inflammatory changes that are the pathological hallmark of pouchitis. Acute inflammation takes the form of an intra-epithelial polymorph infiltrate and this is usually severe although it may be surprisingly focal. Collections of polymorphs are also seen in the lamina propria, but the epithelium appears to be the central focus of acute inflammation and crypt abscesses are characteristic (Fig. 10.8). Ulceration is the second characteristic feature and is usually superficial although often extensive (Shepherd *et al.*, 1987). The overall histological appearances bear a close resemblance to those of ulcerative colitis and are unlike those of Crohn's disease. Using the pathological scoring system devised at St Mark's Hospital (Table 10.1), a variable chronic change score is seen although this is usually high. A score for acute inflammatory change of 4 or more effectively defines pouchitis and correlates with the clinical and endoscopic features of this syndrome (Moskowitz *et al.*, 1986). It would be possible to achieve such high scores in other inflammatory conditions such as ischaemia and Crohn's disease, although this has not been the experience of the authors.

Metaplastic changes are usually present in association with pouchitis, particularly morphological metaplasia (Shepherd *et al.*, 1987; de Silva *et al.*, 1991). Mucin change to colonic-type sulphomucin is also usually seen but in some cases small intestinal sialomucins predominate (Shepherd *et al.*, 1987; Corfield *et al.*, 1990). If metaplastic changes are the basis upon which pouchitis occurs in the pouch, can this apparent lack of large intestinal mucin be explained? In fact, the balance between sialomucins and sulphate-rich mucins is relatively unstable in the face of inflammation and this is particularly well seen in chronic ulcerative colitis, in which sialomucins may predominate in the colonic mucosa when active disease is present or when there is dysplasia (Jass *et al.*, 1986). In a similar way the change from sialomucin to sulphate-rich colonic-type mucin in the reservoir mucosa may be reversed by the active inflammation associated with pouchitis (Shepherd *et al.*, 1987).

Distribution of pathological changes

The success of restorative proctocolectomy with ileal reservoir in terms of function has meant that few pouches have been resected and therefore systematic analysis of the distribution of both chronic and acute inflammatory changes has not been possible. Nevertheless from histological analysis of mucosal biopsies, it is clear that these changes can be very focal both within a single biopsy and between biopsies taken from various sites within the reservoir. Subsequently both inflammation and metaplasia may be much more extensive and more prevalent than single biopsies would suggest. Preliminary data from a prospective analysis of the distribution of chronic inflammatory, architectural and metaplastic changes within quadruple loop (W) reservoirs suggest that these changes are more pronounced in the body and on the posterior wall of the pouch compared with the anterior wall (Fig. 10.9): this may relate to increased contact with static

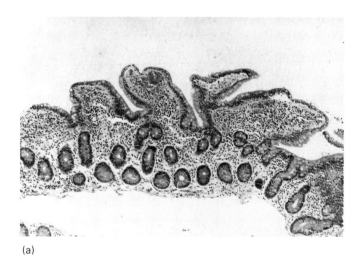

(a)

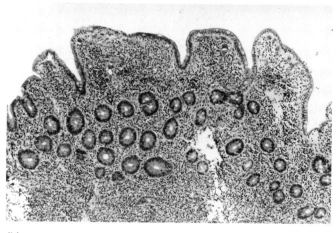

(b)

Fig. 10.9 Mucosal biopsies from (a) the anterior wall, and (b) the posterior wall of a reservoir constructed for ulcerative colitis. Both architectural and chronic inflammatory changes are much more pronounced in the posterior wall biopsy which also shows striking crypt hyperplasia. Both H & E ×40.

faecal residue (Shepherd *et al.*, 1992). To ensure a comprehensive analysis of the pathological changes, we recommend that biopsies are taken from multiple sites during endoscopic assessment (Warren & Shepherd, 1992). These should include both the anterior and posterior walls, the respective sites for mucosal prolapse changes (see below) and the most significant chronic pathological changes. Suture lines should be avoided as these may produce confusing histological appearances.

Mucosal inflammation occurring after restorative proctocolectomy is generally considered to be restricted to the pouch. However inflammation does occur in the normal calibre ileum in association with ulcerative colitis, backwash ileitis (Scott & Phillips, 1989) and proximal to an ileostomy, so-called prestomal ileitis. It has been intimated that the creation of a pouch may lead to inflammatory changes in the ileum proximal to the pouch (O'Connell, 1989). In our prospective analysis of the distribution of inflammatory changes, we have assessed the amount of inflammation in the proximal ileal limb 10 cm proximal to the pouch itself (Shepherd *et al.*, 1992). Our data indicate that the proximal ileum is histologically normal in almost all cases, even in those with active inflammation and pouchitis.

Additional pouch pathology

Preclosure pouchitis

A syndrome of preclosure pouchitis has been described in the two-stage quadruple loop (W) pouch procedure (Warren *et al.*, 1990b). In this syndrome villous atrophy, chronic inflammation and significant active inflammatory change occur in the reservoir mucosa before the temporary ileostomy is closed, and before the faecal stream reaches the reservoir (Warren *et al.*, 1990b). It should be emphasized that this occurs in only a small proportion of cases (certainly much less than 10%). Pathological analysis of these cases has disclosed active inflammatory changes and superficial ulceration, with appearances similar to those of late onset pouchitis. An interesting feature is the predominance of eosinophils in the chronic inflammatory cell infiltrate of the lamina propria (Warren *et al.*, 1990b): this has also been observed as an early phenomenon in the reservoir mucosa after ileostomy closure (Shepherd *et al.*, 1987). It is possible that a few of these cases could represent mucosal ischaemia in the

immediate postoperative period (Shepherd, 1990b) but most lack the characteristic histopathological features of ischaemia. Similarly a recurrence of Crohn's disease could explain some of the features, but none of the cases to date have shown any evidence, either in the original proctocolectomy specimen, in pouch mucosal biopsies or elsewhere in the gastrointestinal tract, to support such a diagnosis.

Perhaps the most attractive explanation for the pathogenesis of preclosure pouchitis is that it represents a form of diversion enteritis. Diversion colitis is a well described phenomenon in the defunctioned large bowel of patients who have undergone faecal stream diversion for various conditions including carcinoma, diverticular disease and chronic inflammatory bowel disease (Editorial, 1989). The histological features of diversion colitis and proctitis may strongly mimic those of chronic inflammatory bowel disease (Editorial, 1989; Komorowski, 1990). The disease is said to relate to a lack of essential short chain fatty acids, including butyrates, required for normal colonic epithelial proliferation and maturation (Harig *et al.*, 1989). The small bowel epithelium may undergo similar inflammatory changes under similar conditions as a consequence of luminal deficiency of necessary nutrients. Why this syndrome is only present in a small proportion of pouch patients remains unexplained. The relationship, if any, between preclosure pouchitis and late onset pouchitis has not been established: the follow-up period of patients with preclosure pouchitis has so far been short (Warren *et al.*, 1990b). Nevertheless a single patient with preclosure pouchitis has developed troublesome recurrent late onset pouchitis although with good response to metronidazole (Warren *et al.*, 1990b).

Mucosal ischaemia

Traction on mesenteric vasculature during the construction of a pelvic ileal reservoir may be sufficient to cause some reduction in blood flow to the pouch mucosa. Localized mucosal ischaemia may also be caused by impairment of the reservoir microcirculation as a consequence of surgery (Tytgat, 1989). In fact, a degree of mucosal ischaemia can be demonstrated both endoscopically (Tytgat, 1989) and histopathologically (Shepherd, 1990b) soon after reservoir construction. Some mucosal ischaemia is to be expected in most surgical procedures but restoration of a normal mucous membrane is almost always rapid and complete.

Nevertheless it has been shown that inflammation in the reservoir mucosa correlates with a reduced mucosal blood flow as assessed by laser doppler measurements soon after pouch construction (Hosie *et al.*, 1989). Some cases of pouchitis may respond to allopurinol, a xanthine oxidase inhibitor: it is suggested that the mechanism of response may relate to reduction of oxygen derived free radicals produced by xanthine oxidase in the ischaemic mucosa (Levin *et al.*, 1990).

Mucosal ischaemia may account for some of the pouch patients who develop high fluid output from the ileal reservoir soon after construction (Hawley PR, personal communication). Nevertheless the pathological evidence indicates that mucosal ischaemia is most unlikely to be a significant cause of chronic relapsing pouchitis. Pouchitis lacks the characteristic features of chronic mucosal ischaemia such as gross crypt atrophy, lamina propria fibrosis and haemosiderin deposition. Furthermore it would not explain the disparity in pouchitis prevalence between ulcerative colitis and polyposis patient groups. We conclude that ischaemia of the superficial epithelium of the reservoir mucosa may cause inflammation and some symptomatology in the immediate postoperative period but we believe that mucosal ischaemia has little or no role in the pathogenesis of chronic inflammatory disorders of the pouch.

Mucosal prolapse

The characteristic clinical and pathological changes of mucosal prolapse are occasionally observed in the ileal reservoir (Shepherd *et al.*, 1987; Warren *et al.*, 1990a). Endoscopically mucosal prolapse manifests as a patch or strip of inflammation affecting the anterior wall of the pouch whilst the rest of the pouch mucosa appears normal. The condition has been called 'anterior strip pouchitis' on account of these endoscopic appearances but this term is to be discouraged to prevent confusion with chronic relapsing pouchitis. Anterior pouch mucosal prolapse has clinical and pathological analogies with the solitary ulcer (mucosal prolapse) syndrome of the rectum (Shepherd, 1990b). Defaecating pouchography can demonstrate radiological evidence of mucosal prolapse and there is evidence that surgery, in the form of a pouchpexy, may alleviate the symptoms and pathological changes (Warren *et al.*, 1990a). Pathologically one observes mucosal inflammation with superficial ulceration, the ulcers often lined by a small cap of granulation tissue. The most charac-

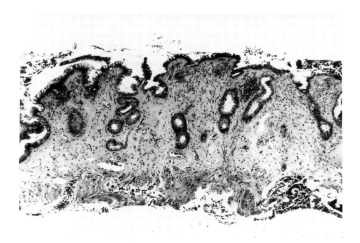

Fig. 10.10 The histological changes of mucosal prolapse in a pouch mucosal biopsy. The lamina propria shows fibromuscular obliteration and the crypt epithelium appears hyperplastic. H & E ×40.

teristic feature is the presence of fibromuscular obliteration of the lamina propria, the smooth muscle fibres appearing to arise from a thickened and splayed muscularis mucosae (Fig. 10.10) (Shepherd *et al.*, 1987).

Mucosal prolapse is perhaps not an entirely unexpected occurrence in the reservoir as some mucosal redundancy is inevitable especially in larger reservoirs. The pathological changes of mucosal prolapse may not be of direct clinical relevance in biopsies taken away from the anterior wall, particularly in voluminous reservoirs. Biopsies taken from suture lines may also show mucosal prolapse changes histologically, and these are also of no clinical significance: suture line biopsies can usually be recognized by the presence of circumscribed defects due to staples or birefringent suture material.

Granulomas and fissures

Granulomas in the reservoir mucosa are a source of diagnostic confusion. These could of course indicate a diagnosis of Crohn's disease, but granulomas are occasionally seen, particularly within lymphoid follicles, in the reservoir mucosa of patients with an indisputable diagnosis of ulcerative colitis (Fig. 10.11) (Shepherd, 1989). Lymphoid follicles of the ileal mucosa have a role in antigen and particulate matter sampling of the luminal contents, and the presence of granulomas at this site suggests that they are a tissue reaction to the altered intraluminal environment or to extraneous material (Shepherd, 1990b). Granulomas are also seen

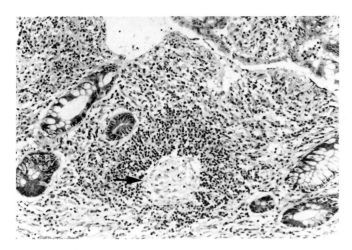

Fig. 10.11 Pouch mucosal biopsy from a patient with an indisputable previous diagnosis of ulcerative colitis on examination of the proctocolectomy specimen. There is a well-formed epithelioid cell granuloma within a lymphoid follicle (arrow). The presence of such granulomas does not necessarily imply a diagnosis of Crohn's disease. H & E ×150.

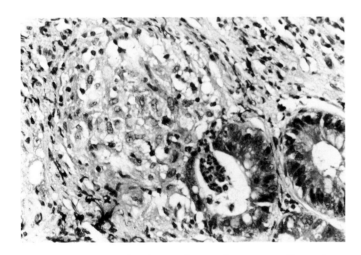

Fig. 10.12 An epithelioid granuloma adjacent to a disruptive crypt abscess in a severely inflamed pouch. Such granulomatous inflammation probably represents a response to released mucins in the lamina propria. H & E ×300.

adjacent to disruptive crypt abscesses in the pouch mucosa of patients with severe active inflammation, particularly pouchitis (Fig. 10.12). These granulomas may represent a tissue reaction to released mucin and should not be taken as definitive evidence of Crohn's disease. Fissures in the reservoir wall are also a source of potential diagnostic error (Tytgat, 1989). Although characteristic of Crohn's disease, they again may be seen in other situations. In the pouch they may be the

result of deep disruptive crypt abscesses in pouchitis, a feature also seen in ulcerative colitis, particularly in association with rectal defunctioning (Warren *et al.*, 1991). Fissures are also seen at anastomotic lines extending deeply and appearing endoscopically as fistulous tracts opening into the pouch (Tytgat, 1989). These defects are usually quick to heal unlike the penetrating lesions of Crohn's disease (Tytgat, 1989). It should be stressed that a diagnosis of Crohn's disease should never be made on the histopathological features seen in reservoir mucosal biopsies alone. Such a diagnosis may have grave consequences for the patient and should always be substantiated by examination of the original proctocolectomy specimen, and by investigation of the remaining gastrointestinal tract.

Polyps in the reservoir

Small polyps are not unusual in endoscopic assessment of the reservoir. These usually represent either hyperplastic lymphoid follicles (Tytgat, 1989) or areas of granulation tissue at the site of anastomotic lines. Some polypoid excrescences may also be seen as a late result of previous ulceration in pouchitis and have the typical histological features of inflammatory polyps. In familial adenomatous polyposis (FAP) patients, adenomas are not infrequently observed in the mucosa of the terminal ileum at the time of total colectomy (Shepherd & Bussey, 1990) and it is therefore not surprising that adenomas have been seen in the reservoir mucosa, both in continent abdominal ileostomies and in pelvic pouches (Beart *et al.*, 1982; Shepherd *et al.*, 1987; Stryker *et al.*, 1987; Hultén, 1989). In some of these cases the adenomas have been multiple and extensive but it is still uncertain whether there is an increased propensity to adenoma formation in the FAP reservoir compared with the normal ileal mucosa.

Specialized laboratory techniques

Immunopathology

Studies of lymphocytic and histiocytic subsets and of major histocompatibility complex (MHC) class II antigen (HLA-DR) expression of the pouch epithelium have added important insights into the pathogenesis of inflammation in the pouch. For instance Meuwissen *et al.* (1989) have demonstrated increased numbers of IgG- and IgA-secreting plasma cells in the lamina propria of biopsies from pouchitis patients, whilst IgM secreting cells are low or normal. These findings are similar to those seen in ulcerative colitis and unlike those of infective colitis (Meuwissen *et al.*, 1989). Characterization of T-cell subsets, specifically CD4 (helper phenotype) and CD8 (suppressor phenotype), has demonstrated no significant differences between normal ileal control, uninflamed pouch mucosa and pouchitis mucosa (de Silva *et al.*, 1990b). Increased numbers of RFD9-positive macrophages, essentially indicating epithelioid and tingible body histiocytes, are seen in pouchitis mucosa and this is a feature of inflammatory bowel disease in general, further supporting an immunopathological link between pouchitis and inflammatory bowel disease (de Silva *et al.*, 1990b).

HLA-DR expression in the small bowel epithelium is usually restricted to fully differentiated epithelial cells in the villi (Bland, 1988). In inflamed pouches, without clinical and pathological evidence of pouchitis, HLA-DR expression is reduced whilst proliferation is increased: the lack of HLA-DR expression probably relates to epithelial immaturity in highly proliferative mucosa (de Silva *et al.*, 1990a). HLA-DR staining is intense in the epithelium in pouchitis patients, and extends into the crypt epithelium (de Silva *et al.*, 1990a). This finding suggests a role for antigen presentation in the pathogenesis of pouchitis.

Proliferative indices

The pouch epithelium shows increased crypt cell proliferation (CCP), in both uninflamed reservoirs and in those with pouchitis, compared to normal ileum controls. This hyperproliferation may be simply disclosed by an increased mitotic index (Fig. 10.13) (Shepherd, 1990b) but has also been demonstrated by use of the monoclonal antibody Ki-67, which recognizes a nuclear antigen expressed in proliferating cells (Gerdes *et al.*, 1984). Using frozen section immunohistochemistry with Ki-67, it has been shown that not only is there increased proliferative activity in the pouch epithelium, more pronounced in the pouchitis patient group, but also such proliferation is inversely related to villous height and directly related to crypt depth (de Silva *et al.*, 1990a). These findings indicate that those reservoirs with most villous atrophy and crypt hyperplasia bearing the closest resemblance to colonic mucosa, are those with the highest proliferative activity.

It has been suggested that changes in proliferative

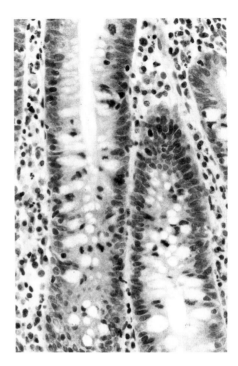

Fig. 10.13 Reservoir mucosa from a patient with pouchitis. Innumerable darkly-staining mitotic figures are seen in the proliferative zone of the crypt epithelium, indicating the greatly enhanced proliferative activity of the pouch mucosa in this condition. H & E ×300.

compartments of the pouch mucosa can be demonstrated such that these more closely resemble those of colonic mucosa than ileal mucosa (Paganelli *et al.*, 1989). Whether increased CCP and the architectural changes are directly related or which precedes the other is uncertain. It could be argued that the architectural changes are the inevitable result of increased CCP and this would help to explain why pouchitis mucosa most often shows subtotal atrophy. Nevertheless some reservoirs show little inflammatory change and relatively low CCP rate in the face of marked villous atrophy and occasional pouchitis cases show only partial villous atrophy. Whilst there is little doubt that CCP and architecture are closely related, the precise nature of their relationship in uninflamed pouches and in pouchitis is still very uncertain and demands further investigation.

Morphometry

Morphometric methods introduce some objectivity into the assessment of the ileal reservoir mucosa, particularly with regard to architecture. Such methods have been more widely used in the assessment of the continent ileostomy reservoir mucosa (Philipson *et al.*, 1975; Nilsson *et al.*, 1980; Helander *et al.*, 1990): these studies have used relatively simple morphometric methods such as point-counting whilst studies of pelvic pouch morphometry have utilized more complex image analysis systems (Nasmyth *et al.*, 1989; de Silva *et al.*, 1991). Nasmyth *et al.* (1989) have shown that villous atrophy, assessed as a ratio of mucosal surface length/lamina propria area on the one hand, and villous height/mucosal thickness on the other (Corazza *et al.*, 1985), correlated significantly with both the number of *Bacteroides* bacteria and with faecal butyrate. These findings suggest that whilst increased numbers of anaerobic bacteria may be involved in the pathogenesis of the chronic inflammatory and architectural changes that occur in the pouch, butyrate may have a protective role upon the pouch mucosa. De Silva *et al.* (1991) have studied architectural changes by image analysis techniques in patients with and without pouchitis. They have shown that the index of villous atrophy (villous height/total mucosal thickness) is significantly lower in pouchitis patients than in those without pouchitis, and that patients without pouchitis showed more villous atrophy and crypt hyperplasia than normal controls. Although these complex methods have enabled some objectivity to be introduced in the assessment of mucosal architectural changes, the results have generally merely substantiated the findings of simple mucosal morphological assessment and have added little to our overall knowledge of the effects of reservoir construction on the ileal mucosa.

Electron microscopy

To date there have been no published accounts of the ultrastructural appearances of the pelvic ileal reservoir mucosa, although we have recently initiated such a study (Bruce *et al.*, 1991). Whilst there appear to be only minor abnormalities in the microvillous architecture, some cells demonstrate basal bodies (Fig. 10.14), an ultrastructural feature not normally seen in small intestinal epithelial cells, but a normal feature of large intestinal epithelium. These observations suggest that colonic metaplasia may also occur at the ultrastructural level. Formal electron microscopic analyses of continent ileostomy reservoir mucosa have been published (Philipson *et al.*, 1975; Helander *et al.*, 1990). These have demonstrated only minor abnormalities in microvillous architecture in reservoir mucosa. Such changes occur soon after reservoir construction and there

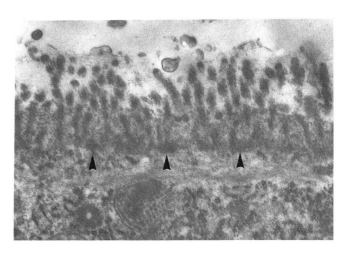

Fig. 10.14 The ultrastructural appearances of the pouch epithelium. The microvilli appear normal but three darkly staining basal bodies (arrowheads) are seen along the basal membrane. EM ×7500.

is evidence that these changes may persist for many years although they appear to be of little clinical significance (Helander *et al.*, 1990).

The potential causes of reservoir inflammation and pouchitis

It is clear to the reader that there are many heterogeneous conditions which have either a definite or potential role in the pathogenesis of inflammation in the reservoir mucosa. Some of these conditions are shown in Table 10.2 together with the authors' views on the likelihood or otherwise of their involvement

Table 10.2 The potential causes of inflammation and pouchitis.

	Cause of inflammation	Cause of pouchitis
Stasis and bacterial overgrowth	+++	−
Specific bacterium or other microorganism	?	?
Mucosal ischaemia	++	?
Mucosal prolapse	+	−
Diversion enteritis	+	?
Crohn's disease	+	−
Ulcerative colitis	++	++

Key to role in pathogenesis: −, no role; ?, possible role but unlikely; +, definitely implicated but only of restricted clinical significance; ++, likely role in pathogenesis; +++, strongly implicated.

in the genesis of inflammation and pouchitis. It is important to reaffirm that chronic inflammation is commonplace, in fact almost universal, in the pouch whilst pouchitis occurs less frequently, the generally accepted prevalence being somewhere between 10 and 20% (Tytgat & van Deventer, 1988; Meuwissen et al., 1989; Nicholls, 1989; Madden et al., 1990; Shepherd, 1990b).

The ileal reservoir functions as a neorectum, and stasis with attendant alterations in faecal flora inevitably occurs. There is good evidence that these new luminal conditions create an environment which leads to the chronic inflammation and architectural changes that characterize the pouch mucosa (O'Connell et al., 1986; Shepherd et al., 1987; Nasmyth et al., 1989). These alterations in intraluminal environment and in pouch mucosal ecology are probably the prerequisite for acute inflammatory changes but do not appear to be the direct cause. For example, the onset of acute inflammatory changes in the reservoir mucosa does not correlate with the type of reservoir, its compliance or with reservoir volume (Dozois et al., 1986; Moskowitz et al., 1986). Furthermore no consistent correlations have been found between bacteriological changes and the development of pouchitis (Nicholls et al., 1981; O'Connell et al., 1986; Luukkonen et al., 1988b; Nasmyth et al., 1989). There is little positive evidence for a role of specific bacteria in the pathogenesis of pouchitis, although many cases do respond to metronidazole, a potent antibiotic against anaerobes (Dozois et al., 1986). However the response to metronidazole need not necessarily be a direct effect on pathogenic bacteria. Metronidazole is known to have immunosuppressive properties. Alternatively the mode of action may be similar to that seen in some cases of colonic Crohn's disease which respond to the drug (Bernstein et al., 1980): its action in this situation relates to an effect on ileal function by reducing bacterial overgrowth and altering bile salt metabolism (Beelsen & Kavich, 1973; Rutgeerts et al., 1981). Our conclusion is that stasis and bacterial change undoubtedly have a role in the acquisition of chronic inflammatory and architectural changes, but that there is currently no compelling evidence to implicate physical or specific bacteriological factors in the aetiology of pouchitis.

As discussed previously, mucosal prolapse undoubtedly occurs in the reservoir and indirectly causes inflammation, but this is not thought to be of significance in the pathogenesis of either chronic inflammation or pouchitis. Mucosal ischaemia could account for some cases of inflammatory pathology in the immediate postoperative period and occasional cases of preclosure pouchitis: a role in the aetiology of pouchitis is much more doubtful. In previous discussion of preclosure pouchitis (see above) we entertained the possibility of a form of diversion enteritis occurring in the reservoir before the temporary ileostomy is closed and the faecal stream reaches the pouch. Diversion colitis and proctitis is a well recognized complication of faecal stream diversion and appears to be caused by a lack of essential short-chain fatty acids, particularly butyrates, normally produced by anaerobic bacteria, which maintain the healthy colonic mucosa (Lusk et al., 1984; Harig et al., 1989). The lack of these fatty acids leads to inflammation in the defunctioned segment and in severe cases the histological appearances of diversion colitis may simulate ulcerative colitis (Komorowski, 1990; Ma et al., 1990). It is possible that these fatty acids may become a potential energy source for the pouch mucosa when colonic metaplasia has taken place and that the lack of these acids may then lead to inflammation. Low concentrations of these fatty acids have been demonstrated in faeces from pouches compared with normal stool (Ambroze et al., 1989; Nasmyth et al., 1989) and there is an inverse relationship between pouch concentrations of butyrate and the degree of villous atrophy (Nasmyth et al., 1989). Could preclosure pouchitis represent a form of diversion enteritis and late-onset pouchitis be the result of a lack of essential nutrients for metaplastic epithelium? Whilst these theses are certainly worthy of further investigation, the lack of response of late-onset pouchitis patients to short-chain fatty acid irrigation is good evidence that the low concentrations of fatty acids are not important in the pathogenesis of pouchitis (de Silva et al., 1989).

The theory that pouchitis is a manifestation of idiopathic chronic inflammatory bowel disease in the ileal reservoir has many attractions. Crohn's disease remains an absolute contraindication for pelvic ileal reservoir surgery but there have been many cases where an erroneous diagnosis of ulcerative colitis has been made, and a reservoir has been constructed in patients subsequently found to have Crohn's disease. In these cases, the outlook for the reservoir has been generally very poor. These cases do not show the characteristic clinical, endoscopic and histopathological features of chronic relapsing pouchitis. Nevertheless it has been suggested that Crohn's disease may develop in the reservoir after proctocolectomy for indisputable ulcerative colitis (Keighley, 1989) and even, that pouchitis may be a manifestation of Crohn's disease (Tanaka & Riddell, 1990).

Great care is advised, however, in making a diagnosis of Crohn's disease based solely on the histopathological features of reservoir mucosal biopsies and even of reservoir resection specimens. All the pathological hallmarks of Crohn's disease, namely granulomas, focal chronic inflammation in the form of lymphoid aggregates and fissures, may be seen in pouches without any clinical, radiological, endoscopic or histopathological evidence of Crohn's disease elsewhere (Tytgat, 1989; Shepherd, 1990b). Evidence against a role for Crohn's disease as a cause of pouchitis is strengthened by the fact that the histological appearances of pouchitis are unlike those of Crohn's disease and that even cases of resistant pouchitis with atypical clinical and pathological features do not appear to reflect underlying Crohn's disease (Subramani et al., 1990).

Despite the undoubted difficulties in the differential diagnosis of idiopathic chronic inflammatory bowel disease and the fact that Crohn's disease has been regarded as an absolute contraindication to pelvic ileal reservoir (Beart, 1988), patients whose colectomy specimens show pathological features intermediate between Crohn's disease and ulcerative colitis, socalled indeterminate colitis, appear to have results as good as those with unequivocal ulcerative colitis and there are no differences in the incidence of pouchitis in these two groups (Pezim et al., 1989).

Having considered all the available evidence, we think it most unlikely that Crohn's disease is the cause of chronic relapsing pouchitis. Could pouchitis represent recurrence of ulcerative colitis in the pelvic pouch which has undergone colonic metaplasia? There is much evidence closely linking pouchitis and ulcerative colitis and the same associations have been observed in the ileitis that complicates continent ileostomy reservoirs (Hultén & Svaninger 1984; Hultén, 1989). Pouchitis, when adequately defined, is relatively more common in ulcerative colitis patients than in those with FAP and indeed may well be restricted to ulcerative colitis patients (Shepherd et al., 1987; Nicholls, 1989) although there is documentation of a single case of pouchitis apparently occurring in a FAP patient (Kmiot et al., 1990). Our pathological scoring system indicates that acute inflammation in the reservoir mucosa, with and without pouchitis, is much more prevalent in ulcerative colitis patients than in

those with FAP (Moskowitz et al., 1986; Shepherd et al., 1987). Patients with extensive colitis at the time of proctocolectomy are more likely to develop pouchitis than those with more restricted disease in the colon, particularly left-sided colitis (Farrands et al., 1988) although there is no relationship between the presence of backwash ileitis in the proctocolectomy specimen and pouchitis (Gustavsson et al., 1987).

Interesting associations have been observed between pouchitis, in both pelvic ileal reservoirs and continent abdominal ileostomies, and the development of clinical conditions, such as arthritis, iridocyclitis and pyoderma gangrenosum, which are characteristic extracolonic manifestations of idiopathic inflammatory bowel disease (Klein et al., 1983; Knobler et al., 1986; Tytgat & van Deventer, 1988). The immunopathological evidence that has already been described in this chapter also supports the thesis that pouchitis is strongly related to ulcerative colitis. The fact that many cases of pouchitis respond well to metronidazole is not well explained by this thesis, but metronidazole does have immunosuppressive as well as antibacterial properties. Pouchitis also responds just as well to other therapeutic modalities of benefit in ulcerative colitis such as sulphasalazine and corticosteroids.

The cause of pouchitis remains obscure and the condition is one of the practising coloproctologist's great enigmas. The weight of evidence is very much against Crohn's disease, mucosal ischaemia and mucosal prolapse as causes of chronic relapsing pouchitis. The thesis that pouchitis results from a process of pouch mucosal metaplasia, possibly as a result of changes in bacterial flora, and the restoration of a colon-like environment which favours the recurrence of ulcerative colitis in the pouch is certainly an attractive one. Clearly much more research is necessary to prove or disprove such a theory. By creating the pelvic reservoir, have we inadvertently also created a very useful human model for the study of the pathogenesis of chronic ulcerative colitis?

Long-term prospects and malignancy risk

The first pelvic ileal reservoir operation was performed in 1976, and very few reservoirs have been in place for more than 10 years. Thus little or nothing is known of the long-term consequences of reservoir construction. The history of Kock's continent abdominal ileostomy reservoir goes back further and it is useful to examine the natural history of these pouches in assessing the long-term prospects for the pelvic pouch. Kock's reservoirs show similar inflammatory, metaplastic and proliferative alterations as pelvic pouches (Philipson *et al.*, 1975; Nilsson *et al.*, 1980; Hultén & Svaninger, 1984; Hultén, 1989) and there is some evidence that these changes may diminish in time with the mucosa of some reservoirs returning almost to normal (Hultén, 1989; Helander *et al.*, 1990). There is little evidence for an increased neoplastic potential in Kock's reservoirs although multiple adenomas have been observed seen in the abdominal reservoirs of FAP patients (Beart *et al.*, 1982; Stryker *et al.*, 1987; Hultén, 1989).

Given the analogies with continent abdominal ileostomy reservoirs, current evidence would suggest that the neoplastic potential of the pelvic ileal reservoir is low. Nevertheless the coexistence of colonic metaplasia and increased proliferative activity in the pouch mucosa does have worrying connotations. Both ulcerative colitis and FAP show hyperproliferation in colonic mucosa and these conditions are associated with very significant dysplasia and malignancy risk (Shepherd, 1990a). As yet no convincing case of epithelial dysplasia has been documented in the pouch of an ulcerative colitis patient. However most cases of colitis-associated dysplasia occur when the history of colitis is in excess of 10 years and very few pouches have been in place for that long. There is a report of a carcinoma arising in the pouch of a colitic patient but in this case the carcinoma was thought to arise not from metaplastic ileal mucosa but from residual mucosa within the rectal cuff (Stern *et al.*, 1990). This situation should become less of a problem with the realization that all rectal mucosa should be diligently removed by mucosectomy at the time of pouch construction (Nicholls, 1987). We have already alluded to the occurrence of adenomas in both Kock's reservoirs and pelvic reservoirs of FAP patients. Adenomas are seen in the ileal mucosa in FAP, although these are much less prevalent than in the colon. Malignancy in the small intestinal mucosa is distinctly unusual in FAP except in the duodenum (Shepherd & Bussey, 1990). The presence of adenomas does not necessarily imply an increased tumorigenesis in the FAP pouch.

What are the long-term prospects with regard to inflammation in the pouch and pouchitis? Most cases of pouchitis seem to occur relatively early in the natural history of the reservoir: we do not know if many of the colitic pouches will develop a form of late onset pouchitis many years later. Could all patients, particularly those with an original diagnosis of ulcerative colitis, eventually develop pouchitis? Are there pathological changes which may predict the onset of pouchitis and allow prophylactic drug therapy to be instituted? These questions remain unanswered. Much more research is required especially with regard to correlation of clinical and pathological features.

We believe that long-term surveillance of all ileal pouches by multiple endoscopic biopsies should be a mandatory part of pouch patient care. It seems likely that only extensive sampling of the mucosa will detect pre-malignant dysplasia in the pouch. The arguments against such surveillance in terms of resource allocation can be countered by the fact that only by such close initial surveillance will we fully understand the malignancy potential and thus divert resources to those most at risk. New technologies have generally been disappointing in the detection of preneoplastic change in the colonic mucosa of ulcerative colitis patients, although there is some suggestion that flow cytometry may have a role: in one large study of patients with ulcerative colitis, aneuploidy in the colonic mucosa was significantly associated with dysplasia and carcinoma elsewhere in the colon (Melville *et al.*, 1988). It is possible that flow cytometric analysis may have a role in pelvic ileal reservoir surveillance. How often patients are assessed is a difficult question, but annual endoscopy and biopsy would seem reasonable until the risks of potential malignant change can be properly assessed.

Summary

Pathological investigation of the ileal reservoir has demonstrated a variety of changes many of which recapitulate pathology seen elsewhere in the intestine. Some of these alterations occur as a result of changes in the intraluminal environment whilst others are the result of functional, mechanical and vascular pathology. Pathological research has helped to further our knowledge of the enigmatic condition of pouchitis and has demonstrated significant differences between the mucosal pathology in patients with ulcerative colitis and familial adenomatous polyposis. Whilst we should remain optimistic about the long-term prospects for patients with a pelvic ileal reservoir, there should be an awareness of the potential risks of many of the pathological changes and for this reason patients should remain in surveillance programmes until we are more knowledgeable about the consequences of ileal reservoir construction on the ileal mucosal microenvironment.

Acknowledgements

We are most grateful to Ms Jill Maybee, Department of Medical Illustration, St Mark's Hospital, for photographic assistance and to Dr Tony Corfield, Department of Medicine, Bristol Royal Infirmary, for advice on mucin biochemistry. Table 10.1 is reproduced with the kind permission of the Editor, *Journal of Clinical Pathology*.

References

Ambroze WL, Pemberton JH, Bell AM, Haddad AC, Phillips SF (1989) Fecal short chain fatty acids after pouch-anal anastamosis. *Gastroenterology* 96:A11.

Beart RW (1988) Proctocolectomy and ileoanal anastamosis. *World J Surg* 12:160–163.

Beart RW, Fleming CR, Banks PM (1982) Tubulovillous adenomas in a continent ileostomy after proctocolectomy for familial polyposis. *Dig Dis Sci* 27:553–556.

Beelsen W, Kavich R (1973) Microbial flora of the upper small intestine in Crohn's disease. *Gastroenterology* 65:390–397.

Bernstein L, Frank M, Brandt L, Boley S (1980) Healing of perianal Crohn's disease with metronidazole. *Gastroenterology* 79:357–365.

Bruce D, Warren BF, Durdey P, Luckett M, Shepherd NA (1991) Ultrastructural appearances of the pelvic ileal reservoir mucosa. *Gut* 32:A1218.

Corazza GR, Frazzoni M, Dixon MF, Gasbarrini G (1985) Quantitative assessment of the mucosal architecture of jejunal biopsy specimens: a comparison between linear measurement, stereology and computer-aided microscopy. *J Clin Pathol* 38:765–770.

Corfield AP, Warren BF, Bartolo DCC (1990) Colonic metaplasia following restorative proctocolectomy monitored using a new metabolic labelling technique for mucin. *J Pathol* 160:170A.

de Silva HJ, Gatter KC, Millard PR, Kettlewell M, Mortensen NJ, Jewell DP (1990a) Crypt cell proliferation and HLA-DR expression in pelvic ileal pouches. *J Clin Pathol* 43:824–829.

de Silva HJ, Ireland A, Kettlewell M, Mortensen N, Jewell DP (1989) Short-chain fatty acid irrigation in severe pouchitis. *New Engl J Med* 321:1416–1417.

de Silva HJ, Jones M, Kettlewell M, Mortensen N, Jewell D (1990b) Subsets of T lymphocytes and macrophages in the mucosa of ileo-anal pouches. *Gastroenterology* 98:1990.

de Silva HJ, Millard PR, Kettlewell M, Mortensen NJ, Prince C, Jewell DP (1991) Mucosal characteristics of pelvic ileal pouches. *Gut* 32:61–65.

de Silva HJ, Millard PR, Prince C, Kettlewell M, Mortensen N, Jewell DP (1990c) Serial observations of the mucosal changes in ileo-anal pouches. *Gut* 31:A1168–A1169.

Dozois RR, Goldberg SM, Rothenberger DA *et al.* (1986) Restorative proctocolectomy with ileal reservoir. (Symposium.) *Int J Colorectal Dis* 1:2–19.

Editorial (1989) Diversion colitis. *Lancet* i:764.

Farrands PA, Shepherd NA, Nicholls RJ (1988) Ileal reservoir inflammation (pouchitis) after restorative proctocolectomy ileal reservoir. *Gut* 29:A1486.

Gerdes J, Lemke H, Baisch H, Wacker HH, Schwab U, Stein H (1984) Cell cycle analysis of a cell proliferation-associated human nuclear antigen defined by monoclonal antibody Ki67. *J Immunol* 133:1710–1715.

Gustavsson S, Weiland LH, Kelly KA (1987) Relationship of backwash ileitis to ileal pouchitis after ileal pouch-anal anastamosis. *Dis Colon Rectum* 30:25–28.

Harig JM, Soergel KH, Komorowski RA, Wood CM (1989) Treatment of diversion colitis with short chain fatty acid irrigation. *New Engl J Med* 320:23–38.

Helander KG, Ahren C, Philipson BM, Samuelsson BM, Ojerskog BO (1990) Structure of mucosa in continent ileal reservoirs 15 to 19 years after construction. *Hum Pathol* 21:1235–1238.

Hosie K, Sachaguchi M, Tudor R, Gourevitch D, Kmiot W, Keighley MRB (1989) Pouchitis following proctocolectomy is associated with mucosal ischaemia. *Gut* 30:A1471–A1472.

Hultén L (1989) Pouchitis – incidence and characteristics in the continent ileostomy. In Pouchitis Workshop. *Int J Colorectal Dis* 5:208–210.

Hultén L, Svaninger G (1984) Facts about the Kock continent ileostomy. *Dis Colon Rectum* 27:553–557.

Jass JR, England J, Miller K (1986) Value of mucin histochemistry in follow up surveillance of patients with long-standing ulcerative colitis. *J Clin Pathol* 39:393–398.

Keighley MRB (1989) Discussion. Pouchitis. (Workshop.) *Int J Colorectal Dis* 4:213.

Klein K, Stenzel P, Katon P (1983) Pouch ileitis: report of a case with severe systemic manifestations. *J Clin Gastroenterol* 5:149–153.

Kmiot WA, Williams MR, Keighley MRB (1990) Pouchitis following colectomy and ileal reservoir construction for familial adenomatous polyposis. *Br J Surg* 77:1283.

Knobler H, Ligumsky M, Okon E, Ayalon A, Nesher R, Rachmilewitz D (1986) Pouch ileitis – recurrence of the inflammatory bowel disease in the ileal reservoir. *Am J Gastroenterol* 81:199–201.

Komorowski RA (1990) Histologic spectrum of diversion colitis. *Am J Surg Pathol* 14:548–554.

Levin KE, Pemberton JH, Phillips SF, Zinsmeister AR, Pezim ME (1990) Effect of xanthine oxidase inhibitor (allopurinol) in patients with pouchitis after ileal pouch-anal anastamosis. *Gut* 31:A1168.

Lusk LB, Reichen J, Levine JS (1984) Aphthous ulceration in diversion colitis. *Gastroenterology* 87:1171–1173.

Luukkonen P, Jarvinen H, Lehtola A, Sipponen P (1988a) Mucosal alterations in pelvic ileal reservoirs. A histological and ultrastructural evaluation in an experimental model. *Ann Chir Gynaecol* 77:91–96.

Luukkonen P, Valtonen V, Sivonen A, Sipponen P, Jarvinen H (1988b) Fecal bacteriology and reservoir ileitis in patients operated on for ulcerative colitis. *Dis Colon Rectum* 31:864–867.

Ma CK, Gottlieb C, Haas PA (1990) Diversion colitis: a clinicopathological study of 21 cases. *Hum Pathol* **21**: 429–436.

Madden MV, Farthing MJG, Nicholls RJ (1990) Inflammation in ileal reservoir: pouchitis. *Gut* **31**:247–249.

Melville DM, Jass JR, Shepherd NA *et al.* (1988) Dysplasia and deoxyribonucleic acid aneuploidy in the assessment of precancerous changes in chronic ulcerative colitis. Observer variation and correlations. *Gastroenterology* **95**: 668–675.

Meuwissen SGM, Hoitsma H, Boot H, Seldenrijk CA (1989) Pouchitis (pouch ileitis). *Neth J Med* **35**:S54–S66.

Moskowitz RL, Shepherd NA, Nicholls RJ (1986) An assessment of inflammation in the reservoir after restorative proctocolectomy with ileoanal ileal reservoir. *Int J Colorectal Dis* **1**:167–174.

Nasmyth DG, Godwin PGR, Dixon MF, Williams NS, Johnston D (1989) Ileal ecology after pouch-anal anastamosis or ileostomy. A study of mucosal morphology, fecal bacteriology, fecal volatile fatty acids and their interrelationship. *Gastroenterology* **96**:817–824.

Nicholls RJ (1987) Restorative proctocolectomy with various types of reservoir. *World J Surg* **11**:751–762.

Nicholls RJ (1989) Clinical diagnosis. Pouchitis. (Workshop.) *Int J Colorectal Dis* **4**:213–216.

Nicholls RJ, Belliveau P, Neill M, Wilks M, Tabaqchali S (1981) Restorative proctocolectomy with ileal reservoir: a pathophysiological assessment. *Gut* **22**:462–468.

Nilsson LO, Kock NG, Lindgren I, Myrvold HE, Philipson BM, Ahren C (1980) Morphological and histochemical changes in the mucosa of the continent ileostomy reservoir 6–10 years after its construction. *Scand J Gastroenterol* **15**: 737–747.

O'Byrne JM, O'Connell PR, Nolan N, Marks P, Tanner WA, Keane FBV (1989) Colonic metaplasia of ileal mucosa: an experimental model. *Gut* **30**:A1477.

O'Connell PR (1989) Discussion. Pouchitis. (Workshop) *Int J Colorectal Dis* **4**:208.

O'Connell PR, Rankin DR, Weiland LH, Kelly KA (1986) Enteric bacteriology, absorption, morphology and emptying after ileal pouch-anal anastomosis. *Br J Surg* **73**:909–914.

Paganelli GP, Biasco G, Lalli AA *et al.* (1989) Cell kinetics of the ileal pouch after pouch-anal anastomosis. In *New Trends in Pelvic Pouch Procedures*, Proceedings of the International Symposium, Bologna, September 1989.

Pezim ME, Pemberton JH, Beart RW (1989) Outcome of 'indeterminant' colitis following ileal pouch-anal anastamosis. *Dis Colon Rectum* **32**:653–658.

Philipson B, Brandberg A, Jagenburg R, Kock NG, Lager I, Ahren C (1975) Mucosal morphology, bacteriology and absorption in intra-abdominal ileostomy reservoir. *Scand J Gastroenterol* **10**:145–153.

Richman PI, Bodmer WF (1987) Monoclonal antibodies to human colorectal epithelium. Markers for differentiation and tumour characterisation. *Int J Cancer* **39**:317–328.

Rutgeerts P, Ghoos Y, Vantrappen G, Eyssen H (1981) Ileal dysfunction and bacterial overgrowth in patients with Crohn's disease. *Eur J Clin Invest* **11**:199–206.

Scott AD, Phillips RKS (1989) Ileitis and pouchitis after colectomy for ulcerative colitis. *Br J Surg* **76**:668–669.

Shepherd NA (1989) The pathology of the ileal reservoir. Pouchitis. (Workshop.) *Int J Colorectal Dis* **5**:206–208.

Shepherd NA (1990a) The pelvic ileal reservoir: apocalypse later? *Br Med J* **301**:886–887.

Shepherd NA (1990b) The pelvic ileal reservoir: pathology and pouchitis. *Neth J Med* **37**:S57–S64.

Shepherd NA, Bussey HJR (1990) Polyposis syndromes – an update. *Current Topics in Pathology. Gastrointestinal Pathology*, GT Williams (ed). Berlin, Springer Verlag. pp. 323–351.

Shepherd NA, Healey CJ, Warren BF, Thomson WHF, Wilkinson SP (1992). The distribution of pathological changes and an assessment of colonic phenotypic change in the pelvic ileal reservoir. *Gut* (in press).

Shepherd NA, Jass JR, Duval I, Moskowitz RL, Nicholls RJ, Morson BC (1987) Restorative proctocolectomy with ileal reservoir: pathological and histochemical study of mucosal biopsy specimens. *J Clin Pathol* **40**:601–607.

Stern H, Walfisch S, Mullen B, McLeod R, Cohen Z (1990) Cancer in an ileoanal reservoir: a new late complication? *Gut* **31**:473–475.

Stryker SJ, Kent TH, Dozois RR (1987) Multiple adenomatous polyps arising in a continent reservoir ileostomy. *Int J Colorectal Dis* **2**:43–45.

Subramani K, Sachar DB, Harpaz N, Bilotta J, Rubin PH, Janowitz HD (1990) Resistant pouchitis: does it reflect underlying Crohn's disease? *Gastroenterology* **98**:A393.

Tanaka M, Riddell RH (1990) The pathological diagnosis and differential diagnosis of Crohn's disease. *Hepatogastroenterology* **37**:18–31.

Tytgat GNJ (1989) The role of endoscopy in pouch monitoring and pouchitis. Pouchitis (Workshop.) *Int J Colorectal Dis* **4**:210–213.

Tytgat GNJ, van Deventer SJH (1988) Pouchitis. *Int J Colorectal Dis* **3**:226–228.

Warren BF, Bartolo DCC, Bradfield JWB (1990a) Pouchitis or prolapse? *J Pathol* **161**:355A.

Warren BF, Bartolo DCC, Collins CMP (1990b) Preclosure pouchitis – a new entity. *J Pathol* **160**:170A.

Warren BF, Shepherd NA (1992) The role of pathology in pouch surgery. *Int J Colorectal Dis* **7**:68–75.

Warren BF, Shepherd NA, Bartolo DCC, Bradfield JWB (1991) The pathology of the defunctioned rectum in ulcerative colitis. *J Pathol* **163**:169A.

Wright NA, Pike C, Elia G (1990) Induction of a novel epidermal growth factor-secreting cell lineage by mucosal ulceration in human gastrointestinal stem cells. *Nature* **343**: 82–85.

Index

References to figures appear in *italic* type and references to tables appear in **bold** type.